CONFIDENTIALITY, PRIVACY, AND DATA PROTECTION IN BIOMEDICINE

International Concepts and Issues

Edited by Edward S. Dove

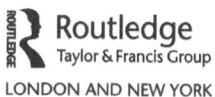

Routledge
Taylor & Francis Group

LONDON AND NEW YORK

First published 2025
by Routledge
4 Park Square, Milton Park, Abingdon, Oxon OX14 4RN

and by Routledge
605 Third Avenue, New York, NY 10158

Routledge is an imprint of the Taylor & Francis Group, an informa business

British Library Cataloguing-in-Publication Data
A catalogue record for this book is available from the British Library

Library of Congress Cataloging-in-Publication Data
Names: Dove, E. S. (Edward S.), editor.
Title: Confidentiality, privacy, and data protection in biomedicine : international concepts and issues / edited by Edward Dove.
Description: Abington, Oxon ; New York, NY : Routledge, 2024. | Includes bibliographical references and index.
Identifiers: LCCN 2024018730 (print) | LCCN 2024018731 (ebook) | ISBN 9781032495866 (hardback) | ISBN 9781032495859 (paperback) | ISBN 9781003394518 (ebook)
Subjects: MESH: Confidentiality | Privacy | Data Management--methods | Internationality
Classification: LCC R728.8 .C6285 2024 (print) | LCC R728.8 (ebook) | NLM WB 291 | DDC 651.02/461--dc23/eng/20240606
LC record available at https://lccn.loc.gov/2024018730
LC ebook record available at https://lccn.loc.gov/2024018731

ISBN: 978-1-032-49586-6 (hbk)
ISBN: 978-1-032-49585-9 (pbk)
ISBN: 978-1-003-39451-8 (ebk)

DOI: 10.4324/9781003394518

Typeset in Sabon
by SPi Technologies India Pvt Ltd (Straive)

CONFIDENTIALITY, PRIVACY, AND DATA PROTECTION IN BIOMEDICINE

Featuring contributions from leading scholars of health privacy law, this important volume offers insightful reflection on issues such as confidentiality, privacy, and data protection, as well as analysis in how a range of jurisdictions—including the US, the UK, Europe, South Africa, and Australia—navigate a rapidly developing biomedical environment.

While the collection of personal health information offers the potential to drive research and innovation, it also generates complex legal and ethical questions in how this information is used to ensure the rights and interests of individuals and communities are respected. But in many ways laws have struggled to keep pace with technological developments. This book therefore seeks to fill a lacuna for legal insight and reflection. Over three parts, the book first explores the conceptual landscape which law and legal institutions must contend, and then turns to examine practical issues such as the GDPR, secondary use of data for research, genomic research, and data trusts.

With cutting-edge analysis drawing on domestic and international case law, legislation, and policy, this comprehensive volume will prove fascinating reading for all students and researchers interested in this evolving and contentious area of study.

Edward S. Dove is a Professor of Law at the School of Law and Criminology, Maynooth University, Ireland.

CONTENTS

CONTRIBUTORS

Heidi Beate Bentzen is a Researcher at the Centre for Medical Ethics, Institute of Health and Society, Faculty of Medicine, University of Oslo, Norway, and at the Cancer Registry of Norway, Norwegian Institute of Public Health, Oslo, Norway.

Jessica Bell is an Assistant Professor in Law at the School of Law, University of Warwick, United Kingdom.

Edward S. Dove is a Professor of Law at the School of Law and Criminology, Maynooth University, Ireland.

Ahmad Haeri Mazanderani is a Clinical Virologist at the Center for HIV and STI, National Institute for Communicable Diseases, a division of the National Health Laboratory Service and Department of Pediatrics and Child Health, University of the Witwatersrand, South Africa.

Graeme Laurie is a Professorial Fellow at the School of Law, University of Edinburgh, United Kingdom.

Safia Mahomed is a Professor at the School of Law, University of South Africa, and an Honorary Associate Professor at the Steve Biko Centre for Bioethics, University of the Witwatersrand, South Africa.

Aisling McMahon is a Professor of Law at the School of Law and Criminology, Maynooth University, Ireland.

Fruzsina Molnar-Gabor is Professor of International Medical and Health Law and Data Protection Law at the Faculty of Law and BioQuant, Heidelberg University, Germany.

Miranda Mourby is a Researcher in Law within the Centre for Health, Law and Emerging Technologies ("HeLEX") at the Faculty of Law, University of Oxford, United Kingdom.

Tanya Murray is a Senior Scientist at the Center for HIV and STI, National Institute for Communicable Diseases, a division of the National Health Laboratory Service and Department of Pediatrics and Child Health, University of the Witwatersrand, South Africa.

Megan Prictor is a Senior Lecturer and Co-Director of the Health, Law and Emerging Technologies programme ("HeLEX@Melbourne") at Melbourne Law School, University of Melbourne, Australia.

Mark A. Rothstein is Director of Translational Bioethics at the Institute for Clinical and Translational Science, University of California, Irvine, United States of America.

Gayle Sherman is a Professor at the Center for HIV and STI, National Institute for Communicable Diseases, a division of the National Health Laboratory Service and Department of Pediatrics and Child Health, University of the Witwatersrand, South Africa.

Ciara Staunton is a Senior Researcher at the Institute for Biomedicine, Eurac Research, Italy and an Honorary Research Fellow at the School of Law, University of KwaZulu-Natal, South Africa.

Mark Taylor is a Professor of Law and Co-Director of the Health, Law and Emerging Technologies programme ("HeLEX@Melbourne") at Melbourne Law School, University of Melbourne, Australia.

David Townend is Associate Dean (Research and Enterprise) and Professor of Health and Life Sciences Law at The City Law School, City, University of London, United Kingdom.

INTRODUCTION

Edward S. Dove

Introducing the world of health privacy law

Plenty has been written and spoken about over the years in relation to the ways in which we want to keep aspects of our personal and social lives private and protected in some way, while also promoting uses of our information for various purposes, including for our direct care and for health research. Ask a stranger on the street what they think each of privacy, confidentiality, and data protection mean, and chances are you will get a relatively thoughtful response—as well as a diverse range of views regarding how private they wish their own health information[1] (and perhaps those of others) to be from access by others, and how accessible they want their health information to be for themselves. After all, the terms "privacy", "confidentiality", and "data protection" are pervasive in our social discourse. Every week, if not every day, we read, hear, or watch a news item that invokes these concepts—be it a massive data breach involving medical records, a hospital staff member seeking access to a famous patient's files, paparazzi snapping photographs of a celebrity in a compromising situation, or efforts proposed by governments or health insurers, pernicious or benign, to make increased use of information provided by us in our interactions with our doctors, banks, employers, revenue service, and even our smartphones.

While almost everyone is likely to have at least a basic understanding of what privacy, confidentiality, and data protection mean, that is quite different from exhibiting a firm grasp of their *interrelationship*, and how they play out in the biomedical domain across different cultures and legal systems. Likewise, it is more difficult to ascertain how the law, and society, can best balance the desire to promote ostensibly beneficial uses of our health-related information (e.g. to reduce health threats, to promote individual and population health, to provide quality healthcare) while protecting privacy—undoubtedly a core human need and condition for living life in dignity and with respect.

DOI: 10.4324/9781003394518-1

This is the overarching objective of this collection. Before getting there, however, it is worth pausing on the importance of meanings. In this volume, we see that each contributor may have their own understanding as to what privacy, confidentiality, and data protection mean to them, reflecting their own socio-cultural and legal traditions. Yet, it is fair to say that in looking across the chapters, we find a family resemblance between meanings, and I would be remiss to not sketch these out in this Introduction. Privacy, in its broadest sense, may be taken to mean a moral, social, and legal construct and a state of affairs that is associated with (but not necessarily primarily about) norms of exclusivity or meaningful control over aspects of one's life. In some countries, it might be a constitutional right, and in others, a human right. Relatedly, confidentiality is a moral, social, and legal construct (the latter through legal codes or case law) that is associated with secrecy and a duty of trust and good faith: protecting information disclosed by one party to another—and sanctioning wrongful disclosure of that information. Finally, data protection is determinedly a legal construct that aims to protect the rights, freedoms, and interests of individuals whose personal data are collected, stored, processed, disseminated, or deleted.[2] The principal purpose of data protection is to facilitate flows of personal data across organizations (and countries) while at the same time ensuring fairness in the processing of data and, to some extent, fairness in the outcomes of such processing. Strong data protection protects some aspects of privacy and preserves many features of confidentiality. The concepts overlap in their meanings and the protections that they offer; an exploration of this interrelationship is a core focus of this volume.

While we may have some sense that privacy is similar yet distinct from confidentiality, and both of which in turn are similar yet distinct from data protection, this does not address the broader question of their linkages. *How* exactly are they similar and distinct? What are their common characteristics, and what are their defining differences? What is the difference between, say, a "duty of confidence" and a "right to privacy" or a "right to data protection"? What are their objectives in law and policy, as well as ethics? How do the courts and regulatory bodies play a role in monitoring or enforcing these duties, rights, and regimes? When must they yield to competing values in society, such as national security and public health? And where does the role of trust, good faith, and respect in the doctor-patient or researcher–participant relationship come into play, to say nothing of the public interest, social good, and public benefit? By asking these fundamental questions, we reveal a significant lacuna in the literature.[3] In this volume, I and the other contributors make a case for why these questions matter, why this lacuna deserves addressing, and why essays on "health privacy law", as I come to call it, can provide a rich contribution to the dual fields of health law *and* privacy law, broadly defined.

Already the rationale for this volume can be gleaned from these introductory remarks. Personal information is one of the most valuable resources in the 21st century, rightly or wrongly sometimes referred to as "the new oil",[4] and this value is particularly recognized and sought for exploitation in the biomedical context. In this domain there is increasing reliance on the collection, sharing of, and access to personal health–related information, often across platforms, systems, and locations. Such information, and linkage of it, holds great potential to drive research breakthroughs and innovations in biomedicine, potentially leading to life-enhancing innovations in the form of diagnostics, therapeutics, vaccines, and devices. As desirable as these benefits are in the abstract, in concrete terms the nature of health information collection and use generate a number of pertinent, complex questions about the legal, policy, and ethical safeguards that ought to be in place to ensure that any collection and use is consensual, safe, and transparent. Law and policy, which this volume focuses on, help ensure that the uses of health-related information are consensual, safe, and transparent, or phrased another way, responsible and conducted in ways that demonstrate trustworthiness, and that protect and promote the rights, interests, and welfare of individuals— and, to a lesser degree at least in most Western cultures, those of groups and communities.

The legal regimes governing health-related information have experienced rapid development in the past several years across much of the globe; Graham Greenleaf's annual review of data protection law, for example, shows that as of 2023 there were at least 162 national data protection laws, and that there were only 36 UN member states with neither acts nor proposed bills in this area.[5] Yet, while many countries across the world have witnessed a tremendous number of new or reformed laws concerning data protection, largely driven by statute, much less attention has been given to other legal regimes in this area that may be based either on common law (by which I mean case law), constitutional frameworks, or penal or regulatory codes—namely the law of confidentiality and the law of privacy. Unlike data protection, privacy and confidentiality as legal regimes often may be less statute-driven (if at all), and to reiterate, to date, this interrelationship has been largely underexplored.

Under-theorizing and failing to give due consideration to this interrelationship can have detrimental impact on clinical practice and research. It also does the academy no favours. The fast pace of legal change and the relative lack of considered reflection of the interplay among these related and at-times overlapping legal regimes leads not only to gaps in legal and policy insight in the local and global economies and in people's lives (as the COVID-19 pandemic has starkly illustrated), but it also contributes to greater uncertainty and risk among those who invariably must at some point participate in biomedicine—from patients to healthcare professionals, and from participants to researchers, and from policymakers to legislators. This is, in other words, too important an area to leave under-explored given the recent and often controversial changes afoot, as reflected in a variety of areas. To take just two examples: what are the implications for health privacy law that arise from the *Dobbs* v *Jackson Women's Health Organization* decision of the US Supreme Court in 2022[6] that effaced a US constitutional right to abortion, and the European Union's proposal for a European Health Data Space in 2022[7] that may fundamentally change how health data is shared across national boundaries and expectations citizens have of increased digital access to and control of their electronic personal health data? These local and regional developments have potential implications for health privacy law globally. It is another core objective of this volume to explore what these might be.

This edited volume seeks to fill these lacunae in our understanding by bringing together original contributions from some of the leading global scholars in health privacy law. Each contributor, as I proceed to summarize below, offers expert reflections on and detailed exploration of all or some these legal regimes in the biomedical context (comprising both healthcare and health research, broadly defined). All offer deep insight into how the law has evolved over time,[8] and how recent changes in law and policy impact, for better or worse, the responsible use of health-related information and what it means for biomedical practice. As such, this volume has at its core two principal objectives: first, to present a critical and original analysis of the core concepts and regimes of confidentiality, privacy, and data protection; and second, to interrogate these concepts and regimes through a variety of methods familiar in legal scholarship, including doctrinal, case study, and theoretical analysis.

The central focus of the volume, as readers will discover and as I have noted above, is the interplay between privacy, confidentiality, and data protection laws, and wider constitutional, legal, and ethical frameworks at the international level. For example, in the United Kingdom (UK) and Europe, this includes national data protection acts, the General Data Protection Regulation (GDPR),[9] national courts case law, European Court of Human Rights jurisprudence concerning Article 8 of the European Convention on Human Rights, the Council of Europe's Convention 108[10]/Convention 108+[11] and other guidelines and recommendations,[12] and even more broadly, the International Covenant on Civil and Political Rights (e.g. Article 17, which states that no one shall be subjected to arbitrary or unlawful interference with their privacy, and that everyone has the right to the protection of the law against such interference or attacks). Each chapter offers cutting-edge analysis and evaluation of this interaction, drawing on a range of sources, including case law, primary and secondary legislation, policy, academic literature, advisory opinions, and domestic and international laws and practices. While there is a strong focus in this volume on the UK and European contexts, contributions from well beyond this region, including South Africa, the United States, and the Asia-Pacific region, offer insights for readers around the globe who are keen to apply themes to their own jurisdictions.

Cross-cutting themes

The volume is divided into three parts over twelve chapters. While each chapter explores a particular aspect of privacy, confidentiality, or data protection in the biomedical domain and often within a jurisdictional focus, at least three cross-cutting themes emerge (and I suspect readers will identify others).

Unease about the path of development of health privacy law

First, each of the chapters documents how we are experiencing a time of profound change in health privacy law and policy. The changes, however, stimulate some degree of unease about future directions; civil society and academics in particular express doubt about where we are going and whether we can say with confidence that we are on a good course. In many cases, these legal and policy developments seek to respond to and address technological developments such as artificial intelligence (AI), Big Data, and biometric devices. In other cases, they are an example of "natural" jurisprudential evolution (or revolution) that reacts to shifting socio-political norms within a country. We recently saw this play out in the UK, for example, which, until Parliament was dissolved ahead of the July 2024 General Election, debated a Data Protection and Digital Information Bill that would have amended the UK GDPR and Data Protection Act 2018 in ways that further de-coupled the UK's data protection regime from the European Union's (EU's) as a post-Brexit goal to spur innovation (and perhaps also to demonstrate to the pharmaceutical industry and life sciences sector that the UK is a "friendly" place to conduct research). We also saw this in the previous UK Government's policy paper *Data Saves Lives*,[13] which indicated that the government was keen to introduce new secondary legislation that would create further exemptions from the common law duty of confidence,[14] raising questions about the precarious balance (another cross-cutting theme noted below) between public interests, as well as the values and other interests, in maintaining confidence in the healthcare and health research systems, and stimulating an innovation-friendly and data-driven economy. Time will tell whether the new UK Government intends to draft new primary or secondary legislation that might spur biomedical research and life sciences innovation in the country, but might also further disharmonize the regulatory environment from the EU and consequently jeopardize international collaboration.

Further comments on such uncertain developments can be found in the chapters from Safia Mahomed on South Africa (covering some of the challenges to privacy as a result of recent statutory developments and the ways in which privacy laws could be managed practically in an increasingly open data-driven society), from me on the uncertain path of the common law in the UK regarding privacy and confidentiality (and specifically the relationship between the causes of action in breach of confidence and misuse of private information), and from Heidi Beate Bentzen on human organoids in the EU (exploring how EU data protection law obstructs personal data transfers to third countries and raises strict obstacles to scientific collaboration between the EU and major third country–based research funders and institutions).

Looking to the United States, as another example, while Mark Rothstein documents in his chapter how there continues to be no comprehensive, national law protecting personal health information (making the United States an outlier on the international stage), and by default, the main applicable law is the limited-in-scope Health Insurance Portability and Accountability Act (HIPAA) of 1996, we nevertheless bear witness to substantial developments impacting health privacy in the country. This includes the enactment in at least 15 US states within the past decade of consumer privacy protection acts, inspired by the GDPR and the perceived need to protect privacy and prevent the non-consensual monetization of online and other consumer information. But biggest development in health privacy law in recent times may well be the *Dobbs* decision, which as both Rothstein and Graeme Laurie note in their chapters, may lead to knock-on effects on the existing protections against the non-consensual disclosure of reproductive health information, information about medication used for abortions, and disclosure of mobile phone geolocation information indicating an individual's proximity to an abortion clinic (so-called geofencing).

So, what we come to see in this volume is that legal developments in the United States, the UK, the EU, South Africa, and beyond may be both positive and negative. The zeitgeist of the 2020s—populism and reactionary politics, protectionist policies, backsliding of liberalism and the liberal international world order, and increasingly autocratic and surveillance-prone regimes—might suggest something other than a Whiggish history of enhanced privacy protection across the globe. Instead, more worryingly, we may be bearing witness to a backsliding of privacy intrusions from the state, state-like, and private actors. Nor is it necessarily the case that new or more law is a net benefit; beyond existing approaches that many commentators see as inadequate (e.g. informed consent, anonymization, international data transfer rules), many in the biomedical community lament what they perceive as a growing thicket of laws, regulations, guidance, and governance that thwart valuable research and innovation, and also hobble the privacy interests of individuals and communities.

Similarly, as we see in the chapters from Megan Prictor; Aisling McMahon and Ciara Staunton; and Miranda Mourby and Fruzsina Molnar-Gabor, recent legal developments across the Asia-Pacific region and EU (respectively) might have the best of intentions to promote a perceived social good (e.g. protecting against data breaches, promoting secondary use of health data for research and innovation). But if they are poorly designed and give too little thought to legal harmonization within and across regions, invariably we will find ourselves if not quite in a legal "square one", then at least in a position from which collectively we ought to have avoided from transpiring at all.

The enhanced voice of patients, participants, and publics

A second theme that one can glean from the chapters is the growing recognition of a role for engagement of and respect for patients and publics, including enhanced means by which individuals can access their own health data. Countries around the world are rolling out apps in which individuals can book GP appointments, request prescriptions, seek medical advice of varying quality, and access their medical files. As much as we might applaud this enhanced "access and control" paradigm as facilitating privacy-related interests, symbolizing perhaps one manifestation of the patients' rights movement and the yearning for greater autonomy, we might also pause to assess both the legal compliance of these technological advances and the longer-term public disbenefit that could accrue if "enhanced access and control" is coded by the state as greater self-responsibilization for health and privatization of healthcare provision. Regardless, enhancing the voices of publics emerges as a core theme in these chapters: not as cacophony leading to anarchical or garbled law and policy, but as pluralistic views leading to richer, more nuanced, and publicly supported, trustworthy law and policy.

We see this theme in Graeme Laurie's chapter calling for a "demosprudence" in privacy law. By this he advocates a pivot away from the "limiting constraints of jurisprudence" and towards more direct engagement with groups that have sought to rely on privacy in the pursuit of a range of political agendas. We also see this in Mark Taylor's chapter, in which he argues that public engagement must not only be about simply understanding what privacy-implicating decision is preferred by the people asked (i.e. the simplistic survey); it must also be a more meaningful activity of ongoing dialogue and mutual understanding that informs

> an understanding of the consequences of action relative to the norms and values held. It [must be an activity that] provides an opportunity for those affected by decisions to check and challenge the reasonableness (if not the rationality) of those decisions relative to their understanding of their own world-view.

And as Taylor says, where the justification withstands scrutiny from the affected public, they are provided with a reason to accept the decision-making process: it conforms with their norms and values (even if they would prefer a different decision had been made).

We also see this theme in Jessica Bell's chapter, in which she argues that data trusts, especially for children in health research, offer promise for increasing involvement and engagement of parents and children, including via respective data subject rights, in longitudinal health research projects like birth cohort studies. Bell cautions, however, similarly to Taylor, that to avoid lapsing into mere tokenistic engagement, in building a data trust, there need to be very clear parameters at the outset and, ideally, *co-design* with those involved. Bell suggests that data trusts have much to learn from the health governance landscape in terms of participatory approaches to data governance, including methods of establishing meaningful channels of engagement between data subjects and trustees.

A precarious balancing of values and interests

A final theme that appears across the chapters in this volume is the precarious balance between the interests of the individual patient or participant, those who make use of their data, and the interests of the public at large. It is of course long known that, say, the duty of confidence is not absolute: a doctor is unlikely to be found liable for warning the police that one of their patient's has demonstrated a clear and present intent to kill their spouse. More recently, in the UK, there has been judicial confirmation[15] that on occasion clinicians may owe a duty of care to people other than their patient, but that such a duty is only capable of arising where there is a close proximal relationship between the claimant and the defendant (i.e. between the non-patient third party and the clinician) and discharging that duty involves appropriately balancing the non-patient third party in being informed of their risk (e.g. a genetic risk) against the patient's interest in preserving confidentiality in relation to their diagnosis and the public interest in maintaining medical confidentiality generally. Examples of this kind of discussion of balance of values and interests can be found in the chapters from David Townend; Aisling McMahon and Ciara Staunton; Miranda Mourby and Fruzsina Molnar-Gabor; Safia Mahomed; and Ciara Staunton and others.

Taken together, however, what the chapters in this volume illustrate is that the balancing exercise itself may mask hidden power structures, and that the balancing exercise itself requires, on occasion, recalibration and reassessment. Quite often, the balance is precarious.

For instance, in his chapter David Townend observes how European data protection law (seen through the GDPR, and before that the Data Protection Directive) creates what he terms "a structural imbalance of power" between the data subject and the data controller, in the latter's favour. As he notes, the rights of the data subject depend upon a stark choice between either accepting the data controller's terms for the processing or not being included, or, where the controller is processing one's personal data without a need for consent, objecting to the processing and being removed from the dataset or the particular processing activity. Either way, the individual patient or participant faces an imbalance of power that law itself may not be adequately addressing, and that organizational policies are unlikely addressing either.

We also observe the theme of balance in other chapters, such as Ciara Staunton and others' chapter on the challenge that the National Institute for Communicable Diseases in South Africa faces in striving to appropriately balance rights to privacy and protection of one's personal information with the wider public interest in delivering on a national HIV programme that protects and promotes public health. Guidance and law seek to protect sensitive health information from unwarranted intrusion, but this information also serves as a treasured resource to be used, shared, and linked with other datasets for the delivery of individual care and also the wider public interest in treatment programmes. Few would advocate guidance and law that absolutely prohibit use of this information for anything other than the direct care of the patient. As ever, though, the devil is in the detail in achieving a reasonable, publicly supported balance between permitting responsible, socially and scientifically valuable uses of this information, and safeguarding it against uses that rub against commonly held social and moral norms. But society (and clinicians and researchers especially) should not operate in a regulatory void. Unfortunately, as Staunton and others argue, the ongoing absence of guidance on the application of South Africa's national data protection law in the context of health has resulted in what they perceive as an unduly restrictive interpretation of the law by health organizations at the expense of public health, even though this restrictive approach does not appear to be matched by the Information Regulator. As a result, Staunton and others worry that the privacy interests of patients and patients' data protection rights may be currently weighted too heavily and not appropriately balanced with the right to health and the state's obligation to protect and promote public health.

Having charted some of the cross-cutting themes in the volume, I now proceed to cover in more detail what each of the 12 chapters offers to readers.

Content and structure of the book

Part I: Conceptual complexities

Diving into the specifics of this volume, Part I opens with a conceptual mapping of several areas of complexity. Here, three contributors look at privacy, confidentiality, and data protection from a higher-plane perspective, questioning in different ways how these concepts and the legal frameworks underpinning them might be reconsidered in ways that enhance protection and the common good. Innovative ideas such as "demosprudence", "reasonable justification", and the injection of the fiduciary duty are proffered here.

Graeme Laurie's opening chapter (Chapter 1) looks at the right to privacy in the backdrop of the US Supreme Court's controversial decision in *Dobbs*, which ruled that the earlier Supreme Court decision in *Roe v Wade* was "egregiously wrong" and as such held that the US Constitution does not confer a right to abortion. Laurie examines the wider and longer-term implications of this turn for privacy itself, particularly as a concept in the United States. Laurie makes the case that privacy's "unending fluidity and malleability" renders it particularly vulnerable to attack, and currently, privacy is under the beginning of an attack through the courts in the United States. Laurie offers an unapologetic defence of privacy as an inescapable and essential part of the human condition and our ethical lives. As he puts it, if a wider view of privacy is adopted, one grounded in "demosprudence" (the study of the relationship between social movements and law in the creation of authoritative meaning within a democratic polity, as developed by scholars Lani Guinier and Gerald Torres), rather than only jurisprudence—and a commitment to understanding the social movements that have coalesced around the very idea of privacy itself—it may be possible that any "wrongness" associated with privacy is in fact a symptom of our failure to get privacy right as a matter of law, rather than in privacy being wrong as something that matters to humanity.

From privacy we then turn to confidentiality. Mark Taylor's chapter (Chapter 2) focuses on the notion of the "public interest" in confidentiality law, specifically as applied to functioning as an enabling device for health data governance to be demonstrably worthy of public trust and capable of maintaining and promoting social licence in relation to health data initiatives. As Taylor argues, current data protection law and common law duties of confidentiality are incapable of either demonstrating trustworthiness or securing social licence, and in turn, that means they are incapable of protecting the public interest in research or public health uses of health information. Like Laurie, though, Taylor remains mostly optimistic. He suggests there is now an opportunity to reorient the protection of health data privacy—away from its current focus on personal data, individual consent, and control—and instead towards the development of conceptual connection between public interest and trustworthiness and a deeper understanding of what is required of public interest decision-making if it is to be deserving of public trust and confidence—namely through the requirement that any decision on (non)interference with medical confidentiality be supported by "reasonable justification". This reorientation, Taylor posits, is vital to protecting the public interest in confidentiality and to enabling research and public health uses of health data in the public interest.

Rounding out the more concept-driven Part I is David Townend's chapter (Chapter 3), which looks at the privacy implications of Big Data research, focusing on the European context. Townend describes his long-standing experiential challenges in reconciling EU data protection law (first the Data Protection Directive and then the GDPR) with potentials for health research using Big Data. As Townend notes, while the secondary processing of already-gathered data is fundamental to recent data science methodology developments in medical research, the established data protection regulatory regime presents conceptual and practical difficulties for new data science methodologies like Big Data. He illustrates this by noting the challenges faced in a multidisciplinary project called SHERLOC (Signs of Health and Risks Looking Out for Cancer). Townend argues that solutions to the difficulties cannot be found within existing data protection law paradigms—a "root and branch reimagining of the paradigm must be considered". Townend makes a case that solutions may be found in the law of confidentiality and in the equitable concept of the fiduciary duty. As he puts it, the duty of confidentiality and the fiduciary duty

> provide both a narrative upon which to address the meanings of the duties expressed in data protection, and a set of enforceable values to establish a relationship between the data subject and data controllers and data processors that reimagines those relationships in a more complete and coherent way.

Part II: Country- and region-specific issues

Following the conceptual complexities charted in Part I, in Part II, and across six chapters, contributors provide country and region-specific analyses, exploring how existing or proposed legal instruments sometimes fail to live up to their potential in achieving their stated aims, or otherwise strive to strike (sometimes with success) a sufficient balance in the interests at stake in biomedicine.

Opening this second part is a deep-dive exploration into the regulatory environment for health data for research and innovation in the EU, written by Aisling McMahon and Ciara Staunton (Chapter 4). They look at the European Union's proposed European Health Data Space (EHDS) Regulation, which provides for a health-specific data environment comprising rules, common standards and practices, infrastructures, and a governance framework, all of which aims to improve Europeans' access to and control over their personal electronic health data. It also enables certain data to be reused for public interest, policy support, and scientific research purposes. McMahon and Staunton question whether the proposed Regulation adequately balances and protect the breadth of rights and interests at stake. They argue that regulatory frameworks, including the proposed EHDS Regulation, need to account for and engage with these competing motivations and interests, and must also ensure that benefits arising are accessible to stakeholders in an equitable manner. McMahon and Staunton argue that data protection and re-identifiability are not the only concerns relevant here, and that both the GDPR and proposed EHDS Regulation fail to fully consider the wider social and ethical concerns in this space. Ultimately, they propose that a more holistic approach is needed—

> one that is underpinned by transparency and by respect for individuals and a broader range of communities and publics involved—which seeks to maximize the benefits from health research that may arise, without disproportionately affecting or harming individuals and the collective interests at stake.

Retaining a European focus, Miranda Mourby and Fruzsina Molnar-Gabor's chapter (Chapter 5) also critically assesses the proposed EHDS Regulation, and in particular the proposal's second dimension: to make health data available for "secondary uses" such as medical research and developing health-related algorithms. As they note, much of this controversy revolves around the degree of control patients should have over secondary uses of their information. Mourby and Molnar-Gabor compare the UK and Germany to analyse their differing legal approaches to the secondary use of health data and as a means of critiquing the proposed EHDS Regulation, including its unlikelihood of enabling patients' informational control through creation of an "opt-in" system for secondary uses of health data. Yet their analysis suggests that the requirements of both the UK and German legal cultures could be satisfied by an EHDS system with "opt-outs" from secondary uses of health data, which they are broadly supportive of. Their concern lies primarily with the European Commission's suggestion that the question of individual autonomy versus secondary uses is best left to Member States, which allows scope for multiple derogations at the Member State level, resulting in obstacles to sharing health data across national boundaries. They advocate therefore for the consistent availability of "opt-outs" across the EHDS and call for further research into the creation of accessible opt-outs for patients in all EU Member States, complemented by enhanced public engagement.

Moving from Europe to South Africa, in Chapter 6, Safia Mahomed explores the post-transition evolution of privacy in the healthcare context in South Africa, charting the numerous changes to legislation and ethical frameworks that impact the interplay of privacy, confidentiality, and data protection in the country. As Mahomed notes, with the advent of the Constitution of the Republic of South Africa, 1996 and increasing awareness of research participant protections, the "right to privacy", a concept that was predominantly interpreted by the common law beforehand, is now governed by various pieces of legislation and ethical guidelines, and influenced by international laws. Her chapter emphasizes that South Africa has made many legislative and ethical strides over the past 30 years in protecting patients and research participants' fundamental right to privacy, from its inception within the Bill of Rights, to its emphasis on protecting personal information under the Protection of Personal Information Act, 2013 (also known as POPIA). Mahomed speculates that South Africa will need to further legislate and craft sensible policies in the coming years to address current challenges. These include AI and protection against local data breach incidents, particularly in the healthcare setting. As Mahomed puts it, "any practical data management tool that is developed to regulate data flows should be adapted in line with appropriate safeguards that respect the dignity of people, particularly considering the pre-democratic South African context".

From South Africa we then move to the United States, where in his chapter (Chapter 7), Mark Rothstein explores the costs and benefits of health privacy through considering an array of health information technology, healthcare systems, legal provisions, and societal attitudes. He asks whether health privacy is "worth the cost", tracing the history of health privacy and the related concepts of confidentiality and security and assessing the consequences of various methods of protecting privacy. From his survey, Rothstein draws two main conclusions. First, he finds that there are significant social and economic transactional costs associated with health privacy—as well as inadequate legal protection of it (at least at the federal level). He advocates the need for policies that address health privacy, including its myriad financial and non-financial costs along with the tangible and intangible benefits. Second, he finds that the question of whether health privacy is "worth the cost" is complicated by the numerous circumstances in which it arises. As Rothstein notes:

> [o]n a societal level, the answer depends on the overall risks and benefits of disclosing certain types of health information, including to whom, in what form, and for what purpose. On a personal level, the answer may depend on the individual's age, health status, socioeconomic position, cultural background, psychological disposition, and risk tolerance.

In the end, Rothstein is doubtful that comprehensive health privacy laws will be enacted in the United States (again, at least at the federal level) unless there is a public consensus that the cost of safeguarding health privacy is a reasonable price to pay for living in a society that respects the dignity, autonomy, emotional wellbeing, and personal space of every individual. Yet even enactment of more modest, limited measures can, in his view, still make a vital and significant improvement to health privacy protection in the United States, and in the end, then, health privacy is worth the cost because there is so much more at stake than just economics.

In Chapter 8, I provide an English law doctrinal analysis of the relationship between the cause of action in breach of confidence and the recently established cause of action in misuse of private information (MOPI). I make two substantive contributions in this chapter. First, I rationalize the law to show a way through what hitherto has remained an elusive, complex private law muddle that has befuddled even academic scholars in privacy law and medical law (comprising what I call a "decade of jurisprudential confusion" from roughly 2005 to 2015). I make the case that breach of confidence should continue to be grounded in equity, meaning a duty of trust and honour, and a duty to be of good faith that fastens on the conscience of a party which often (but not absolutely) arises out of their relationship with the confider, whereas MOPI ought to be viewed and classified as a tort arising out of the common law. My second contribution is to unpack MOPI to analyse where legal gaps might remain. I argue that both the MOPI tort and an emerging common law right of privacy (in Scotland) as additional forms of legal protection may be partially welcomed as "gap-filling" measures to address long-standing concerns about lack of full coverage from the other legal regimes, and this is especially valuable in a health context given the general sensitivity of much information generated, collected, and used in this area. I also suggest that there is need for further common law development: courts across the UK ought to expand the existing contours of privacy law to afford protection to violations equivalent to an intrusion upon seclusion or solitude (which remain under-protected), and grant scope for a "third party interests doctrine" to afford better legal protection to groups and communities whose privacy interests may be adversely affected by information misuse and intrusions upon seclusion.

The final chapter (Chapter 9) in Part II comes from Megan Prictor, who undertakes a comprehensive survey of laws across the Asia-Pacific region. Prictor reminds us that health data breaches are ubiquitous and show no signs of dissipating. Poor cyber-security practices and increasingly sophisticated hackers are causing significant harm to patients as well as data custodians. Health data breaches can cause severe, negative impacts of loss of personal privacy given the sensitive nature of this information, which may relate to, for example, drug and alcohol misuse, mental ill health, sexually transmitted and other communicable diseases, and pregnancy termination. Prictor looks across a plethora of notifiable data breach (NDB) statutory schemes to assess how well these laws respond to and seek to remedy health data breaches. With a view to informing the development of improved measures to address this substantial and growing issue, Prictor finds that the region is experiencing a rapid growth of NDB schemes and increasing alignment around GDPR-like provisions, particularly in relation to reporting timeframes (which she welcomes). Yet further reform is likely. Beyond calling for further research on the effects and effectiveness of NDB schemes, and specifically, the act of notification itself, Prictor argues that growing sophistication of cyber-attacks on health data require an enhanced NDB framework *across* the region (i.e. broad alignment between national schemes) "whose design is more strongly connected to its underpinning aims, with more robust harm mitigation measures that accommodate diverse types of breached data, and based upon greater evidence of the impacts of notification on those affected".

Part III: Acute challenges

Rounding out the volume, the concluding Part III looks at what we might call more "acute" challenges in privacy, confidentiality, and data protection as applied to biomedicine, and how novel solutions could address those challenges, be it through new tools or reforms to the law.

Jessica Bell's chapter (Chapter 10) opens this final part by looking at the challenges and opportunities that data trusts provide for health research. Data trusts, which can be broadly defined as a legal structure based on trust law that provides independent stewardship of data, are increasingly seen as a viable mechanism for creating a trustworthy environment for data sharing and rebalancing power asymmetries in data exchanges. Bell's chapter focuses on the UK context to explore the extent to which legal mechanisms and principles associated with a data trust may help protect interests in, and address some of the challenges associated with, data governance for health research in the future. While noting that the concept of a data trust is still novel, and introducing the trust model into the health research setting raises many complex issues, she nevertheless posits that "there are a number of possibilities for data trusts to add value to existing approaches that would benefit both those seeking to use health data and those being asked to provide it". To this end, she endorses several pilot projects that are currently underway that seek to move data trusts from theory to practice and that will provide valuable insights into whether the benefits of data trusts are realizable and can shed light on some of the outstanding issues to be addressed.

Heidi Beate Bentzen (Chapter 11) then investigates a perennial question that has largely eluded policymakers and regulators for years and shows no sign of resolution as applied to new technologies: are human organoids, which are stem cell-derived mini organs, "things or data"? The consequences of that answer are profound with respect to potentially overlapping regulation of human biological samples and personal data, and in turn for the possibility for international collaboration and scientific progress in the organoid field. Focusing on the European context, Bentzen argues that both the legislation pertaining to human biological samples and personal data apply to organoid research. Although flawed, the legislation is quite adequate to cover the current state of organoid research. This does not address, however, more serious problems that organoids cause, because they are not *mere* things. Organoids are models of human development and may in the future become sufficiently similar to human embryos to acquire their own unique moral status. As Bentzen writes,

> [w]hen we can implant an organoid into a human uterus and it will survive, or we can make organoids that develop consciousness and sentience, classifying organoids merely as artefacts or things or biological material will no longer adequately capture their nature.

The binary question must give way to a deeper, more complex consideration that this is a hybrid category, situated between human biological material and personal data, and between a thing and a person. As such, Bentzen argues that sector-specific legislation may then become necessary, particularly if we need to consider the protection and rights of the hybrid itself. And, linking to the wider themes of the volume, Bentzen suggests that inspiration for sector-specific legislation may be drawn from confidentiality law and privacy law, which, in contrast to data protection law, capture a wider scope than just data and speak deeply to protecting human dignity. "Lifting the regulation of organoid research up a level in a similar sense", she writes, "may be useful to capture all hybrid elements worthy of protection".

The final chapter (Chapter 12), co-authored by Ciara Staunton, Ahmad Haeri Mazaderani, Tanya Murray, and Gayle Sherman, looks at the South African National Institute for Communicable Diseases (NICD). This NICD has a legislative role in the surveillance, management, and research into HIV in South Africa, which means it routinely collects, stores, uses, re-uses, and shares large quantities of health personal information, including consolidated lists of HIV-related laboratory results that require clinical action. The authors describe how the coming into effect of the country's POPIA (covered in-depth in Safia Mahomed's earlier chapter) led the NICD Paediatric HIV Surveillance Team to establish whether its current management of individual personal information related to HIV surveillance was POPIA-compliant. As they note, the team experienced a number of challenges in complying with POPIA while also striving to meet their HIV reporting objectives. Learning from this experience, among other things, they call for sector-specific guidance in the delivery of healthcare and treatment programmes in South Africa and high-light how vital institutional and sectoral leadership is for public health institutions to ensure a successful approach towards complying with new, complex data protection laws such as POPIA. The final chapter in this volume puts into stark relief the difficulty public health organizations around the world face in balancing patients' rights to privacy and data protection on the one hand, and the public interest in ensuring individuals are provided with optimum care on the other. In many ways, the chapter allows us to read the chapters in Part I in complementary light, such as Taylor's call for decisions that might interfere with privacy, data protection, or medical confidentiality to be supported by "reasonable justification" as means of protecting and promoting trustworthiness and the public interest in endeavours such as of the NICD Paediatric HIV Surveillance Team and the management of HIV in South Africa.

Concluding thoughts

It is my aim that this volume, beyond filling the lacuna of stimulating more reflection and discussion about the interrelationship between privacy, confidentiality, and data protection in biomedicine, will encourage practitioners, legal scholars, and students alike from around the globe to interrogate further some of the key concepts, rules, and functions of these laws and legal regimes across multiple jurisdictions. Paraphrasing Taylor, Floridi, and van der Sloot in their excellent edited collection on group privacy,[16] it is not my intention, nor those of the contributors, to offer anything like final answers or solutions to enduring questions about these legal regimes, their interrelationship, and their application to the biomedical domain. And paraphrasing William Lowrance in his groundbreaking book some years ago, this volume cannot resolve all of the issues; "no-one has, and no book could".[17] But I hope—we hope—that each chapter can be seen as engaging in a dialogue with the others and pointing towards some intriguing and exciting new ways of thinking about this emerging and increasingly significant field of health privacy law. As Christopher Kuner has remarked: "It should never be forgotten that scholarship can play an important role in strengthening the position of data protection and privacy, which is constantly under threat from governments, companies, law enforcement agencies, and others".[18] In this volume, we aim to provide a necessary crucial and analytical lens to exploring and operationalizing these fundamental concepts. To put it another way, this volume initiates a conceptual and practical discussion of where we came from, where we are, and most importantly, where we ought to go.

Notes

1 In this Introduction, I use the terms "health information" and "health data" interchangeably.
2 Data protection law may also be known in different jurisdictions as privacy law or personal information protection law. Nonetheless, the contributors in this book, and scholars more generally, contrast data protection law from privacy law in that the former (often through statute) governs the collection, use, and disclosure of personal data by various entities (be they public or private), while privacy law may comprise a mix of constitutional law, human rights law, and common law (or civil code) that protects different aspects of one's private life, a scope that transcends the regulation of personal information (which also may not be private per se).
3 And one that I am grateful that Russell George and the fantastic team at Routledge also recognized. I must also acknowledge several excellent books that have broken ground in this emerging field of health privacy law, albeit generally without a focus on the interrelationship of privacy, confidentiality, and data protection. These include: Chris Clark and Janice McGhee (eds), *Private and Confidential? Handling Personal Information in the Social and Health Services* (Policy Press 2008); William W Lowrance, *Privacy, Confidentiality, and Health Research* (Cambridge University Press 2012); Aris Gkoulalas-Divanis and Grigorios Loukides (eds), *Medical Data Privacy Handbook* (Springer 2015); Christina Munns and Subhajit Basu, *Privacy and Healthcare Data: 'Choice of Control' to 'Choice' and 'Control'* (Routledge 2015); Maria Tzanou (ed), *Health Data Privacy under the GDPR: Big Data Challenges and Regulatory Responses* (Routledge 2021); Ahmed Elngar, Ambika Pawar, and Prathamesh Churi (eds), *Data Protection and Privacy in Healthcare: Research and Innovations* (CRC Press/Routledge 2021); Carolyn Adams, Judy Allen, and Felicity Flack, *Sharing Linked Data for Health Research: Toward Better Decision Making* (Cambridge University Press 2022); and Thierry Vansweevelt and Nicola Glover-Thomas (eds), *Privacy and Medical Confidentiality in Healthcare: A Comparative Analysis* (Edward Elgar 2023).
4 Jon Suarez-Davis, "Data Isn't 'The New Oil'—It's Way More Valuable Than That" (12 December 2022) The Drum, available at: https://www.thedrum.com/opinion/2022/12/12/data-isn-t-the-new-oil-it-s-way-more-valuable.
5 Graham Greenleaf, "Global Data Privacy Laws 2023: 162 National Laws and 20 Bills" (2023) 181 *Privacy Laws and Business International Report* 1.
6 597 US 215 (2022).
7 European Commission, "Proposal for a Regulation of the European Parliament and of the Council on the European Health Data Space" COM (2022) 197 final, available at: https://eur-lex.europa.eu/legal-content/EN/TXT/?uri=CELEX%3A5 2022PC0197.
8 This volume thus answers in part the call from Christopher Kuner, former Editor-in-Chief of the journal *International Data Privacy Law* (of which I am an Editor), that

> Data protection law would also profit from a historical turn in which scholars would look back over 30, 40, 50 years or more to understand how concepts, rules, and institutions arose, what their original purpose was, and how they have developed.
>
> See Christopher Kuner, "Some Parting Remarks, With a Hopeful Glance Towards the Future" (2024) 14 *International Data Privacy Law* 1.

9 Regulation (EU) 2016/679 of the European Parliament and of the Council on the protection of natural persons with regard to the processing of personal data and on the free movement of such data (General Data Protection Regulation) 2016.

10 Council of Europe, Convention for the Protection of Individuals with Regard to the Processing of Personal Data (CETS No. 108) (1981), available at: https://www.coe.int/en/web/conventions/full-list?module=treaty-detail&treatynum=108.

11 Council of Europe, Convention 108 +: Modernised Convention for the Protection of Individuals with Regard to the Processing of Personal Data, CM/Inf(2018)15-final (2018), available at: https://search.coe.int/cm/Pages/result_details.aspx?ObjectId=09000016807c65bf.

12 See e.g. Council of Europe, Recommendation No. R (97) 5 on the Protection of Medical Data (1997); Council of Europe, Recommendation CM/Rec(2019)2 on the Protection of Health-Related Data (2019).

13 Department of Health and Social Care (UK Government), *Data Saves Lives: Reshaping Health and Social Care with Data* (June 2022), available at: https://www.gov.uk/government/publications/data-saves-lives-reshaping-health-and-social-care-with-data/data-saves-lives-reshaping-health-and-social-care-with-data.

14 Ibid. ("We will amend [The Health Service (Control of Patient Information) Regulations 2002] to ensure that they facilitate timely and proportionate sharing of data, engaging with stakeholders and the public by the end of 2022 to make sure that changes are implemented transparently—delivery date subject to Parliamentary processes.").

15 *ABC v St George's Healthcare NHS Trust & Ors* [2020] EWHC 455 (QB).

16 Linnet Taylor, Luciano Floridi, and Bart van der Sloot, "Introduction: A New Perspective on Privacy", in Linnet Taylor, Luciano Floridi, and Bart van der Sloot (eds), *Group Privacy: New Challenges of Data Technologies* (Springer 2017) 11.

17 Lowrance, n 3, xiii.

18 Kuner, n 8, 1.

PART I

Conceptual complexities

1

IS PRIVACY EGREGIOUSLY WRONG? REFLECTIONS ON A CONCEPT THAT CAN MAKE OR BREAK CONSTITUTIONS

Graeme Laurie

Introduction

This chapter asks whether privacy is "egregiously wrong". This framing is adapted from the emotive language of the United States (US) Supreme Court in *Dobbs v Jackson Women's Health Organization*,[1] which controversially overturned the decision laid down in *Roe* v *Wade* that the Constitution of the United States confers a right to abortion.[2] The finding in *Roe* was based on the right to privacy. The chapter is not, however, about abortion or access to abortion services. Many others have written elsewhere and far more expertly on these crucially important topics.[3] Indeed, *Dobbs* was not about privacy per se because the constitutional framing had moved on since *Roe* when the right to privacy was central to securing the constitutional right to an abortion. Nonetheless, as will be shown, the nature of the US constitutional right to privacy and its judicial lineage mean that private decisions to seek termination of pregnancy are inherently tied to a wealth of other decisions in the private realm. These are currently protected by the Constitution as a direct result of the prior success of arguments about privacy as a necessary and inherent part of the Bill of Rights. Thus, what has happened to the right to abortion in *Dobbs* invariably will have consequences for other rights grounded in privacy, past and future. In other words, the work done by privacy may come to be the undoing of privacy itself. It is imperative that we understand how this might come to pass and what it says about the concept. This also provides a platform to ask deeper questions about the nature of the concept of privacy embedded in many Western constitutions, written and unwritten.

Many have tried to articulate the "true" nature of privacy, with varying degrees of success. Principal among these has been the legal scholar Ruth Gavison, whose 1980 *Yale Law Review* article remains a tour de force in privacy literature.[4] It engages privacy both as a US constitution concept and as a social construct of immeasurable utility to many. Gavison's article was

DOI: 10.4324/9781003394518-3

written in the wake of *Roe* v *Wade* but was also set against a much broader and longer sweep of jurisprudence that engaged with privacy. It is fruitful to revisit her insights in the wake of *Dobbs* and to refresh our collective memories about the history of privacy before *Dobbs* and *Roe*, notably to return to the US Supreme court decision of *Griswold* v *Connecticut*,[5] which saw its 50th anniversary in recent years. As will be shown, doing so reveals that privacy is richer and more expansive than the more recent reproductive jurisprudence would suggest.

Equally, it is important to hold a healthy scepticism about privacy and its utility. Very recent campaigns have sought to re-interpret privacy in an attempt to deny or restrict citizens' rights, as has happened in the context of the rights of transgender persons. This reminds us that privacy—both legally and socially—is far from an unqualified good. Few matters are immutable in the realm of privacy, making it a dangerous axiom in constitutional lore.[6] It also raises fundamental anxieties about what privacy is and what it can be used for. It is important to articulate these anxieties in an attempt to better understand them and privacy itself.

The majority of the Supreme Court in *Dobbs* said repeatedly that the previous ruling that the Constitution of the United States confers a right to abortion was "egregiously wrong". And, if one accepts that decisions such as the abortion decision rightfully lie within the private realm—irrespective of whether one agrees that they should be legally or constitutionally protected—then the labelling of egregious wrongness to a constitutional right to abortion might equally be attached to privacy in many of its guises. It is suggested herein that indeed, this is what will happen in the US with respect to the Constitutional Right to Privacy. But whether that label is attached with any legitimacy cannot be decided by looking at court jurisprudence alone. For a multiplicity of reasons, court decisions are not a good place to start when seeking to understand fundamental human constructs like privacy. Rather, we require an approach that builds on the privacy case law and seeks to go beyond it to understand the socio-political and *ethical* meaning-making that has surrounded privacy.[7] In turn, this takes us far beyond the US socio-political scene because a similar exercise could be constructed in Europe with the European Convention on Human Rights (ECHR) in respect of Article 8,[8] and indeed in any country which has privacy at the heart of its constitutional protection of citizens' rights.

If we are to understand meanings of privacy—and if we are to make privacy more meaningful beyond the ways it has been interpreted in the confines of the courtroom—it is suggested that this kind of socio-politico-ethical approach is required because it allows us to revisit three dimensions of privacy that have created enduring anxieties about privacy, namely, as to its definition, its scope, and its function. By these means, it is the central aspiration of this chapter to contribute to on-going debates about privacy, its utility and disutility, and its role in our constitutions and in our lives.

The chapter is structured as follows: Part 1 uses the recent decision of the US Supreme Court in *Dobbs* as a gateway to examine privacy as a constitutional concept. It demonstrates that the origins of the constitutional right to abortion laid down in *Roe* v *Wade* not only inherently tied the abortion choice to the right to privacy, but that through those ties there are strong reasons to suspect that *Dobbs* is but the beginning of an attack through the courts on wider privacy-related rights in the US. This section examines privacy at a conceptual and constitutional level to explain why this is so. Part 2 develops the analysis further by examining privacy and its anxieties. Judicial pronouncements and scholarly attention are replete with a range of consternations about privacy and its nature and meaning. This section offers an original tripartite analysis of these anxieties around privacy: (i) as to its definition, (ii) as to its scope, and (iii) as to its function. This reveals a deeper understanding of what is at stake when privacy is invoked, while at the same time leading us to question how far jurisprudential analysis of privacy through a constitutional lens can deliver full explanatory power. To supplement jurisprudential analysis, in Part 3 an approach is advocated that is grounded in "demosprudence", i.e. the study of power dynamics between law-making and social movements.[9] This allows us to capture understandings about the highly political and polarizing forces behind privacy. It is shown how this approach to understanding privacy lays bare its strengths and its weaknesses as a tool in the constitutional armamentarium. This framing offers a basis for an answer to the central question of this chapter: Is Privacy Egregiously Wrong? Unsurprisingly, such a crude interrogation is rejected. The chapter is an unapologetic defence of privacy as an inescapable and essential part of the human condition and our ethical lives. Our inability as a society to get privacy "right" through the courts does not mean that we should ever accept that privacy itself is invariably or egregiously "wrong". There are good reasons to be concerned that a constitutional attack on privacy in the US is but the thin edge of a wedge that potentially will be riven in Western societies more widely. The basis of this concern is laid out below, followed by a proposal for the protection of privacy itself.

Privacy as a constitutional concept

In June 2022, the Supreme Court of the United States overruled the landmark ruling of *Roe* v *Wade* (1973) on the eve of its 50th anniversary. This chapter is written in 2023 on the advent of that anniversary. Famously, *Roe* v *Wade* secured the right to abortion as part of the Constitutional Right to Privacy, interpreted out of various amendments[10] to the US Constitution and its Bill of Rights. This right was construed as part of a penumbra of rights contained in the Bill of Rights itself.[11] The recognition of such a right was held to be necessary to secure the "fundamental" and "ordered liberty" of citizens as "… a guarantee of certain areas or zones of privacy".[12]

The focus of this chapter is the concept of privacy *simpliciter*—which was central to the judicial reasoning in *Roe*—and which paved the way for multiple further instances of judicial and socio-political recognition of the right to privacy and its role in Western society. In this section, I trace what happened to the right to privacy after *Roe*, and I revisit the judicial history leading up to *Roe*. The picture that emerges is fuzzy, not least because the direct link between abortion and privacy was subsequently broken after *Roe* by the Supreme Court in *Planned Parenthood of Southeastern Pennsylvania* v *Casey* (hereafter *Casey*).[13] Indeed, the *Dobbs* decision overruling *Roe* is not ostensibly about privacy at all. Nonetheless, as will be shown, arguments about the nature of any putative right to abortion, or indeed about reproductive rights in general, are inherently linked to arguments about the nature and protection of the private realm that citizens inhabit. Thus, if the primary purpose of a constitution—in whichever form it manifests—is to protect citizens in their relationship with the state, then we must explore and understand how constitutions create and protect the private realm, often re-enforcing what is socially constructed without the force of law. An examination of *Roe*, and its antecedents and precedents, serves us well in such an analysis.

Roe was overruled by *Dobbs*.[14] This last case involved a challenge to Mississippi's Gestational Age Act, passed in 2018 and which provided that

> …[e]xcept in a medical emergency or in the case of a severe fetal abnormality, a person shall not intentionally or knowingly perform … or induce an abortion of an unborn human being if the probable gestational age of the unborn human being has been determined to be greater than fifteen (15) weeks.

Manifestly, this was contrary to the right laid down for women in *Roe* and confirmed in *Casey*. The Supreme Court held, however, "the Constitution does not confer a right to abortion. *Roe* and *Casey* must be overruled, and the authority to regulate abortion must be returned to the people and their elected representatives".[15]

It is impossible to speak or write about the decision in *Dobbs* in a dispassionate fashion. It is disingenuous to claim otherwise even when the decision is stripped down to its constitutional bones of legal arguments about substantive due process, the nature of precedent (stare decisis), and the vagaries of judicial activism. It is therefore incredulous to read Justice Kavanaugh:

The *Roe* Court took sides on a consequential moral and policy issue that this Court had no constitutional authority to decide. By taking sides, the *Roe* Court distorted the Nation's understanding of this Court's proper role in the American constitutional system and thereby damaged the Court as an institution...The Court's decision today properly returns the Court to a position of judicial neutrality on the issue of abortion, and properly restores the people's authority to resolve the issue of abortion through the processes of democratic self-government established by the Constitution.[16]

The overt moral and political proselytizing of the majority in *Dobbs* is revealed by the fact that it stated no fewer than nine times that *Roe* was "egregiously wrong". It is a genuine conundrum how any court could reconcile claims that a decision protecting one of the most intimate decisions in a person's life was "egregiously wrong" with any credible notion of "judicial neutrality". The dissenting judges in *Dobbs* recognized this and feared for the rule of law itself:

> In the end, the majority says, all it must say to override *stare decisis* is one thing: that it believes *Roe* and *Casey* "egregiously wrong."[17] That rule could equally spell the end of any precedent with which a bare majority of the present Court disagrees.[18]

The same fear sits at the heart of this chapter. It is a fear about citizens' and human rights and most notably about the right to privacy. In the remainder of this section, the substance of this concern will be laid out using the privacy precedents that led up to and stemmed from *Roe*.

Roe[19] involved a constitutional challenge to a Texas criminal law that prohibited procuring or attempting an abortion except on medical advice for the purpose of saving the mother's life. Blackmun J spoke for the entirety of the Supreme Court, except for two brief and thin dissents, in finding that the abortion decision formed part of the Constitutional Right to Privacy. As such, the Texas law was struck down as unconstitutional. Moreover, because this decision was recognized to be in the realm of fundamental rights, regulation of abortion was only permissible when there was a compelling state interest to do so. This, in turn, gave rise to the controversial trimester approach where no state interference was initially justified and only upon viability of the foetus could prohibitions be imposed.

Roe was immediately the focus of moral, social, political, and constitutional attack.[20] Its full weaknesses have been well explored elsewhere.[21] Our interest for present purposes lies in the Supreme Court's focus on privacy. Why was an issue that is ostensibly about autonomy—i.e. a right to self-determination over one's body and life choices—framed as a privacy issue? Indeed, why was privacy invoked at all when an appeal to liberty prima facie had far more resonance in the context of a constitutional debate? The answer to these questions in a US context is highly complex and convoluted, but there are two strands of legal precedent that—when analysed—reveal important insights that explain a turn towards privacy in the framing of issues such as abortion. First, it is important to understand that by the time *Roe* was decided, judicial treatment of liberty had acquired a very poor reputation. Indeed, the constitutional meaning and scope of liberty had proved to be a battle ground for a power struggle between the Supreme Court and legislatures almost since the signing of the Constitution itself. The notorious watershed case of *Lochner* v *US*[22]—striking down legislation to limit workers' hours in the name of freedom of contract—came to represent all that was wrong with judicial activism in relying on substantive due process (Fourteenth Amendment) to declare unconstitutional legislative acts to which the Court took objection. Albeit that the *Lochner* era cases were primarily concerned with economic rights, the taint on liberty as a constitutional tool for an activist Court was deep and potentially poisonous.[23]

Secondly, for a Court deliberating in the politically charged early years of the 1970s, a more fruitful avenue had been emerging in the immediate prior decades. *Roe* drew heavily on *Griswold*,[24] which is, in fact, hailed as the landmark decision that ushered in the Constitutional Right to Privacy. *Griswold* is commonly cast as the contraception case—is it constitutional for a state to attempt to limit access to contraception for married couples? Delivering the majority ruling and a negative answer to this question, Douglas J was at pains to distance the decision from *Lochner*, both as to substance and approach: "[o]vertones of some arguments suggest that *Lochner*...should be our guide. But we decline that invitation..."[25] Eschewing any perception of a role as a super-legislature, the Court accepted arguments that the case was essentially about the intimate relations of a husband and wife and the implications for the relationship of a state statute making it a crime for any person to use any drug or article to prevent conception. In carving out the Constitutional Right to Privacy to strike down such a statute, Douglas J invoked the notion of penumbras cast by various amendments to the Constitution throwing protection to citizens in the form of recognition of zones of privacy into which the state could not intrude without strong justification.[26] Such a device was necessary because the US Constitution makes no explicit mention of privacy per se. The metaphor of shadowlands of protection is both helpful and unhelpful. Conceptually, it invokes and has strong resonance with the very human intuition that a sphere of private life exists and is important. The notion of a shadow of existence, hidden from public view, is powerful (and potentially oppressive).[27] Constitutionally, the idea is hopelessly vague and open to attack for lacking legal foundation. For such reasons, Goldberg J in *Griswold* preferred to find a concrete basis for the right to privacy in the Ninth and Fourteenth Amendments, while Harlan J (concurrence White J) expressly found that the Due Process clause of the Fourteenth Amendment protected the right to privacy. Dissents from Black J and Stewart J could find no basis in the Constitution for any such right.

Griswold begat *Eisenstadt v Baird*[28] (in which the same protection, namely, access to contraception, was recognized for unmarried couples) and both begat *Roe*, which extended privacy protection to the realm of access to abortion services and physical autonomy over the abortion decision.[29] Indeed, the history of right to privacy cases as "sex" cases is well traced by Rubenfeld[30] throughout the 1970s and 1980s. He notes, however, that any intuition that sex and sexuality are rightly and inherently privacy matters into which the state has no right of intrusion was thwarted by the ruling in *Bowers* v *Hardwick*[31] relating to the constitutionality of sodomy laws. In that case, the Supreme Court explicitly rejected an argument that the right to privacy protected "...all private sexual conduct between consenting adults".[32] In inflammatory language, the Court decreed that there was no "...fundamental right to engage in homosexual sodomy ..." in much the same way that the *Dobbs* Court ruled that ordered liberty and the Fourteenth Amendment do not protect the "right to an abortion" in the US Constitution. As to sexuality, however, *Bowers* was later overruled in *Lawrence v Texas*,[33] in which the Supreme Court affirmed the line of precedents carving out a realm of private life, albeit that the Constitutional foundation had shifted somewhat. Thus, we have Kennedy J for the majority:

> The petitioners are entitled to respect for their private lives. The State cannot demean their existence or control their destiny by making their private sexual conduct a crime. Their right to liberty under the Due Process Clause gives them the full right to engage in their conduct without intervention of the government. "It is a promise of the Constitution that there is a realm of personal liberty which the government may not enter." [citing *Casey* at 847]. The Texas statute furthers no legitimate state interest which can justify its intrusion into the personal and private life of the individual.[34]

Scalia J, for the dissent, warned of the inevitable moral ruin that would ensue if such a reading of substantive due process were permitted (yet to materialize), and Thomas J—a long-standing opponent of inclusive interpretation of substantive due process—reflected the reasoning of the dissents in *Griswold*:

> ...just like Justice Stewart, I "can find [neither in the Bill of Rights nor any other part of the Constitution a] general right of privacy," ibid., or as the Court terms it today, the "liberty of the person both in its spatial and more transcendent dimensions," ante, at 562.[35]

Notwithstanding, in *Obergefell* v *Hodges*,[36] a majority of five (with four dissenting judges) ruled that state bans on same-sex marriage were unconstitutional and in violation of the Fourteenth Amendment (due process and equal protection). In resonant language from *Lawrence*, the Court referenced the constitutional promise of liberty to all for rights that "...extend to certain personal choices central to individual dignity and autonomy, including intimate choices that define personal identity and beliefs". Tellingly, the Court rejected the respondent states' framing of the issue as a "right to same sex marriage". The matter fell to be considered as the right to marry "in its comprehensive sense".

Before commenting on this line of authority, it is important to add one final piece to the puzzle that is privacy, namely the judgment in *Casey*.[37] This case represented the culmination of controversies that followed *Roe* in terms of testing the limits of when, where, and how a state could impinge on a woman's abortion decision. *Casey* was a direct challenge to key provisions of the Pennsylvania Abortion Control Act of 1982 that contained requirements such as a waiting period, notice to a spouse, and parental consent before a minor could undergo an abortion procedure. The Supreme Court upheld *Roe* to the extent that a right of access to abortion was preserved, but constitutionally it shifted the goalposts. The decision was no longer framed in terms of the right to privacy as such; rather, the plurality opinion focused on the "essential holding" of *Roe* that relied on substantive due process in the Fourteenth Amendment. This had a number of consequences, including that the trimester model was abandoned in favour of a viability approach—allowing greater state latitude for interference—and the standard for judging state action moved from strict scrutiny requiring a compelling interest to a lower undue burden test, meaning that some elements of the Pennsylvania law would stand.

In order to make sense of all of this, it is helpful to differentiate between two key perspectives: the constitutional and the conceptual. This is not to suggest that these elements are not inherently linked; rather, it is important to be clear about issues that are about the vagaries of US constitutional and judicial reasoning and the larger human enterprise of making meaning about the role of privacy in our lives.[38]

Constitutionally, in the US, the abortion decision became disentangled from the idea of a constitutional right to privacy. The legal grounding came to be anchored more overtly in substantive due process. Moreover, just as *Roe* can be traced back to *Griswold* and the line of authority extended forward to *Lawrence* and beyond, it is also possible to witness a constitutional shift in the framing of the issues at stake—away from an express right to privacy and towards claims emerging from the nature and meaning of substantive due process. This matters very much for the constitutional rights of citizens in the US. In *Dobbs*, when overruling *Roe* and *Casey*, the Supreme

Court went to extreme lengths to distinguish the "right to abortion" as a special case because of the implications for human life. The majority argued feverishly that the precedent being set related only to the absence of a "right to abortion" in the US Constitution and the lack of any history of protection thereof before *Roe*. But *Griswold* was also about personal decisions that have implications for future human life. And none of the rights recognized under the penumbra of privacy—now linked to substantive due process—have the kind of history the majority in *Dobbs* would require to secure their sustained constitutional protection. One need only read the concurring decision of Thomas J, which is an overt attack on any kind of inclusive reading of substantive due process, to realize that *Dobbs* is not, and will not ever only be, about abortion. Indeed, in order to overrule *Roe* and *Casey* the *Dobbs* Court had to dismantle the principle of stare decisis itself. No existing case is safe.[39] The private realm itself is now laid bare.

It is tempting to understand the US Constitutional Right to Privacy as relating primarily to sexual intimacy, reproduction, and sexuality.[40] It would, however, be a mistake to do so. On the 50th anniversary of *Griswold* in 2015/16, a spate of new scholarship revisited the decision and was able to analyse the ruling relative to the subsequent decisions that built upon it and against the broader sweep of socio-political influences that gave rise to the case itself.[41] Both constitutionally and conceptually, a deep understanding of *Griswold* is key to realizing the aims of this chapter.

First, the caricature of *Griswold* as dealing with intimacy in the marital bedroom must be challenged. This framing is accurate only to a degree and it was certainly strategically crucial in getting the case to the Supreme Court and in securing the outcome that was delivered. However, as Reva Siegel deftly demonstrates, *Griswold* and its precedents[42] entrenched the right to privacy precisely because the decision reflected and captured ongoing and wider social struggles about personal autonomy and liberation more generally.[43] The breadth of those social struggles extended far beyond the bedroom, as illustrated by Franklin, who reminds us that *Griswold* was about a public clinic committed to serving low-income women.[44] *Griswold* was as much, if not more, about poverty as privacy. It was about securing access for citizens who were disadvantaged in their private lives by systemic structural injustices.[45] Moreover, there was no imperative to frame *Griswold* in terms of privacy at all.[46] As explained above, socio-political factors meant that a liberty framing was unpalatable at the time, but the nature of the issues being addressed could just as easily have lent themselves to an examination within an equality paradigm[47] and on multiple other grounds.[48]

But if we extend our historical lens even further back in time, there are good reasons that explain why the Supreme Court settled on the language of privacy in *Griswold* and, indeed, perhaps why Douglas J invoked the notion of penumbras. It is a cliché that the 1960s were the decade for revolutions of all kinds, and it can be easy to forget about the origins of such revolutions in preceding years. Private morality and public (in)tolerance were central feature of social and academic debate in the 1950s, most notably focused on the British Wolfenden *Report of the Committee on Homosexual Offences and Prostitution* published in 1957.[49] The recommendation that homosexuality be decriminalized in Britain turned on the most famous quote from the report:

> Unless a deliberate attempt is to be made by society, acting through the agency of the law, to equate the sphere of crime with that of sin, there must be a realm of private morality and immorality which is, in brief and crude terms, not the law's business.[50]

The profound social implications of this statement and the full report were felt on both sides of the Atlantic. In the United Kingdom,[51] it gave rise to the (in)famous Hart-Devlin debate about the relationship between law and morality, known to every law student as "Jurisprudence 101". And those actors and that debate crossed to the US, the history of which is recounted by David Minto in his persuasive account of the influences leading up to *Griswold*.[52] The suggestion is that the idea embodied by a private realm is reflected in the rhetoric of protection afforded by penumbras from the US Constitution in *Griswold*.[53]

Conceptually and constitutionally, it matters very much how we talk about privacy. In *Griswold*, "...the majority held that in the 'penumbras' of the U.S. Constitution's stated protections—in the light-dark interplay of 'emanations from those guarantees that help give them life and substance'—lay 'a right of privacy older than the Bill of Rights.'"[54] But, when the claims about our private lives are reduced to specific, putative *rights*—such as a right to abortion or a right to homosexual sodomy—they become immediately vulnerable to attack in a constitutional setting where the text never foresaw future context. Much of the judicial discussion in *Dobbs* and *Bowers* is about the absence of any "deep rooted history" of protection for abortion and sodomy. And, on such framing, it is easy to find absence. Just as there will be an absence of protection for access to contraception, or same-sex marriage, or any technological claim about assistance in, or protection for, our private lives.[55]

If, however, we shift thinking and discourse from rights to realms, the notion of a realm of privacy—a sphere of protection for the citizen—we immediately highlight the centrality of privacy at the heart of constitutional deliberation. All international human rights instruments recognize this in some form or another; indeed, the influence of post–World War II human rights discourse on US judicial decision-making has already been the subject of analysis elsewhere,[56] albeit that the Supreme Court has made no direct reference to human rights in the development of its jurisprudence. In contrast, and in the context of the ECHR, Article 8(1) provides: "Everyone has the right to respect for his private and family life, his home and his correspondence." This, in essence, recognizes and protects the private realm. Any intrusion is only justifiable when the strict terms of Article 8(2) are met and it is demonstrably necessary and in accordance with the law. The realm of "private and family life" has enjoyed an expansive development in the 70+ years since the ECHR came into force, but it is by no means unfettered.[57] Constitutionally, it has served to police the state–citizen boundary seeking equipoise in response to constantly shifting social circumstances.

In contrast, the Right to Privacy in the US has both over-promised and under-delivered. It has served to secure some of the most personal and intimate protections any citizen could aspire to, but it has also been politicized and exploited on all sides to the point where it has been stripped of any core authentic meaning. Two examples illustrate this. In her book *Beyond Abortion: Roe v Wade and the Battle for Privacy*, Ziegler provides a history of privacy politics in the US, demonstrating how *Roe* has been relied upon by various social movements—including sexual politics, medical consumer rights, informational privacy, mental health, and death and dying—to pursue and advance their agenda.[58] At the same time, *Roe* came to be seen in many quarters as a modern *Lochner*—a vehicle for unbridled judicial activism, and this in the end is what sounded its death knell in *Dobbs*.[59] Most recently, a coalition of Christians, Republicans, conservative legal organizations, right-wing foundations, and trans-exclusionary radical feminists have sought to redefine the right to privacy in service of anti-transgender politics. The movement is a blatant attempt to weaponize privacy within anti-transgender politics.[60]

In light of all of this, we must ask: is privacy itself egregiously wrong? Does a concept that is so malleable, polarizing, and so amenable to weaponization have any rightful place in our constitutions? Equally, we must consider: is privacy wrong or is it that we have got privacy wrong? I address these questions in the following sections.

Privacy and its anxieties[61]

In this section I confront what is wrong with privacy; or rather, I analyse why it is so difficult to get privacy right as a matter of law and more broadly in society. The approach is to examine privacy and its anxieties. The previous section has revealed judicial consternation about privacy in a US constitutional context, but the anxieties generated by privacy extend far beyond the legal domain. This is revealed by the extensive literature on privacy that spans myriad disciplines. The terrain is vast and some navigation is required. A first beacon is found in the legal scholarship of Ruth Gavison, who wrote about privacy, conceptually and constitutionally, in the late 1970s and 1980s. Her work remains pioneering among academic understandings of privacy and for its advocacy to move beyond law. Second, I humbly offer my own analysis of the anxieties of privacy through an original tripartite analysis, exposing and explaining anxieties as to (i) definition, (ii) scope, and (iii) function. The argument is made that we must go beyond jurisprudence to demosprudence, as explained below, and with respect to each of these facets of privacy if we are to have any hope of getting to grips with our anxieties about privacy itself. Section 3 offers some signposts in this regard.

Ruth Gavison wrote "Privacy and the Limits of Law" in 1980, and it opens with the following observation:

> Anyone who studies the law of privacy today may well feel a sense of uneasiness. On one hand, there are popular demands for increased protection of privacy, discussions of new threats to privacy, and an intensified interest in the relationship between privacy and other values, such as liberty, autonomy, and mental health.[62]

Truly, it seems that nothing has changed. If anything, our uneasiness is only heightened both about privacy and for privacy in the light of *Dobbs*. Indeed, the *Dobbs* decision proves Gavison to be right in her scholarship in three important respects.

First, Gavison makes the astute observation that privacy is rarely protected on its own. Invariably, when a remedy for invasion of privacy is given, there is another interest at stake, such as liberty, autonomy, property, and reputation. This explains why so-called reductionists are quick to dismiss the value of privacy itself, arguing that core concerns can just as easily be protected by existing legal means. This is one explanation of the jurisprudence on the US Constitution Right to Privacy culminating in *Dobbs*. For Gavison, however, this is misleading and misses the point: "…it does not follow from this that the presence of privacy in a situation does not serve as an additional reason for protection".[63] This speaks to the core function of privacy in society. Gavison advocates that we must first seek a neutral understanding of privacy before we imbue any value to it.

Secondly, Gavison cautions against seeking a deeper understanding of privacy by looking merely at the case law. As with all jurisprudence, cases come to court through haphazard, unpredictable, serendipitous, and opportunistic means. Precedents are merely a patchwork of circumstances sewn together by judicial threads that could be unpicked or broken at any time. Again, this is illustrated all too clearly by *Dobbs*. For Gavison, starting with the jurisprudential domain will tend to support reductionist accounts of privacy both because parallels interests will be invoked and because the patchwork will prove to be full of holes over time, i.e. the overall picture will appear incoherent as to the core values at stake. She concludes: "[s]tarting from the extra-legal concept of privacy enables us to avoid these pitfalls".[64] This is not, however, tantamount to simply asking people why or whether privacy is important. It requires a more sophisticated engagement with manifestations of privacy across multiple domains, and it also speaks to the need for a meaningful and coherent definition of privacy. Ultimately, for Gavison privacy is composed of three elements: secrecy, anonymity, and solitude.[65] These are related, but distinct, notions protecting connected dimensions of a person's private life. They are linked through the common notion of accessibility.

Finally, Gavison warns that:

> [a]djudicative techniques may cause the coherence of legal concepts to blur. For example, an early case may establish a "right to privacy". This "right" will be invoked in later cases, and as long as the situations are analogous the invocation is proper and illuminating. If a court relies on this right in situations that are significantly different from the early ones, however, it will be for different reasons than those that impelled the original court to grant recovery.[66]

This speaks to the appropriate scope of privacy claims. For Gavison, abortion and liberty-related claims are not appropriately part of a coherent constitutional concept of privacy. She defends the bounded view of privacy as a concern with accessibility against literature at the time that examined, variously, privacy as a right to be let alone,[67] privacy as an aspect of human dignity,[68] and privacy as a shield to protect nefarious and unacceptable behaviour.[69]

The insights from Gavison endure to this day. Her entreaty to approach privacy neutrally in the first instance provides a level *tabula rasa* to begin discussions about the concept. While there are many reasons to value privacy, it is equally undeniable that the private sphere hides many ills. Privacy is not a self-evident good, and this must be fully acknowledged. Equally, as the above analysis of her work reveals, there are anxieties about privacy that endure to this day as to its definition, as to its scope, and as to its function. The remainder of this section addresses each of these.

Learning lessons from anxieties about definition, scope, and function of privacy

Gavison sought an extra-judicial basis for her definition of privacy as linked to inaccessibility and distinguished it from multiple other conceptualizations. In doing so, she found distinctive value in understanding and protecting privacy in its own right. Contrariwise, she identified the presence of reductionists in the literature who would either deny anything distinctive about privacy and who would herald any attempt at definition as futile or misguided, or who would seek to define privacy in the narrowest of terms. An excellent example of this is the work of William Parent.[70] In true philosophical broom-sweeping style, he reveals a taxonomy of ten concepts that are often subsumed within our everyday understanding of privacy.[71] These are: (i) privacy, (ii) liberty, (iii) autonomy, (iv) peace, (v) health, (vi) property, (vii) solitude, (viii) solitude, (ix) seclusion, and (x) anonymity. Parent argues that it is a mistake to define privacy as a "complex" of one or more of these concepts, as done by Gavison. He preferred a definition of privacy related to "the absence of undocumented personal knowledge about a person". However, in later work he goes further to question whether privacy is indeed an essential component of our "moral inviolability" and deserving of protection at all, having shown how concerns about privacy are all vulnerable to philosophical critique.[72]

This kind of work goes beyond mere anxiety about producing a workable and defensible definition of privacy. It reveals how anxiety about definition is inherently and invariably bound up with anxieties about function and scope. Parent sought to limit a definition of privacy to a scope that made it distinguishable from other concepts that we value. He was unapologetic about its narrowness and his retort to critics is that other values and concepts can do the heavy lifting to protect concerns such as access to abortion or rights to same-sex marriage. But a rejoinder to this is that while Parent's exercise might be philosophically robust, its social worth is far more questionable if the definition of privacy that is provided does not have resonance with citizens' understandings of why privacy is important and valuable to them. In other words, privacy is meaningless and worthless outside of its social context.

The exactitudes of philosophical inquiry or judicial reasoning ought not to dictate how we address our *social* and *ethical* anxieties about privacy. Reductionists cannot explain why new appeals to privacy constantly occur. Technological change is one obvious source of new threats, but so too are democratic threats represented by rulings in cases such as *Dobbs*. Equally, we must not fall into the obvious trap of conceiving of privacy solely in individualistic terms—as Cohen has said, there has been too much scholarship that conceptualizes privacy "…as a form of protection of the liberal self".[73] This renders privacy "reactive and ultimately inessential".[74] And, even if the answer to conundrums about privacy does not lie in constitutional salvation, we must persist in asking deep questions about privacy, its anxieties, and its social value.

For my part, I would like to offer my own contribution to the debate about these anxieties about privacy. I have studied and written about privacy for more than 30 years, and I share many of the anxieties;[75] however, I would humbly suggest that my own research can offer some novel insights on each of the elements of privacy identified above, namely, as to its definition, its scope, and its function.

As to definition, I am firmly in the Gavison camp in believing that we should be cautious not to impute any value to privacy before we have an understanding of what it is, ontologically, and which functions it serves, sociologically. Thus, to speak prematurely of a right to privacy or an interest in privacy, or even to use the language of a claim to privacy, runs the risk of assuming and assigning a value that might not be merited (and certainly not be shared in a wider community). For these reasons, I have argued elsewhere that first and foremost we should understand privacy to be a state of separateness from others.[76] This can encompass a physical separateness from others, a psychological separateness from others, and/or a separateness of intimate aspects of ourselves, such as personal data or information. Intrusion occurs when that state of separation is broken down, as with physical access to the body, the unsolicited disclosure of information to a person, and/or when unauthorized access occurs to personal data or information. To recognize such acts as "intrusion" is not to imbue the private state with any prima facie normative value as such; it is simply to acknowledge that a division between public and private has broken down. This permits the private to exist while we are in the public realm (consider the plight of celebrities) and requires that we understand context and values in play. Contextual integrity requires us to recognize and maintain a boundary between sense of public and private in any given situation, and to acknowledge incursion from one realm into the other as having human consequences for those who inhabit the private sphere. Whether we wish then to make such an intrusion actionable, in law or otherwise, is a separate step that requires us to reflect on why we might think a state of separateness could be valuable for those who inhabit it. But this speaks to content and function, and these are related by distinct considerations.

As to scope, I would argue that a definition based on separateness from others speaks to the very heart of what privacy is. Its meaning is fundamentally tied to our understanding of publicness. Without the public sphere—without others—privacy has no valid meaning. We are not in a state of privacy if I am stranded on a desert island. There is no "other" in such a situation. This is isolation, not privacy.[77] By the same token, this is not to suggest that privacy can only be enjoyed by the individual. As the work of Cohen,[78] Murray,[79] and Skinner-Thompson[80] has shown, the notion of group privacy is socially, ethically, and politically fundamental to any meaningful and defensible conceptualization of privacy. Rather, for present purposes, the point is that to understand privacy or private life we need also to include an understanding of publicness and public life. Not only do the two co-exist, but these human spaces are in a constant state of flux relative to each other. This explains in large part why attempts at definitive definitions frequently fail. The scope of privacy and private life is malleable, transient, and contingent. For these reasons, I find considerable appeal in the conceptualization of *realms* of privacy—or zones of privacy to use the early US Constitutional language. The European human rights jurisprudence has far fewer problems than its US counterpart in carving out a sphere of separateness under the imperative to show "respect for private and family life", the scope of which has shifted considerably in the last 70 years.[81] An advantage to this is that the inherently changeable nature of privacy is captured; the serious downside is that it makes full articulation and protection a never-ending exercise. But why is this necessarily problematic if this understanding accurately reflects what privacy does for most citizens?[82]

This brings us to the function(s) of privacy. As the above discussion of the literature demonstrates, there have been myriad attempts to pin down the core functions that privacy has in our lives. It is certainly true that a concept that is potentially expansive enough to include concerns about press intrusion, access to abortion services, access to artificial reproduction for homosexual couples, claims to support same-sex marriage, and which can be turned against marginalized groups such as transgender persons to deny them other fundamental rights[83] is conceptually questionable and functionally problematic because there is no apparent core coherence to how appeals to privacy are made. Once again, this is a principal driver behind reductionist accounts, and it also explains the writings of scholars such as Parent who seek to narrow the function and scope of privacy to carve out a distinct and workable definition. My concern with such attempts is that they miss something vital about the role of privacy in our lives. In our attempts to distil privacy into a neat and functioning concept, we can easily ignore the work that it has already done in countless human lives. The language of the Wolfenden Report in identifying a "realm of private morality" was recognition that privacy functions for the people when they are away from the public glare; it recognizes that public and private spheres are inherently connected. Public morality shifts with time and so too does our understanding of privacy. Of course, privacy cannot, and should not, be used to obscure or legitimate acts that are abhorrent, but this begs the very question that sits at the heart of privacy: who decides what is socially abhorrent and how does society accommodate divergent views and behaviours? This is an eternally unanswerable question. It cannot be decided by courts alone, and the recent experiences in the US with *Dobbs* suggest that the conversations about privacy as a constitutional right are set to be shut down. But this is all the more reason to recognize the enduring fact that privacy is important in our lives[84]—and that its function and scope shift over time with the endlessly shifting sands of public morality. A zone of privacy is particularly important for the protection of marginalized groups.[85] A society committed to equality, diversity, and inclusion has little hope of success without commitment to robust protection of privacy. If it is indeed the end of the constitutional road for privacy in the US, this must be seen as a mere crossroads for the ongoing discussions about privacy and its value (including its non-value in many contexts). But how, then, should we proceed from here?

Is privacy egregiously wrong?

As I have already indicated, Gavison urges us to look beyond jurisprudence to make sense of privacy. Thus, even if the future for privacy looks bleak in the US constitutional context, it does not follow that privacy itself is egregiously wrong. So, where and how are we to look for alternative ways to think about, speak about and—where appropriate—to mobilize privacy in defence of citizens' rights or to finally sound its death knell?

One answer emerges from the social contextualization of the Right to Privacy as recounted by Ziegler, above.[86] It will be recalled that the Right to Privacy has been mobilized by multiple social movements in the pursuit of wider recognition of civil and social rights. We do not fully understand why this particular kind of mobilization has occurred. Yet, an enquiry into such a phenomenon has been styled *demosprudence* by Guinier and Torres, being

> the study of the dynamic equilibrium of power between lawmaking and social movements … [it] is the study of the relationship between social movements and law in the creation of authoritative meaning within a democratic polity.[87]

As a method, demosprudence can be contrasted with jurisprudence, the latter being concerned with the work of judges in formal judicial settings. Instead, demosprudence involves the examination of the ways in which the action of peoples—especially marginalized groups—can effect legal changes in the personnel and/or actions of law-making bodies as well as in the environments in which law is made. There are a number of advantages to this approach when applied to privacy. First, it frees our enquiry from the ivory towers of the courts and plants it firmly in the fields of grassroots action. Second, it considerably expands the legal territory in which change can occur. Thus, in the present context, we are no longer constrained by judicial pronouncements from a supreme judicial body presiding over the contours of a constitution. Instead, legal change might occur far more extensively and effectively at the local level, for example, at the site of state legislatures whose make-up and political agenda might be more open to influence from social movements.[88] Third, this approach can adopt a stance with its core objective to reveal understandings as to "democracy-enhancing" and "meaning-making capacity" of social movements across the political spectrum. As its proponents claim:

> demosprudence is not a philosophy of the left or the right. Neither is it the philosophy of unmediated preference gathering (like the populist initiative process or the market). Rather, demosprudence represents a philosophical commitment to the lawmaking force of meaningful participatory democracy.[89]

So, what could demosprudence do for privacy? Freed from the limiting constraints of jurisprudence, this approach could be deployed to engage directly with groups that have sought to rely on privacy in the pursuit of a range of political agendas. The questions asked about privacy by scholars for decades could provide a rich basis for such research. Examples might include:

- What are the motivations driving a particular social movement?
- What is the appeal of privacy as an idea that embodies the social end that it sought?
- In what ways is the notion of privacy more apt than similar ideas, such as liberty and/or autonomy?
- What does a protected zone of privacy represent in terms of regulating the relationship with others and the state?
- Ideally, what would be protected in the daily lives of the members of the social movement by a legally enforceable right to privacy?

Furthermore, demosprudence invites empirical, comparative, and historical analyses of social movements—their successes and failures—by focusing on understanding the power relationships at stake and how these have had influence on the content of law (or not).

Such an approach could produce new insights into the politics and practice of privacy. More specifically, it would provide a rich evidence base for renewed conversations about the definition, scope, and function of privacy in a democratic society.[90] Much work remains to be done, but in one crucial respect it would provide a means for us to come to terms with our anxieties about privacy.

But it is important to examine the potential of demosprudence and social movements more closely. Building on the work of Guinier and Torres, more recent work by Akbar, Ashar, and Simonson has made the case for a new approach of *movement law*.[91] This has been presented as a new methodology for scholars and lawyers to work alongside social movements to co-produce ideas and strategies for social and legal change. The entire ethos is about praxis and experimentation in collaboration with social movements in and around law. At the same time, the approach is informed by theories such as critical legal studies and feminist legal theory, particularly in the focus on the lived experience of individuals and groups and the exposing of structural injustices. As the authors state:

> ...movement law scholars work to understand the strategies, tactics, and experiments of resistance and contestation. By studying these strategies, tactics, and experiments—including but not limited to law reform

campaigns—scholars engage pathways and possibilities for justice often obscured within legal scholarship.[92]

Movement law requires engagement with communities involved in social action and affected by it. It implies an accountability to those groups to capture, retell, and mobilize on the accurate recounting of their experiences, narratives, and motives. Regarding privacy, the above questions would represent a solid foundation for this kind of engagement. But many further questions arise from the prospect of embarking on such an endeavour in an effort to make meaning for privacy and its future relationship with law and legal institutions.

Who should be engaged?

This chapter began with a discussion of the Supreme Court ruling in *Dobbs* as it has fundamentally changed the law of abortion in the United States. However, as the ensuing analysis has hopefully demonstrated, the effects of this decision are likely to be considerably more far-reaching, especially under the rubric of privacy as a basic human need and as an amorphous legal concept. Indeed, the historical account reveals that the breadth of social injustices brought with the purview of privacy are very extensive and extend to many groups that have traditionally been marginalized, discriminated, and abused within prevailing social norms. As a result, when we ask, which social movements about privacy ought to be engaged?, the answer is rich, diverse, and expansive. The answers to the above questions about privacy will reflect this and will doubtless be challenging to reconcile in terms of developing clear and potentially effective next step strategies about privacy. For example, should the struggle for access to abortion be cast only as an issue affecting women and their bodies or is there merit in trying to develop cross-cutting strategies from the experiences of other groups and from which all groups might ultimately benefit?

There are important considerations on both sides. On the one hand, the scholarship of Siegel has shown—using the example of the Equal Rights Amendment defeat—how effective alliances can emerge from apparently diametrically opposed political positions to effect change.[93] On the other hand, there is the contribution from Blackhawk who has examined equity outside the courts, and who has argued that the United States has a strong tradition of (marginalized) groups turning to the legislature when denied justice through the courts on the application of general law. Where successful, this has resulted in specificity of law to accommodate a given group's rights and interests. This phenomenon has attracted criticism in many quarters from legal scholars who favour generality of law as a fundamental tenet of the appropriate operation of Rule of Law. As a counter, Blackhawk argues strongly that this kind of strategy can indeed deliver a novel form of equity that is both legitimate and necessary in a pluralistic society:

> Recognition of the value of equity outside the courts and its longstanding and integral role within American legislatures could begin a conversation on how best to distribute, design, and facilitate public engagement with the lawmaking process and, thus, processes of equity within lawmaking—now that we finally accept that the process fulfills an integral role of representation within legislatures.[94]

This might suggest a strategy of focusing on particular groups affected by privacy decisions and attention to what local legislatures could do to protect and advance their specific interests and rights. More broadly, however, Blackhawk draws on the work of Eskridge[95] to make the point that this wider search for equity could lead to a reimagining of equal protection within the courts themselves and could represent a shift towards empowerment of social groups. This would require the courts to examine the law-making and interpretation processes forensically and to scrutinize, in particular "...lack of deliberation and exclusion, and substance—oppression and subordination".[96] In other words, it would lead courts to ask: how has a denial of recognition of the value of the private realm led to injustices? This brings us to the next question on the potential role of movements and demosprudence.

Where should the attention of social movements be directed?

There is no single answer to this question, nor should there be. As the above examples illustrate, it is not because the courts have failed us that we should give up any hope of influencing their future approach. Equally, it does not follow that the success of one group in persuading a legislature to support their agenda means that other successes with a legislature cannot follow for other groups. Nor does it mean that social movements should direct their attention solely at the political sphere rather than the legal domain. Indeed, the advocates for movement law (above) talk about the need for a "constellation of efforts" to bring about social change.

By the same token, there are risks. Cummings has charted many social movement initiatives and has argued forcefully that the shift of attention to a predominantly political domain of action can impoverish legal scholarship and can ignore potential action that is still focused on law and legal institutions.[97] Engagement with groups about their experiences, motives, needs, and aspirations can risk replacing one unacceptable situation arising from activist courts delivering decisions with which we disagree (counter-majoritarianism) with another equally problematic scenario (crude majoritarianism). Self-evidently, law is political, but it should not be reduced to politics. No advocate of demosprudence or movement law supports vocal groups simply receiving what they shout loudly for. Rather, such approaches are designed to gather and mobilize evidence of both experiences and the wider impacts of law—some would say the "violence of law"[98]—as these have occurred to date. Any violence of law must be exposed. The integrity of law matters, and the character of law matters even more. Fundamentally, concerns about character are concerns about ethics. And so, how might we fold all of this into some lessons about preserving the ethics of privacy law?

How can we imagine an ethical future for privacy law?

In supporting a shift of our attention from jurisprudence to demosprudence, I do not mean to suggest an abandonment of law or legal institutions; indeed, my intention is quite the opposite. Rather, I seek means to deepen and enrich our understandings of the importance of privacy in human lives. As the discussion has demonstrated, demosprudence (and its sister concept of movement law) are methodologies or approaches to understanding law in practice and to strategize about what we do about law in the future. Quite what we do with the evidence that is gathered is an entirely different matter, but no matter what we do we must proceed ethically. The ethical heart of the law lies with justice. Any attempt to gather evidence about law ought to seek out injustices and any social movement ought to commit to putting them right. In this regard, the ethical concept of intersectionality can greatly enrich the task. The term originates from the scholarship of Crenshaw, who was concerned about how anti-discrimination law disadvantaged Black women because there was no means to argue simultaneously about the cumulative effects of discrimination based on both race *and* sex.[99] For her:

> Intersectionality is a metaphor for understanding the ways that multiple forms of inequality or disadvantage sometimes compound themselves and create obstacles that often are not understood among conventional ways of thinking.

This metaphor enriches any approach to gathering an evidence base about privacy (or the denial thereof) because it exposes unequal power dynamics in society, forces us to confront structural injustices, and requires us to examine the multiple ways in which these phenomena conspire to compound inequality. Intersectionality is not about identity per se. As such, it suggests that a holistic exercise is required in how we understand the injustices that arise from privacy protection, or rather the lack of protection. Multiple injustices can and do exist for myriad groups. An authentic commitment to justice for and through privacy requires that all be revealed and addressed.

To paraphrase the words of AC Grayling, "[t]o understand a phenomenon such as [privacy], we learn much by examining what we lose in losing it".[100]

There is a repertoire of strategies available to us to test and begin to answer the question: is privacy egregiously wrong? It would be fruitless, presumptuous, and hubristic to attempt a definitive answer here. Rather, what this chapter offers are good reasons to force such a question in the first place and to suggest sound and ethical ways to explore its contours. If intuition counts for anything, I wager that yet further and robust examination of privacy and its vagaries will yield crucial insights to both the human condition and the future role of law in privacy protection.

Conclusion

Privacy is not solvable precisely because it is inherently malleable. It is not fully describable precisely because it is ethereal, subject to the vagaries of subjective interpretation, and inherently tied to shifting public mores. But privacy is real in a very profound human sense because it makes sense to each and every one of us. It is no surprise that appeals to privacy have manifested in so many ways through attempts to protect private spheres of life. This should be celebrated, not denigrated, because it reflects our inherent human condition. Our inability to capture and articulate the complexity of what is happening when we appeal to privacy is no reason to deny the value of privacy itself. Legally, however, it suggests that all of our attempts to protect privacy will fail on some or multiple levels. But, as in life, we must learn to live with our (legal) anxieties. We cannot give up trying to address those anxieties. It might be that—as a matter of narrowly interpreted US constitutional law—a right to privacy is egregious wrong. But the arguments in support of such a view stem almost exclusively from jurisprudence. When a wider view is adopted—perhaps one grounded in demosprudence and its commitment to understanding the social movements that have coalesced around the very idea of privacy itself—I wager that the wrongness of privacy lies in our failure to get it right as a matter of law, rather than in privacy being wrong as something that matters to humanity.

Acknowledgements

I wish to thank Mark Taylor and Jennifer Wagner for their insightful comments on a previous draft of this chapter. The usual disclaimer for any errors applies.

Notes

1 *Dobbs* v *Jackson Women's Health Organization*, 597 US 215 (2022).
2 410 US 113 (1973).

3 Aliza Forman-Rabinovici and Olatunde CA Johnson, "Political Equality, Gender, and Democratic Legitimation in Dobbs" (2023) 46 *Harvard Journal of Law and Gender* 81; Risa Kaufman and others, "Global Impacts of *Dobbs v. Jackson Women's Health Organization* and Abortion Regression in the United States" (2022) 30 *Sexual and Reproductive Health Matters* 22; and Neil Siegel, "The Wages of Crying Roe: Some Realism About *Dobbs v. Jackson Women's Health Organization*" (2024) 2 *Journal of American Constitutional History* 101.
4 Ruth Gavison, "Privacy and the Limits of Law" (1980) 89 *Yale Law Journal* 421.
5 381 US 479 (1965).
6 There are parallels with the concept of dignity and attempts to manifest it in law and policy. See e.g. Deryck Beyleveld and Roger Brownsword, "Human Dignity, Human Rights, and Human Genetics" (1998) 61 *Modern Law Review* 661; see also Tim Caulfield and Roger Brownsword, "Human Dignity: A Guide to Policy Making in the Biotechnology Era?" (2006) 7 *Nature Review Genetics* 72.
7 Mary Ziegler, *Beyond Abortion: Roe v Wade and the Battle for Privacy* (Harvard University Press 2018).
8 European Convention on Human Rights (1950, as amended).
9 Lani Guinier and Gerald Torres, "Changing the Wind: Notes Toward a Demosprudence of Law and Social Movements" (2014) 123 *Yale Law Journal* 2740.
10 For example, for the First Amendment, see *Stanley* v *Georgia* 394 US 557 (1969); for the Fourth and Fifth Amendments, see *Terry* v *Ohio* 392 US 1 (1968), *Katz* v *United States* 389 US 347 (1967), *Boyd v United States* 116 US 616 (1886), and *Olmstead* v *United States* 277 US 438 (1928); for the Ninth Amendment, see *Griswold* v *Connecticut* 381 US 479 (1965); and for the Fourteenth Amendment, see *Meyer* v *Nebraska* 262 US 390 (1923). Ultimately, as the Court said in *Roe* v *Wade*, n 2, at 77:

>   This right of privacy, whether it be founded in the Fourteenth Amendment's concept of personal liberty and restrictions upon state action, as we feel it is, or, as the District Court determined, in the Ninth Amendment's reservation of rights to the people, is broad enough to encompass a woman's decision whether or not to terminate her pregnancy.

11 *Griswold*, n 10, 484–485.
12 *Roe* v *Wade*, n 2, 76.
13 *Planned Parenthood of Southeastern Pennsylvania* v *Casey* 505 US 833 (1992).
14 N 1.
15 Ibid., 292.
16 Ibid., 346–347.
17 Ibid., 231.
18 Ibid., Breyer, Sotomayor and Kagan, JJ., dissenting, 390.
19 Accompanied by *Doe* v *Bolton* 410 US 179 (1973) challenging a Georgia criminal law.
20 John Hart Ely, "The Wages of Crying Wolf: A Comment on *Roe v. Wade*" (1973) 82 *Yale Law Journal* 920.
21 See Ely, n 20, and most recently in the same vein, Jonathan Mitchell, "Why Was *Roe v. Wade* Wrong?", in Geoffrey Stone and Lee Bollinger (eds), *Roe v. Dobbs: The Past, Present, and Future of a Constitutional Right to Abortion* (Oxford University Press 2024) 51–66.
22 198 US 45 (1905).
23 See further Jed Rubenfeld, "The Right to Privacy" (1989) 102 *Harvard Law Review* 737, 741–744.
24 381 US 479 (1965).

25 N 24, 481–482.
26 See *Dobbs*, n 1, 263ff for a recent account of the key penumbra cases and how the Supreme Court distinguished these from the right to abortion in the instant case. See also 286ff for cases that built on *Roe*.
27 See Scott Skinner-Thompson, *Privacy at the Margins* (Cambridge University Press 2020) for an excellent critique of individualistic conceptualizations of privacy at the expense of understanding its value in challenging oppression of marginalized groups and potentially in protecting those groups from such attacks.
28 405 US 438 (1972).
29 David Garrow, *Liberty and Sexuality: The Right to Privacy and the Making of Roe v. Wade* (University of California Press 1994), 196–229.
30 N 23.
31 478 US 186 (1986).
32 Ibid., 191.
33 539 US 558 (2003).
34 Ibid., 578.
35 Ibid., 606.
36 576 US 644 (2015).
37 N 13.
38 This is not to ignore the political which is omnipresent. For a good discussion of the politicization of privacy and other rights, such as disability rights, to thwart access to abortion, see Nina Roesner and colleagues, "Reason-Based Abortion Bans, Disability Rights, and the Future of Prenatal Genetic Testing" (2022) 48 *American Journal of Law & Medicine* 187.
39 Ian Loveland, "After *Dobbs*: Can *Obergefell* Survive?" (2023) 4 *European Human Rights Law Review* 354.
40 Leigh Ann Wheeler, *How Sex Became a Civil Liberty* (Oxford University Press 2014), 93–119.
41 See also, Mary L. Dudziak, "Just Say No: Birth Control in the Connecticut Supreme Court Before *Griswold v. Connecticut*" (1990) 75 *Iowa Law Review* 915.
42 Douglas NeJaime, "*Griswold*'s Progeny: Assisted Reproduction, Procreative Liberty, and Sexual Orientation Equality" (2015) 124 *Yale Law Journal Forum* 340.
43 Reva B. Siegel, "How Conflict Entrenched the Right to Privacy" (2015) 124 *Yale Law Journal Forum* 316.
44 Cary Franklin, "*Griswold* and the Public Dimension of the Right to Privacy" (2015) 124 *Yale Law Journal Forum* 332.
45 Similarly, on access to abortion services in the wake of *Griswold* and before *Roe*, see: Roy Lucas, "Federal Constitutional Limitations on the Enforcement and Administration of State Abortion Statutes" (1968) 46 *North Carolina Law Review* 730.
46 See Catherine G. Roraback, "*Griswold v. Connecticut*: A Brief Case History" (1989) 16 *Ohio Northern University Law Review* 395, 399–400; Thomas I. Emerson, "Nine Justices in Search of a Doctrine" (1965) 64 *Michigan Law Review* 219 (discussions of multiple alternative grounds on which *Griswold* could have been decided).
47 Melissa Murray, "Overlooking Equality on the Road to *Griswold*" (2015) *Yale Law Journal Forum* 324;
Neil S. Siegel and Riva B. Siegel, "Contraception as a Sex Equality Right" (2015) *Yale Law Journal Forum* 349.
48 Emerson, n 46.
49 Home Office and Scottish Home Department, *Report of the Committee on Homosexual Offences and Prostitution*, Cmd 247 (1957), henceforth "The Wolfenden Report".

50 Wolfenden, n 49, [61].

51 Deborah Cohen, *Family Secrets: Shame and Privacy in Modern Britain* (Oxford University Press 2013); David Vincent, *Privacy: A Short History* (Polity Press 2016).

52 David Minto, "Perversion by Penumbras: Wolfenden, *Griswold*, and the Transatlantic Trajectory of Sexual Privacy" (2018) 123 *The American Historical Review* 1093.

53 See also in the wake of *Roe*, Louis Henkin, "Privacy and Autonomy" (1974) 74 *Columbia Law Review* 1410.

54 Minto, n 52, 1093.

55 See NeJaime, n 42, for an argument that *Griswold* could serve as a basis for claims to access to artificial reproductive technologies for same-sex couples.

56 Mark Philip Bradley, *The World Reimagined: Americans and Human Rights in the Twentieth Century* (Cambridge University Press 2016).

57 Moreham offers an analysis into five categories involving three "freedoms from" and two "freedoms to". See Nicole A. Moreham, "The Right to Respect for Private Life in the European Convention on Human Rights: A Re-Examination" (2008) 1 *European Human Rights Law Review* 44. More recently, see Päivi Hirvelä and Satu Heikkilä, *Right to Respect for Private and Family Life, Home and Correspondence: A Practical Guide to the Article 8 Case-Law of the European Court of Human Rights* (Larcier-Intersentia 2022). See also Martin Buijsen, "On Interpretation and Appreciation. A European Human Rights Perspective on *Dobbs*" (2023) 32 *Cambridge Quarterly of Healthcare Ethics* 323.

58 Ziegler, n 7.

59 David S. Cohen, Greer Donley, and Rachel Rebouché, "The New Abortion Battleground" (2023) 123 *Columbia Law Review* 1.

60 Joanne Wuest, "A Conservative Right to Privacy: Legal, Ideological, and Coalitional Transformations in US Social Conservatism" (2021) 46 *Law & Social Inquiry* 964.

61 I borrow and adapt this terminology from Minto, n 52.

62 Gavison, n 4, 421.

63 Ibid., 463.

64 Ibid., 462.

65 Cf., Woodrow Hartzog, "What Is Privacy? That's the Wrong Question" (2021) 88 *University of Chicago Law Review* 1677–1688, who argues we should move beyond existential angst about the nature of privacy and focus instead on the functions it serves and the values it reflects. This builds extensively on the contribution of Daniel J. Solove, "I've Got Nothing to Hide and Other Misunderstandings of Privacy" (2007) 44 *San Diego Law Review* 745.

66 Gavison, n 4, fn 47.

67 William L. Prosser, *The Law of Torts* (4th edn, West Publishing Company 1971), 804.

68 Edward J. Bloustein, "Privacy as an Aspect of Human Dignity: An Answer to Dean Prosser" (1964) 39 *New York University Law Review* 962.

69 Richard A. Posner, "The Right of Privacy" (1978) 12 *Georgia Law Review* 393; Richard A. Epstein, "Privacy, Property Rights, and Misrepresentations" (1978) 12 *Georgia Law Review* 455.

70 See also Daniel J. Solove, "A Taxonomy of Privacy" (2006) 154 *University of Pennsylvania Law Review* 477.

71 William A. Parent, "Recent Work on the Concept of Privacy" (1983) 20 *American Philosophical Quarterly* 341.

72 William A. Parent, "Privacy: A Brief Survey of the Conceptual Landscape" (1995) 11 *Santa Clara High Technology Law Journal* 21.

73 Julie E. Cohen, "What Privacy Is For" (2013) 126 *Harvard Law Review* 1904, 1905.
74 Ibid., 1905.
75 Graeme Laurie, *Genetic Privacy: A Challenge to Medico-Legal Norms* (Cambridge University Press 2002); Graeme Laurie, "Personality, Privacy and Autonomy in Medical Law", in Niall Whitty and Reinhard Zimmermann (eds), *Rights of Personality in Scots Law: A Comparative Perspective* (Edinburgh University Press 2009); Graeme Laurie, "Recognizing the Right Not to Know: Conceptual, Professional, and Legal Implications" (2014) 42 *Journal of Law, Medicine & Ethics* 53.
76 Laurie, *Genetic Privacy*, n 75.
77 I must credit this example to the literature and to deep memory. I am unable to locate the source, but it is most certainly not me.
78 N 73.
79 N 47.
80 N 27.
81 See Moreham, n 57.
82 See Hartzog, n 65, and associated text and references.
83 See Wuest, n 60, on this last point.
84 Vincent, n 51.
85 Gavison also recognized this: n 4, 452–459.
86 N 7.
87 N 9, 2750.
88 See Mitchell, n 21, and the Honorable Gregory C. Cook, "The Rising Importance of State Courts" (2023) 27 *Harvard Journal of Law & Public Policy Per Curiam* 1.
89 Guinier and Torres, n 9, 2751.
90 Mary Ziegler, "Should Constitutional Rights Reflect Popular Opinion? Interpreting *Dobbs v. Jackson Women's Health Organization*" (2023) 6 *Modern American History* 88.
91 Amna A. Akbar, Sameer M. Ashar, and Jocelyn Simonson, "Movement Law" (2021) 73 *Stanford Law Review* 821.
92 Ibid., 848.
93 Reva B. Siegel, "Constitutional Culture, Social Movement Conflict and Constitutional Change: The Case of the de facto ERA" (2006) 94 *California Law Review* 1323.
94 Maggie Blackhawk, "Equity Outside the Courts" (2020) 120 *Columbia Law Review* 2037, 2113.
95 William N. Eskridge Jr., "A Pluralist Theory of the Equal Protection Clause" (2009) 11 *University of Pennsylvania Journal of Constitutional Law* 1239.
96 Blackhawk, n 94, 2116.
97 Scott L. Cummings, "The Social Movement Turn in Law" (2018) 43 *Law & Social Inquiry* 360.
98 Akbar, Ashar, and Simonson, n 91, 851.
99 Kimberlé W. Crenshaw, "Demarginalizing the Intersection of Race and Sex: A Black Feminist Critique of Antidiscrimination Doctrine, Feminist Theory and Antiracist Politics" (1989) *University of Chicago Legal Forum* 139.
100 Grayling is talking about love, but his words have particular resonance also in the current context. See Anthony C. Grayling, *Philosophy and Law* (Penguin/Random House 2023), 188.

2

PUBLIC INTEREST AND TRUSTWORTHINESS

Connecting the concepts through reasonable justification for (non)interference with medical confidentiality

Mark Taylor

Introduction

In the trial of the Duchess of Kingston for bigamy, reported in 1776, the surgeon to the Duchess initially refused to answer questions about what he may, as surgeon to one or both, have heard of the Duchess' marriage to Lord Bristol. Lord Mansfield, cross-examining Mr Caesar Hawkins, conceded that "if a surgeon was voluntarily to reveal these secrets, to be sure he would be guilty of a breach of honour, and of great indiscretion".[1] However, he continued, "but, to give that information in a court of justice, which by the law of the land he is bound to do, will never be imputed to him as any indiscretion whatever".[2] The value and significance of medical confidentiality has long been recognized but the law has never recognized a health professional's duty to preserve confidentiality to be absolute.

The limits of confidentiality are no longer determined by questions of "professional honour" nor understanding what would be imputed by others to be an indiscretion. Now, more typically (though not exclusively),[3] the extent of the duty and its limits are characterized around the world by reference to the concept of the public interest. The concept of public interest has been employed as both a justification for upholding confidentiality and a justification for overriding it. I will argue here that there may be merit in reconnecting with the values expressed in 18th-century England: not to the idea of professional honour, but to the idea that there are normative expectations held reasonably by patients and publics more generally of health professionals (and others such as academic researchers in whom they confide health information) that may help to enliven a modern understanding of the concept of public interest. An advantage of doing so is that it may (re)connect the

DOI: 10.4324/9781003394518-4

concept with the idea of "trustworthiness": enriching our understanding of the public interest but also, crucially, making explicit what is required for public interest decision-making to contribute toward justifying trust in medical confidentiality—even when the decision is to permit a breach of confidence. In other words, it will help us to understand the proper role of the public interest in trustworthy health data governance.

The concept of trustworthiness is expanded on more fully below but put most briefly, "trustworthiness" is a property possessed by people or things worthy of trust. "Trust" itself is an attitude (expressed in behaviour). When people trust other people, they rely upon an expectation; that the person possesses some quality or character that will lead them to perform in a particular manner. They are trusted to behave in a certain way. People trust healthcare professionals to try to make them better. They choose to give confidential information to them because they trust they will use the information for some limited purposes (e.g. delivering safe and effective care) and not others (e.g. selling to a newspaper or gossiping with neighbours). In a modern healthcare system that trust needs to extend, beyond an attitude toward healthcare professionals, to all aspects of the system judged relevant to risk. If people do not think the healthcare system will use information only in ways they consider appropriate (for I leave aside here the question of whether you can trust someone or something to do the *wrong* thing), then they will not trust the system with their information. Of course, this does not mean they will not provide the information. People may choose to surrender information to a system they do not trust, but a failure of trust will count against full disclosure and likely lead to sub-optimal function of the system itself. People may censor their story and not share details where *they* judge the risks outweigh the significance of the information to their care. Any healthcare system that seeks to promote candour will aspire to the trust of those using it. It should also, unless it aims to solicit misplaced trust, aspire to the trustworthiness needed to merit it. Importantly, for the argument I make, this should extend to any decision to permit an interference with medical confidentiality.

The argument advanced is that a robust conception of public interest can contribute to trustworthy data governance, but—perhaps rather obviously—that contribution is dependent on public interest decision-making satisfying justificatory conditions connected with the idea of trustworthiness. I will suggest that it is common to both demonstrating trustworthiness and justifying public interest decision-making that persons can be offered a reason for accepting the vulnerability to which they are exposed. People voluntarily expose themselves to a vulnerability when they choose to trust. People are exposed, involuntarily, to a vulnerability when a public interest decision-making process weighs in favour of permitting the disclosure of their confidential information. If that decision-making is to be worthy of trust, then it must be possible to justify the decision reached in terms that persons have reason to voluntarily accept. In other words, I argue (1) there is value in recognizing trustworthiness to be a minimum requirement of a public interest justification for interference with medical confidentiality, and (2) this requires that persons are exposed to the vulnerability that disclosing confidential information incurs, only when any risk can be sufficiently justified in terms *they* value.[4] If sufficient justification can be made to those affected (and to whom justification is directed) for them to (have reason to) accept the vulnerability, then I shall suggest this equates to—from the perspective of those affected—"reasonable justification". The requirement that any decision on (non)interference with medical confidentiality be supported by reasonable justification places a constraint on public interest decision-making. It is a constraint that may be needed to promote and protect public confidence in modern data sharing initiatives. Moreover, it is what is required for public trust to be well placed in those who determine whether a duty of confidentiality is to be overridden.[5]

People must be able to trust that the professionals, to whom they confide private information, will treat it with due regard to the vulnerabilities created. Decisions about (non)disclosure of confidential information based on the public interest ought to demonstrate that professionals behave in this way and that the system permits them to do so, i.e. that they, and the system, is worthy of trust. When Mr Hawkins attempted to stonewall the House of Lords by asking, "I do not know how far any thing that has come before me in a confidential trust in my profession should be disclosed, consistent with my professional honour",[6] he was not only attempting to protect his friends. He was also seeking to protect the integrity of his position and the confidential trust placed in the health professionals by their patients. If there is no public confidence that the system will protect information, then trust in healthcare professionals' ability to maintain confidence will be undermined. Having demonstrated the value of recognizing how a requirement for "reasonable justification" may connect the ideas of trustworthiness and public interest, I move to suggest that there are reasons to doubt current conceptions of the public interest, whether expressed through judicial dicta or statutory language, recognize this connection, or require it to be practically demonstrated. To illustrate the point, I give a single example of a statutory definition of public interest at work in Australia today which I suggest misses this opportunity.

I offer this argument with hope that it might contribute to an understanding of what is required of public interest decision-making if it is to be deserving of public trust and confidence. My observation is that we too often fall short of this standard. Adopting and applying a concept of public interest, as currently enshrined in law, may not protect health professionals, academic researchers, and the health service more generally, from the imputation of indiscretion: to put it more plainly, it does not protect them from the perception that they have done something wrong. There is, however, an opportunity to reconsider how the concept of public interest is relied on in decision-making and the opportunities for the concept to contribute toward trustworthy health data governance.

This chapter has three unequal parts. In part one, I consider judicial recognition of the public interest in medical confidentiality and how it is weighed in a balancing operation by the courts against other public interests. I consider the different kinds of constraint that might be applied to such an operation to avoid arbitrary decision-making and relate one constraint in particular, the requirement of reasonable justification, to the ideas of social licence to operate and social legitimacy. In part two, I apply this analysis to the concept of trustworthiness with a view to identifying how reasonable justification is common to the justificatory process. I will suggest this connection may be recognized in public interest decision-making by the courts but also, and perhaps in some circumstances more readily, by other kinds of public interest decision-making bodies. In part three, I provide an example of a statutory definition of public interest that does not feature this constraint on decision-making. I suggest that, unless this is addressed, there is a risk that the concept of public interest within such regulatory regimes may do nothing to support the trustworthiness of a decision-making process and, when information is originally collected in a healthcare context, may even undermine the public interest in medical confidentiality.

The duty of confidence, medical confidentiality, and the public interest

The nature of the public interest in medical confidentiality was indicated by Rose J in *X Health Authority* v Y:[7]

> In the long run, preservation of confidentiality is the only way of securing public health … confidentiality is vital to secure public as well as private health: for unless those infected come forward they cannot be counselled and self-treatment does not provide the best care.[8]

In *Campbell* v *MGN*,[9] Baroness Hale of Richmond favourably cited the European Court of Human Rights in *Z* v *Finland*:[10]

> Respecting the confidentiality of health data is a vital principle in the legal systems of all the Contracting Parties to the Convention. It is crucial not only to respect the sense of privacy of a patient but also to preserve his or her confidence in the medical profession and in the health service in general. Without such protection, those in need of medical assistance may be

deterred from revealing such information of a personal and intimate nature as may be necessary in order to receive appropriate treatment and, even, from seeking such assistance, thereby endangering their own health and, in the case of transmissible diseases, that of the community.[11]

The public interest in medical confidentiality has thus—in this context at least[12]—been understood by the courts to be a confluence of (at least) three different interests shared by members of the public: (1) an interest in being able to confidentially seek healthcare, (2) an interest in others (particularly those with transmissible disease) being able to (confidentially) seek healthcare, and (3) an interest in the appropriate protection of individual privacy interests. This may not be an exhaustive account of the interests that the public hold in medical confidentiality,[13] but that does not matter for the argument offered, so long as they are among the interests that are protected and promoted. The point to be made initially now, and expanded upon later, is that (at least) the first two require individuals to trust that the information they confide to others will not be used in ways that they do not want or value: if we are to realize the benefits of medical confidentiality, then it matters what people think and feel about how confidentiality is respected and protected.

As has already been recognized, it has never been the case that a duty of confidentiality is absolute. In the case of *W* v *Egdell*,[14] Lord Justice Bingham remarked that:

> The decided cases very clearly establish: (1) that the law recognises an important public interest in maintaining professional duties of confidence; but (2) that the law treats such duties as not absolute but as liable to be overridden where there is held to be a stronger public interest in disclosure.[15]

If public confidence in medical confidentiality matters, then it matters whether any breach of confidence can be justified to the relevant public. There are two fundamental points here. The first is that there is something about public interest decision-making in this context (at least) that requires consideration of public opinion; otherwise, this risks the individual and social benefits that trust in medical confidentiality can deliver. The second is that there is not only a public interest in medical confidentiality, but also a public interest *in the balancing operation* itself. If people have no confidence in the balancing operation, then they have no reason to trust medical confidentiality and the public interest(s) in confidentiality will be jeopardized.

The balancing operation

In *W* v *Egdell*, a health professional was found to be justified in sharing patient information against the express wishes of the patient: there was a public interest recognized in medical confidentiality but also a public interest in safeguarding public safety.[16] In the circumstances, the court found that the competing public interests should be resolved in a way that supported disclosure. The principle limiting the duty of confidence, and the process by which that limit is determined, was described by Lord Goff in *A-G* v *Guardian Newspapers Ltd (No 2)*:[17]

> [A]lthough the basis of the law's protection of confidence is that there is a public interest that confidences should be preserved and protected by law, nevertheless that public interest may be outweighed by some other countervailing public interest which favours disclosure. This limitation may apply [...] to all types of confidential information. It is a limiting principle which may require a court to carry out a balancing operation, weighing the public interest in maintaining confidence against a countervailing public interest favouring disclosure.[18]

In *A-G* v *Guardian*, the balance was between the public interest in preserving confidentiality and freedom of expression. In *Z* v *Finland*, confidentiality was weighed against investigating the public interest in investigating and prosecuting crime and in the publicity of court proceedings.[19] There is judicial obiter to indicate that, in some circumstances, the public interest in health research and management may override the public interest in confidentiality.[20] The NHS Scotland Public Benefit and Privacy Panel for Health and Social Care regularly carries out this balancing operation on behalf of those holding NHS Scotland controlled data. One aim of the panel is

> to ensure the right balance is struck between safeguarding the privacy of all people in Scotland and the fiduciary duty of Scottish public bodies to make the best possible use of the health and social care data collected.[21]

It is worth explicitly noting at this point, it is not always necessary to strike a balance. It can be possible to preserve confidentiality *and* achieve other public interest objectives. In the context of health research, a breach of confidence can be avoided by asking a research participant for consent to the use of confidential information or by anonymizing information. Furthermore, when there is an unavoidable opposition, and a balance must be struck, the relevant balancing operation is not always carried out by courts or within a legal setting. Where there is no consent, and anonymization is inappropriate or impractical, then, as Schaefer and others note, "a small but growing number of jurisdictions that have a public interest or equivalent criterion for granting consent waivers".[22] This criterion may function within the context of a statutory gateway (e.g. setting aside the common law duty of confidentiality) or as a requirement for lawful processing (e.g. within a data protection regime).[23] The function may be discharged by an Institutional Review Board, an Ethics Committee, as part of a portfolio of responsibilities or a specifically constituted body like the Public Benefit and Privacy Panel in Scotland[24] or the Confidentiality Advisory Group in England and Wales.[25] Wherever the function is performed, to the extent that it invokes the concept of "public interest" to justify (non)disclosure of confidential health information, the argument offered here is intended to apply.

Alongside the diversity of institutional setting, there is also a diversity in the source of relevant obligation: medical confidentiality is not only protected by law. Professional standards and guidance also protect privacy and confidentiality in healthcare settings. Across different contexts, with different methods for striking a balance embedded differently in different regulatory regimes and frameworks, the point is that the public interest is regularly called upon to perform some normative heavy lifting and, via some kind of "balancing operation", justify an interference with medical confidentiality. This balancing operation may be performed by a health professional personally or, increasingly likely, by another person or entity (such as those mentioned immediately above) invested with that responsibility. Ultimately, however, these decisions—across different contexts—must be defensible at law. This offers the law's application of the concept of public interest a privileged position: the legal contours of medical confidentiality will cascade through other decision-making contexts.

While the argument offered here is largely agnostic between different regulatory contexts (e.g. legal, professional ethics, regulatory guidance), there is one way in which it is quite specific. The argument is only of any critical significance where opposition is unavoidable, a balance must be struck, and an individual or entity is responsible for striking that balance. Across the various loci of decision-making, I will suggest the law does not go as far as it might—or should—to constrain decision-making processes and require deciding makers to meet particular requirements with regard to justifying the balancing operation: the law does not do enough to require those exercising the discretion that balancing implies to demonstrate others have reason to trust the decision. It is the nature of that balancing operation—and its justification to those affected by (non)interference with medical confidentiality—that I now turn to consider.

The balancing operation, when one public interest is weighed against another, cannot be a straightforward mathematical calculus: it is a normatively driven evaluation. The value-laden nature of the operation, and the risks introduced, were described by Gummow J at first instance in *Smith Kline and French Laboratories (Australia) Ltd* v *Department of Community*

Services and Health.[26] Commenting negatively on what he saw as a recent trend in English authority, Gummow J opined that,

> an examination of the recent English decisions shows that the so-called "public interest" defence is not so much a rule of law as an invitation to judicial idiosyncrasy by deciding each case on an ad hoc basis as to whether, on the facts overall, it is better to respect or override the obligation of confidence.[27]

In contrast with such an invitation for uninhibited discretion, he supported the view that:

> equitable principles are best developed by reference to what conscionable behaviour demands of the defendant not by "balancing" and then overriding those demands by reference to matters of political or social opinion.[28]

Gummow J does not explain how reference to the demands of "conscionable behaviour" avoids judicial idiosyncrasy. I suggest that there may be value in expressly recognizing that political and social opinion, or at least a decision-maker's perception of it, may in fact be centrally relevant to an understanding of what conscionable behaviour demands. As Sorbie says, when discussing related themes, there is

> the long established "intellectual tradition" within the law of inventing fictional persons to provide a barometer of what "reasonable" members of the public might think, feel or expect in a given situation.[29]

When Lord Mansfield reflected on whether Caesar Hawkins' testimony would "be imputed to him as any indiscretion", he surely had the opinion of not only the House of Lords but also Mr Hawkins' colleagues and other patients in mind. Surely, beyond his immediate legal jeopardy, those were the views most significant to Mr Hawkins himself. I suspect that, in this context at least, conscionability may be closely associated with reasonable justification, but exploration of this relationship would be tangential (although not irrelevant). So instead, I move to consider more closely the relationship between the balancing operation, matters of political or social opinion, and the justificatory requirements of public interest decision-making. I will show how, far from inviting idiosyncrasy, it may be through requiring those conducting the balancing operation to have reference to such matters, at least as expressions of the general and social norms of an affected public, that the idiosyncrasy Gummow J observed may be avoided. Indeed, I will later suggest that it may be necessary if the system is to be worthy of the trust of those voluntarily sharing confidential information and exposing vulnerability to the balancing operation.

Substantive and procedural requirements

To rely upon the public interest in the context of an act or decision is self-evidently to claim that a decision or act may be justified (at least in part) by reference to it. (The alternative is to concede the claim to be indefensible or that the public interest does absolutely no work in the justification.)

This raises some obvious questions about how different public interests are to be reconciled in case of conflict. As previously described, this is often described as a "balancing exercise" and, in the context of healthcare research and an interference with medical confidentiality, the exercise may be given focused consideration in the context of a decision on whether to waive a requirement for consent to research use of data. Schaefer and others suggest that this enquiry encompasses two levels:

> the substantive question of whether a given study is in fact in the public interest; the procedural issue of how systems (local, institutional or even national) should be designed to legitimately and reliably evaluate the public interest criterion.[30]

In relation to the former, substantive question, they suggest it is possible to construct a criteria-based framework a decision-making body could apply. Candidate criteria include whether the application addresses a health priority, scientific robustness, open access, non-patentability/copyright, and translatability.[31] They recognize such criteria are context-dependent and an exhaustive list may not be possible.[32] I will return to these criteria later, but it should be noted that while they may contribute to an understanding of the public interest in health research use of confidential information, they do not determine whether any interference in medical confidentiality is justified (not even for this specific use). They contribute to an understanding of how heavily weighted one side of the scale is, but not to whether there is a public interest in how the scales are balanced.[33]

To address this limitation, the authors[34] suggest supplementing the substantive criteria with procedural considerations—in particular, those focused on ensuring that the decision-making process is "fair, consistent and relevantly informed".[35] These are said to include ensuring decision-making practice is congruent with policies that are themselves "transparent, reasonable, and accountable". Each of these considerations is important and the authors spend time explaining each. For the purposes of this argument, however, I explore further the constraint put upon a decision-making process, and the associated "balancing operation", by a requirement that the process conform to a "reasonable" policy. This may seem to be substituting one notoriously uncertain idea (public interest) for another (reasonableness). Indeed, one of the reasons that public interest decision-making can appear opaque is that even when the public interests engaged are well characterized, there is disagreement over what is in fact a reasonable trade-off or balance between competing interests.[36] William Zarecor once remarked:

> It would be perfectly plausible to interpret the history of political theory as a series of attempts to formulate the best possible method of serving the public interest. Considered from this point of view, the various forms of political theory can be explained in terms of varying interpretations of the term "public interest".[37]

No one thinks their own political theory unreasonable. No judge thinks their own conception of what a reasonable person might think or feel to be *un*reasonable. Thus, reasonableness might seem to offer little promise of substantively constraining decision-making. Indeed, this may be why Schaefer and others consider this a procedural consideration (rather than a substantive criterion). However, if we take the requirement of reasonableness seriously in the context of a justification of a decision to others, then I think we will find it does place some significant constraints upon the decision-making process and what one can justify as being "in the public interest". Moreover, I suggest reasonable justification may also provide the nexus for both conceptual and practical connection with the concept of trustworthiness.

Reasonable justification

Anyone relying upon "the public interest" to explain and defend an act or decision must consider it capable of justifying that act or decision, either alone or in concert with other justifying reasons. This extends to justifying any negative impact on others. The work being done by reference to the public interest will extend to justifying any "balancing operation": "weighing" different public interests and reaching a decision on (non)interference with medical confidentiality. In this context, it is useful to briefly consider three things: (1) *to whom* any justification is directed (and is to be satisfied with it), (2) any constraints placed upon the nature of the justification by the "public interest" nature of the claim, and (3) how one can tell if a public interest justification is "sufficient" in the circumstances.

The answer to these questions will vary by context. It has already been noted that it is not only the courts that will consider issues of public interest, nor will they consider them only in relation to medical confidentiality. Other institutions, organizations, and individuals, when making public interest determinations, may find their reasoning appropriately shaped and constrained by their specific constitution, function, and circumstance. Nevertheless, in each case, if one is making a "public interest" decision, then specific forms of constraint will be imposed by any requirement that the decision can be justified as not only lawful but also reasonable to others.

In the context of a legal argument, the answer to the first question—who is to be satisfied with the legality and reasonableness of a public interest justification—will be dictated by the roles of those involved, e.g. judge, counsel, appellate authority. Similarly, the answer to the second question—the nature of any constraints on the nature of permissible justificatory argument—will be shaped by the norms of contestation in, and construction of, legal knowledge. Precedent, case law, constitutional requirement, and statutory obligation all play a part. Relevant legal norms will likely be drawn from privacy and data protection law as well intellectual property, international law, and human rights. The sufficiency of the argument will be determined by its acceptance and adoption by officials in the relevant legal system. It will only be adopted if it is accepted, all things considered, to be reasonable in their worldview.[38]

Legal officials are not, however, the only relevant audience. Given what we have previously noted about the significance of public confidence in confidentiality, we should recognize the consequences if patients and publics affected by decisions are not also considered to also be an important audience. If much of the value of medical confidentiality is only realized if people perceive confidentiality to be adequately protected, then we should value the adequacy of any justification *to them*. This implies different answers to the second and third questions posed above. Regarding the second question: the public nature of the interest demands that the reasons for interference are accessible and intelligible to the relevant publics. Intelligibility requires appeal to interests, values, or norms that make sense *to them*: resonate with their politics, values, and normative commitments (which may be tied to individual and group identity). When discussing the procedural constraint of "congruence with a reasonable policy", Schaefer and others suggest:

> Reasonableness is understood as being justifiable to stakeholders regardless of their personal parochial views; any accepted notion of the public interest must in this way appeal to values that are, in turn, of appeal to the general population, and not just a subset.[39]

While not necessarily understanding why the values appealed to must—according to "any accepted notion of the public interest"—apply to "the general population", I would certainly agree there to be a value in a *public* interest justification appealing to values accepted by the publics to whom the justification is addressed: referencing what is held in common between them, whether parochial or not. I have previously suggested that, for our purposes, plausible candidates for such commonly held interests, valued by all persons are interests in both health(care) and medical confidentiality.[40] The implications of this are more fully considered shortly.

Regarding the third question: where there is unavoidable conflict between public interests, and a balance implies an interference with at least one, then the sufficiency of the justification is also to be judged from the perspective of the affected public. However, to protect public confidence in confidentiality it is not enough that the reasons for any interference appeal to values they hold. To be a sufficient justification, the appeal must override the perceived vulnerabilities. Only by considering *the balancing operation* from the perspective of those affected by the decision can one assess whether the balance is one they have reason to voluntarily accept. While I consider the concept of trust more fully below, I foreshadow that this is tantamount to determining if they have reason *to trust* the decision-making process. If sufficient justification can be made to those affected (and to whom justification is directed) for them to (have reason to) accept the decision, then this equates to a "reasonable justification" from their perspective. There are at least two different ways in which the reasonableness of a justification may be assessed. Both operate from the perspective of the affected public, but understanding the difference will show how the idea of a reasonable justification for the balance may connect public interest decision-making with the idea of social licence to operate (which, in turn, may be connected to the idea of public "trust") and social legitimacy (which, in turn, may be connected to the idea of "trustworthy" decision-making).

Social licence to operate

There is an important method by which one may determine if stakeholders consider a balancing operation to be reasonable: by asking them. Does empirical testing reveal that people are willing to accept,[41] as a matter of fact, the interference in question? Clearly there will likely be differences of opinion expressed. There is also not likely to be a clear or consistent answer to the question of what cohort or percentage of people *need* to regard a position to be reasonable in order for a justification to be "sufficient". This will vary according to the nature of the "need" in question. Here we may identify a relationship between a reasonable justification with what is described as a "social licence to operate":

> The concept of social license is used to describe a privilege granted to an occupation or profession to do things other members of society are not allowed to do and which may not be morally acceptable in the wider society.[42]

The relevant privilege needs to be granted by enough of society for the activity to be effectively allowed. The significance of a social licence to operate can be most evident when withdrawn. The consequences of a lack or loss of social licence might range from an activity becoming effectively impossible, to it merely being more challenging. Success will be prevented if voluntary participation is a necessary element and social licence is entirely withdrawn. An example here could be a research activity which is impossible to success-fully undertake if it depends on the voluntary participation of people who find the research unacceptable. The impacts of a lack or loss of social licence might manifest one step removed from the activity itself. For example, people choosing to no longer seek healthcare, or no longer being candid when doing so, could impact on research reliant on secondary use of information con-fided in the healthcare setting. A lack or loss of social licence for that research might similarly affect how people act in that healthcare setting: affecting what people tell their doctors. Other activity such as lobbying, advocacy, and protest directed at partner organizations, regulators, media, and funders may or may not be fatal to an activity but could certainly contribute to an envi-ronment hostile to success.[43] The point is that a social licence to operate may manifest in different ways, with varying effects, but it can form an important, sometimes essential, public dimension of the necessary authorizing environ-ment for an activity.

A willingness to support an interference with medical confidentiality for the purpose of health(care) research is likely to be informed by, as Allen, Adams, and Flack suggest, "the community understanding of and belief in the value of research".[44] If that understanding and belief in the underlying value proposition is lacking, or is lost, then disclosure for research (or public health) purposes may be associated with the undesirable consequences already described: the benefits associated with public confidence in medical confidentiality may be undermined. It is only where people recognize the risks associated with a decision on (non)disclosure to be reasonably justified that they have reason to voluntarily accept the vulnerability that the decision implies. We might note here, by way of aside, that this is how a reasonable justification may conceptually connect trust and social licences in the context of public interest decision-making: both require that persons *perceive* suffi-cient reason for accepting the vulnerability to which they are exposed. Both social licence and a public's trust require people to voluntarily accept risk. A reason to trust others to do something that would not otherwise be allowed is necessary for a social licence to operate.

This is then one way in which one might assess whether a public interest decision-making process, determining (non)disclosure of confidential infor-mation, is reasonably justified from the perspective of the public: is there, as a matter of fact, a social licence to operate. If there is not, then this will undermine any activity dependent on social support. However, this is not the only relevant perspective from which we can or should assess the sufficiency of any justification for public interest decision-making. Public trust and will-ingness to accept relevant risk may be an important dimension of the authorizing environment, but there is a difference between being granted a social licence and deserving one. It can make a tremendous practical difference if the balancing operation is accepted by the people with the power to disrupt an activity, but if that were the only thing that mattered, then it would be irrelevant if a social licence were granted due to misunderstanding or deception. If the ambition is to be worthy of any social licence, and to be worthy of the trust this may imply, then the reasonableness of a justification cannot just be demonstrated empirically by acceptance in fact. It requires, instead, assessment of what might be labelled, not social licence, but social legitimacy.

Social legitimacy

The term "social legitimacy" has been defined in various ways over the years. Deephouse and Suchman offer an overview and usefully summarize some of the alternatives.[45] They start their history in the 1970s with Weber's writing on the subject, noting it suggested that "legitimacy can result from conformity with both general and social norms and formal laws".[46] While more recent uses of the would appear to overlap much more considerably with the idea of "social licence to operate", through an emphasis on the "role of the social audience in legitimation dynamics",[47] I seek instead to use the term more in line with Weber's original approach. Lipset associated social legitimacy with "the capacity of the system to engender and maintain the belief that the existing political institutions are the most appropriate ones for the society".[48] I adopt that understanding only to the extent that the belief is based on a genuine ability of the system. I am thus using the term "social legitimacy" to imply actual conformity with not only formal legal but also, and here in particular, general and social norms: the capacity to engender a *well-founded* belief in the appropriateness of a system for a relevant public. Although this may vary from some contemporary uses of the term "social legitimacy", I adopt it to establish clear water between it and the idea of a "social licence to operate". Just as members of the public may have the power to disrupt a data initiative by withholding or withdrawing a social licence to operate, it may be that an organization or individual has the ability to ride roughshod over any pockets of dissent: exercising a de facto power to interfere with medical confidentiality. Enough of society may allow that interference, in practice, due to impotence, indolence, or ignorance. The kind of hollow permission that power may coerce does not, and cannot, render interference socially legitimate (in the way I am using the term): even if it may, as noted above, furnish (at least temporarily) a simulacrum of social licence. It may help sharpen the distinction, and the reason for emphasizing it, if I note now that this idea of social legitimacy may be connected with the idea of trustworthiness in a similar, but contrasting, way to the idea of social licence may be connected to the idea of trust.

If one is interested in determining if a balancing operation can be justified in terms of social legitimacy (or if one wants it to be *worthy* of a public's trust) then what kinds of reason for (non)interference with medical confidentiality are relevant? Note we are not here concerned with offering a practical reason, a reason for action, but a metaphysical reason: a reason for a belief. What reason can be offered for a belief that interference with medical confidentiality is reasonable: that the balancing operation affected through the decision-making process is appropriate for an affected public? The answer can only be provided with reference to other deeply held beliefs as, fundamentally, legitimacy is no more or less than concordance with relevant norms. Norms themselves may be drawn, even within a single public, from many different sources. Ultimately, for an interference with medical confidentiality to be one that a person has reason to accept, the justificatory argument must be consistent with their own world-view and the normative commitments of the public with which they identify. If one seeks to construct an understanding of what a "reasonable person" would have reason to accept, then one's starting point may be more or less abstract: appealing to normative commitments associated with features of human experience that are more or less generic.

At one end of the spectrum, a rationalist moral philosophy would find legitimacy, and the possibility of reason requiring acceptance of an interference with medical confidentiality (on pain of self-contradiction) dependent on concordance with a supreme moral principle or categorical imperative.[49] This may require socially legitimate public interest decision-making to protect certain generic features of action and the possibility of viable human agency.[50] While a dialectically necessary argument may offer a practical reason to accept certain fundamental normative commitments, and may require no more than an attribution of agency to members of a particular public,[51] it is both controversial and unnecessary if one can find more proximate common ground to support relevant argument.

Toward the other end of the spectrum, but not yet at the point where norms are irreconcilable across different publics, is a position that would seek to universalize from other shared features of human experience. While not as universal as mere agency, I have already noted that I have previously argued,[52] including with a colleague,[53] that the kind of metaphysical reason we seek may be found by analysing the implications of recognizing members of the relevant public to share common interests in health(care) and medical confidentiality. My position is that if one adds to this combination of common interests a common value in (and normative commitment to) persons being respected as free and equal, then this implies a particular kind of justificatory requirement: namely, that one must recognize an obligation to justify interfering with either common interest in a way that accords with the dictates of public reason: the justification for any balancing operation must be accessible, impartial, and acceptable to the affected public.[54] It also implies that, unless such a justification can be offered, an individual's autonomy to determine the proper balance for themselves ought not to be interfered with: hence, my own proposed "triple test" of public-interest decision-making. Any decision in the public interest ought to be for reasons that persons have reason to expect, to accept, and which respects their own expressed preferences in all but the most exceptional circumstances.[55]

However, if even this relatively modest idea of what might be universally required of public interest decision-making in this context is rejected (or found incompatible with the general and social norms and formal laws of a particular public), then social legitimacy would require it to give way to a justification that *was* compatible with the affected public's general and social norms. This is still different from securing a social licence to operate because it requires a justification that people can be demonstrated to have *reason to accept*. It is a reason for a belief, rather than a belief. It does not require and is not dependent upon the belief's empirical confirmation or public acceptance, in fact, of any particular decision. As an example, we might here recall that one of the aims of the NHS Scotland Public Benefit and Privacy Panel makes reference to the "fiduciary duty of Scottish public bodies to make the best possible use of the health and social care data collected".[56] A fiduciary duty requires one party to act in the best interests of another. This is the kind of reason for acting that one might plausibly claim a beneficiary has reason to accept, without confirmation through empirical testing. This is not to dismiss the role of empirical enquiry. When it comes to understanding the norms, values, or best interests of an affected public, then there may still be a very important role for public engagement and involvement.[57] The engagement here, however, is not simply to understand what decision is preferred by the people asked—there is no intent to translate public opinion uncritically into action. Rather, it is to inform an understanding of the consequences of action relative to the norms and values held. It provides an opportunity for those affected by decisions to check and challenge the reasonableness (if not the rationality) of those decisions relative to their understanding of their own world view. Where the justification withstands scrutiny, the affected public are provided with a reason to accept the decision-making process: it conforms with their norms and values (even if they would prefer a different decision had been made).[58] I will suggest it is through the justificatory requirement implicit in this approach that one may be able to identify a conceptual connection between public interest decision-making and trustworthiness.

Trust, trustworthiness, and public interest decision-making

In her article on Regulatory Trust, Bratspies notes that

> even without a clear definition, most scholars seem to agree that trust embodies a willingness to accept vulnerability under conditions of uncertainty.[59]

"Trust" is thus an attitude commonly, perhaps necessarily,[60] expressed in behaviour. As such, it represents a position or viewpoint that may be held more or less deliberately and may be influenced by an individual's overall disposition and life experiences. Whether or not an individual does trust another person or thing in any given circumstance will, of course, be a result of many different considerations. Mayer, Davis, and Schoorman suggest that contributing toward any willingness to accept relevant vulnerability is likely to be a perception that the party being trusted possesses the characteristics of ability, integrity, and benevolence.[61] If one is trusting another to do something, there must be a belief that they are able to do that thing to an acceptable standard: they are competent. This aspect of trust may be task-specific, but it may also be relatively unspecified. This will depend on the context and nature of the relationship. You may trust someone to give health advice but not cook an important meal; you may trust a close friend to do both and many other things besides (but to different extents). If one puts this in the context of public interest decision-making, then one must trust those making the decision to make a sequence of *different* judgements, all oriented—more or less—towards the trust that has been placed. If making decisions regarding (non)interference with medical confidentiality, then there is a need to competently assess the public interest in confidentiality and to assess the conflicting public interest, such as the public interest in health research, and to then be able to competently balance them. These may require different competencies, but each is relevant to the balancing operation overall: one cannot properly balance what one has not properly weighed.

Even if one focuses on the balancing operation as a single aspect of an entity's functions, there is, of course, an important distinction to be drawn between trust and trustworthiness.[62] Whether a balancing operation, and those carrying it out, is trusted may, as a matter of fact, have little to do with trustworthiness. Trust may be given, or withheld, inappropriately. For example, one may form a view of competence based on incomplete or misleading information. Attempts to demonstrate trustworthiness might even, perversely, undermine it.[63] However, if trust is invited without trustworthiness being established, then those who trust are exposed to unjustified vulnerabilities. This is an important relationship between trust and trustworthiness. Trustworthiness justifies exposing those who trust to the vulnerability that trust implies. If we are concerned with what it means to be *worthy* of trust in this context, then we may recall the substantive criteria articulated by Schaefer and others in relation to assessment of the public interest in health research.

Schaefer and others offer a series of considerations relevant to determining the substance and degree of public interest in use of health data for research purposes. This is about determining the value of the research and is only one of the first in the sequence of judgements that must be made. It may be difficult to describe equivalent criteria to assess the *significance* of the breach of medical confidentiality that the use represents in order to competently balance the different interests. One might consider the numbers of people involved, the nature and extent of the disclosure (to whom, where, how, etc.), and the nature of the data, with even health data occupying a sliding scale of sensitivity. However, the significance of each of these things, for the people whose data is to be used, may be hard to assess by an independent entity or court. The cultural, social, and personal significance of different kinds of data may be obscure to someone who does not share the characteristics, experience, or community of the people involved.

Here we may see the value of applying what Sorbie describes as a processual lens to the balancing operation and the construction of a public interest determination.[64] Sorbie argues that a flexible and processual approach requires that public engagement inform an iterative evolution of an understanding of what the public interest requires: through dynamic engagement with "the messy realities and subjectivities, both of the law, as broadly conceived, and of evidence of actual publics in a pluralistic society".[65] Through such an approach, one may demonstrate an understanding of what an interference with medical confidentiality would really mean for an individual and a community. It may also provide the opportunity to understand, and demonstrate an understanding of, how to balance different public interests in a way that affected persons have reason to accept. If the reasonableness of the justification (for the balance and the vulnerability implied) is demonstrated by conformity with the norms and values that engagement has revealed, then one can provide a reason for the affected persons to trust the balancing operation: respect for general and social norms is one aspect of demonstrating trustworthiness. For reasons provided earlier, it may also be associated with the social legitimacy of the balancing operation. Respect for, and conformity with, social and general norms contributes to demonstrating that the trustor has reason to trust that the trustee is capable of paying due regard to their vulnerabilities. In fact, it demonstrates more than mere competence to conduct the balancing operation; it contributes also to demonstrating at least one other relevant characteristic of trustworthiness described by Mayer and others.

As well as a belief in relevant competence, a willingness to expose oneself to vulnerability will depend upon a belief that the party will not take improper advantage of the vulnerability. Trustworthiness will depend upon that belief being well placed. The belief is formed from not only an understanding of the entity's competence (i.e. their ability to do the thing) but also a perception of their motivations and values; these are the characteristics that Mayer and others describe as integrity and benevolence. They describe benevolence as "the extent to which a trustee is believed to want to do good to the trustor

[...] the perception of a positive orientation or attitude toward the trustor".[66] They describe integrity as "the trustor's perception that the trustee adheres to a set of principles that the trustor finds acceptable". Mayer and others offer the following as examples of factors that might be relevant to an evaluation of integrity:

> consistency of the party's past actions, credible communications about the trustee from other parties, belief that the trustee has a strong sense of justice, and the extent to which the party's actions are congruent with his or her words.[67]

We might note here that conformity with a set of acceptable principles, as presumably at least aligned if not grounded in general and social norms, continues to resonate with the posited idea of social legitimacy, while the *perception* of integrity resonates with the idea of social licence to operate. As trust is a willing exposure to some kind of vulnerability, it makes sense to suggest that one will not willingly invest trust in a person or process unless there is some confidence that doing so will actually yield a desired outcome. This extends beyond a trustee's competence to do the wanted thing to an all-things-considered evaluation: including such things as, will they actually do what they are capable of doing? Will they take the opportunity also to do something unwanted? The trust*worthiness* of the balancing operation thus depends on its actual conformity with relevant social and general norms and not just the perception of integrity. It may be clear how an ability to take due regard of a public's vulnerabilities demonstrates not only competence but also integrity, but what is the significance of Mayer and others' characteristic of benevolence?

I suggest that, in this context at least, it may not be so significant whether an entity intends to "do good" for the affected public. This may be one of many potential circumstances in which an individual can have good reason[68] to willingly accept risk even though there are weak or no reasons for thinking that the trusted party wants to do good to the trustor.[69] Even a temporary alignment of interests may be sufficient to give a person reason to think another is motivated to act only in the way that is valued and wanted. Estranged partners may trust each other not to reveal the other's indiscretions to their child, not due to any residual good feeling toward each other, but a mutual understanding this would hurt the child in a way that neither of them want. A common purpose—a normative alignment—may be sufficient to ground trust in an entity's actions. In other words, it may not be a requirement that the entity intends to do good *for* the affected public so long as they intend to do good *according to* that public. O'Neill points out that we regularly trust others whom we may not have any reason to think wish us well, noting, for example, that we regularly trust complete strangers to abide the rules of the road. However, she also notes that

> Trust is most readily placed in others whom we can rely on to take our interests into account, to fulfil their roles, to keep their parts in bargains.[70]

In this light, the relationship between trustworthiness and public interest decision-making, at least in the context of decisions on (non)disclosure of confidential health information, becomes a little clearer. A public interest decision-making process should be able to demonstrate how the interests of the affected persons are (at least sufficiently) taken into account to offer those persons a reason to accept the decision as a reasonable one: to accept as justified (by reference to their own normative commitments) the vulnerability that the decision inevitably exposes. We have considered how this will invariably involve an appeal to common values and interests if it is to resonate with affected publics. If this is done through the kind of processual approach described by Sorbie, then it is the very reasonableness of the decision (relative to values and norms held by that public) that justifies the public interest determination and, incidentally, demonstrates the trustworthiness of the entity making that decision. Through its conformity with the general and social norms of the affected public, meeting this justificatory requirement of trustworthiness contributes also to demonstrating the social legitimacy of the decision-making process. That the interference is *perceived* to be justifiable will be fundamental to trust in the decision-making process and will be associated with granting a social licence to operate.

Before moving to consider how this might be applied in practice, it may be useful to briefly summarize and recap the argument thus far:

1   the public interest in medical confidentiality has been recognized to manifest in things, such as enabling care and treatment of communicable disease, that depend upon persons having confidence that confidentiality is appropriately protected;
2   this extends to the balancing operation that determines whether medical confidentiality is overridden by another public interest in the circumstances;
3   there is value in the public interest decision-making process, and associated balancing operation, satisfying procedural and substantive requirements that include being able to provide a reasonable justification for any (non)interference with medical confidentiality;
4   "reasonable justification" may be assessed via different methods, as perceived by the affected public (granting a social licence), or by

demonstrating actual conformity with the general and social norms (establishing social legitimacy);

5   there is a distinction between trust, which is an (enacted) attitude, and trustworthiness, which is a property or combination of characteristics;

6   if trust is invited without trustworthiness being established, then persons are exposed to an unjustified vulnerability;

7   trustworthiness includes the competence and integrity to conduct the balancing exercise sensitive to the vulnerabilities in play and normative commitments of those affected by a decision;

8   while relevant normative commitments may be derived from universal features of human experience, or understood to be particular to specific publics, an understanding of the significance of an interference for a particular public (especially if the decision-making entity is somehow distinct from the affected public) may only be obtained through meaningful public engagement;

9   a public interest decision-making process should be able to demonstrate how the interests of affected persons are (at least sufficiently) taken into account to offer those persons a reason to accept the decision to be reasonable in the circumstances: to accept the vulnerability and trust the process;

10   if that reasonable justification is not perceived then persons have no reason to trust the balancing operation or grant the decision-making process a social licence; and

11   if that reasonable justification is not present, then not only does the public interest decision-making process jeopardize the benefits of medical confidentiality, but the balancing operation lacks social legitimacy and is not worthy of trust.

A practical example of an underutilized public interest requirement

In Australia there is a Data Availability and Transparency Act 2022, which provides the legislative framework for what is known as the DATA (Data Availability and Transparency Act) Scheme. The DATA Scheme authorizes federal government ("Commonwealth") bodies to share public sector data with accredited users. As the webpage explaining the scheme notes:

Australian Government data encompasses all data lawfully collected, created or held by a Commonwealth body, or on its behalf. Data can include a wide range of topics, from data dealing with the weather, personal and business data, through to freight and traffic movements, and agricultural yields.[71]

The sharing, collection, and use must be consistent with the data sharing principles as defined by the 2022 Act and for the defined data sharing purposes. The latter include (a) the delivery of government services, (b) informing government policy and programmes, and (c) research and development. The Act has five objects. These include, listed first, to "serve the public interest by promoting better availability of public sector data". They also include to "build confidence in the use of public sector data". The argument here is that the latter ("building confidence") could be better served by a particular interpretation of the former ("public interest"). However, this is not an interpretation that is expressly required by the Act or supplementary material.

The data sharing principles laid out by the 2022 Act parallel what are commonly referred to as the 5-safes and include the project principle, the people principle, the setting principle, the data principle, and the output principle. Each must be satisfied before data can be shared under the scheme. There are other controls, including a number of precluded purposes, such as enforcement-related purposes. It is not necessary to consider further these controls. The aim here is not to suggest that the DATA Scheme will support inappropriate sharing. There are many safeguards built into the Scheme that are not here discussed and the Scheme is overseen by an independent Data Commissioner with responsibility for "overseeing the Scheme as its regulator, holding participants accountable to robust standards of privacy, security and transparency".[72] An independent regulator may be well placed, arguably better placed than the courts, to engage in the kind of work that may be associated with demonstrating trustworthiness. I reiterate that the aim here is not to question the DATA Scheme and its operation overall. The aim is only to question the work that is specifically being done by the concept of a public interest test operating in the context of the Scheme and to ask whether, in light of earlier analysis, there might be opportunity to further develop the test to more directly require reasonable justification for any decision on (non-) interference with confidentiality.[73]

Reference to public interest is most significantly contained within the "project principle" which expressly requires the project "be reasonably expected to serve the public interest".[74] Section 6 of the Data Availability and Transparency Code 2022 distinguishes between the purposes of "delivery of government services", "medical research or statistics analysis etc. relevant to public health or safety", and "other projects for the purposes of informing government policy and programs or research and development". If for the first purpose ("delivery of government services"), then there is a presumption that the project can reasonably be expected to serve the public interest.[75] If for the second purpose (medical research or statistics analysis etc. relevant to public health or safety), then there is a presumption that the project can reasonably be expected to serve the public interest if existing standards are met, e.g. "the data custodian is sharing the data in the course of medical research within the meaning of the Privacy Act 1988 and in accordance with guidelines made under section 95 of that Act".[76] Such guidelines would, among other things, permit the disclosure of confidential patient information without individual consent on the basis of a consent waiver approved by a human research ethics committee.[77] If for the third purpose (other projects for the purposes of informing government policy and programmes or research and development), and the second purpose does not apply, then the project can only be determined to be in the public interest (and consent waived) if the entity "concludes that the arguments for the project serving the public interest outweigh the arguments against the project doing so".[78]

The Commissioner must make a data code addressing, among other things, the principles that participating entities must apply in determining if a project is necessary or "in the public interest".[79] There is opportunity within the code to more fully describe how the public interest test is to be understood and applied. There are projects that the code finds would not satisfy the public interest. These include those that would only serve the benefits of another nation, or the people of another nation, or a commercial benefit to an entity other than an Australian entity.[80] Outside these exclusions, the code provides guidance regarding the matters that an entity must consider, and those which an entity may consider, when reaching a decision on the relative weighting of "the public interest" arguments. In the "must" consider column there are matters such as:

(i) the public interest in promoting better availability of public sector data (see paragraph 3(a) of the Act);
(ii) any benefits to individuals or groups of people, including commercial benefits, that can reasonably be expected to result from the project;
(iii) any benefits to Australian citizens, permanent residents and other people in Australia that can reasonably be expected to result from the project;
(iv) if the data sharing purpose of the project is or includes informing government policy and programmes—the desirability of government policy and programmes being informed by evidence that can reasonably be expected to result from the project;
(v) any adverse impacts on individuals or groups of people, including impacts related to privacy, that can reasonably be expected to result from the project;
(vi) if the data sharing purpose of the project is or includes research and development—whether, and when, output of the project will be released.

Even without considering what is in the "may consider" column, there are a number of notable things that may already be said about the approach taken to public interest decision-making. The first is that the balancing exercise is to be carried out by the body sharing the data.[81] The Scheme applies to

Commonwealth Government bodies who control public sector data (unless specifically excluded). Each body will be responsible for making its own decision on whether the public interest test is satisfied. There is to be a public register that must contain certain details, including not only how those participating give effect to the data sharing principles but also, specifically, "how the project serves the public interest".[82] The data sharing agreement between the disclosing and receiving entities must also describe how the public interest is served by the project.[83] This requirement for transparency does not, however, expressly extend to the balancing operation itself: there is a risk that it may be understood to be sufficient to describe the arguments *for* the project serving the public interest, not also the arguments against *and* the reasons for finding one to outweigh the other.

The code provides a couple of examples of projects that would be considered to be in the public interest. This includes guidance that

> [a] project can reasonably be expected to serve the public interest even if adverse impacts on some people, or on groups of people, can reasonably be expected. This is possible as long as other matters that must or may be considered under this subsection mean that, overall, the benefits that can reasonably be expected outweigh the adverse impacts.[84]

There is no suggestion there that the parties adversely affected by the disclosure would themselves have any reason to accept the disclosure to be appropriate. Although adverse impacts on individuals or groups are to be considered, there is nothing to suggest that *these individuals or groups* are reasonably to be expected to benefit from the disclosure or even that justification itself should appeal to reasons that are impartial and common to all affected persons or publics. There is no requirement for the kind of processual lens that Sorbie advocates. There is nothing to require that the individuals or groups have reason to expect or accept the disclosure or that they will have an opportunity to express a preference. There is no merits-based review by the Commissioner in case of any complaint that the entities got the balance wrong or were wrong to balance according to what might be considered a relatively simplistic utilitarian equation.

Noting that decisions on (non)interference with medical confidentiality may not be subject to this test (as the second purpose may apply rather than the third), this nevertheless represents a lost opportunity to embed a requirement for reasonable justification in a public interest decision-making that could have applied to any use under the arrangements established by the 2022 Act. Schemes, such as the DATA scheme, present the opportunity through the establishment of an independent commissioner for an open public-interest decision-making process—or processual lens—capable of supporting *both* social licence and legitimacy in data sharing. There is still an opportunity for the code to reflect justificatory requirements that would engage relevant publics and impose obligations to explain decisions in ways that were tested and found to be reasonable by them. This could extend to an ongoing public conversation: demonstrating what has been learnt from previous applications of the test and showing the benefits justifying the disclosure. Not only would this show the decision-maker to be (increasingly) competent to make those decisions, it would also demonstrate the common purpose necessary to promote public trust and demonstrate trustworthiness.

If an organization can make such public interest decisions internally, without application of the constraints of reasonableness being tested in the ways described, then it is at risk of being significantly out of step with public opinion and, moreover, lacking trustworthiness. This might not happen with the Australian DATA Scheme, but the point is that there is little in the public interest test to guard against it. There have been instances where the relatively nebulous concept of public interest has been used by organizations in other contexts to pursue their own idiosyncratic idea of the public interest—without sufficient challenge in terms of acceptability to those affected—and public trust in both medical confidentiality and the process of decision-making has been damaged as a result.[85]

Conclusion

It matters what people think and feel about how medical confidentiality is respected and protected. We will only realize the benefits of medical confidentiality if individuals believe that the information they confide to healthcare professionals will only be used in ways they value. The decision-making process must be able to offer a reasonable justification, for the vulnerabilities implied by decisions on (non)interference with medical confidentiality, to the people affected by those decisions. This is a justificatory requirement of a robust conception of public interest and necessary to promote public trust in the decision-making process. If a reasonable justification cannot be offered, then the decision-making process is not trustworthy.

Where there is an unavoidable conflict between the public interest in medical confidentiality and other public interests, then systems tend to permit an interference with confidentiality only following a "balancing operation" performed by either a court or other empowered entity. When the public interest in medical confidentiality conflicts with another public interest, such as the public interest in health research, this balancing operation may take place in the context of a decision on whether to waive a requirement for individual consent to the use the confidential information. If this is to be more than an invitation to idiosyncrasy, then substantive and procedural constraints must be placed around the public interest decision-making process. If the benefits of public confidence in medical confidentiality are to be protected, then these constraints must protect public trust in the balancing operation and offer sufficient justification for the balance struck to different audiences. Given the privileged position of law within society, the balance must be consistent with a legal obligation acceptable to legal officials. If constraints are to protect and promote public confidence in the decision-making process—and what has been described as the social licence to operate—then affected persons must also perceive the balancing operation to provide sufficient justification for the vulnerability implied (if only by the existence of the balancing operation itself).

In other words, to protect the benefits of medical confidentiality, persons affected by a decision on (non-)interference must see the use of the data enabled to be worth the vulnerability implied by allowing the interference. If people are not to be invited to accept that which they should not—according to their own normative commitments—then the decision should also be *worthy* of their voluntary acceptance and granting of social licence. The balancing operation should actually conform not only with formal legal rules but also their general and social norms: it should be socially legitimate. This is about the balancing operation being defensible in terms that resonate with normative commitments of persons affected by decisions on (non-)interference with medical confidentiality; it is not about abdicating responsibility for a decision to a populist process. There is value in being able to justify a public interest decision as socially legitimate. Flathman describes it thus:

> The individual citizen may be obligated to obey governmental actions which conflict with his interests, but government is expected to justify its decisions and actions in terms of a standard appropriate to the position which requires those decisions, its position as a public agent. The function of the concept of "public interest" is to provide such a standard, and its logic corresponds to that function.[86]

The point here is that a balancing operation will necessarily involve an interference with one or more interests. Without a reasonable justification providing a relevant standard for that interference, this interference—while named as "in the public interest"—will not be demonstrated to be socially legitimate to the persons affected by the decision. The logic for adoption of that standard is avoidance of soliciting an unjustified social licence: imposing a vulnerability that cannot be normatively justified. Public interest decision-making is only worthy of public trust if people are not exposed to vulnerabilities that cannot be justified in terms of their own normative commitments.

It is through the requirement of a reasonable justification that one can connect the concepts of public interest and trustworthy governance. A public interest decision on (non-)interference with medical confidentiality exposes affected persons to vulnerabilities. Trust involves a voluntary acceptance of risk under conditions of uncertainty. A reasonable justification for the exposure to vulnerability thus may serve not only to demonstrate social legitimacy, and to promote social licence, but also as a reason to trust the decision. Reasonable justification may also, however, require some degree of social engagement. It may be crucial to understanding whether a decision will conform with the general and social norms of those affected by a decision.

The DATA Scheme in Australia represents a lost opportunity to embed this kind of concept of public interest requirement into the regulatory landscape. This does not mean the Scheme cannot operate in a way that is trustworthy; it means only that the operative concept of public interest is not doing what it might to support demonstration of trustworthiness. The concept of public interest operating in the Scheme at present does not go as far as it might to enable the National Data Commissioner to require reasonable justification from decision-makers for the public interest balance they strike. It is only one example. Too often the concept of public interest is left disconnected from the justificatory requirements necessary to trust and trustworthiness. Of course, justifying a balancing operation is not sufficient to protect trust or demonstrate the trustworthiness of a system overall. It should, however, be recognized to be a necessary part from the perspective of those affected by a decision on (non-)interference.

Unless one is able to demonstrate why the effects of a particular public interest decision on (non-)interference with medical confidentiality ought to be accepted as appropriate by affected persons, then one will not be able to demonstrate how the concept of public interest contributes towards trustworthy health data governance. Recognizing the conceptual connection between public interest and trustworthiness may place substantive and procedural limits around public interest decision-making, but such guardrails should ultimately only serve to promote public trust and confidence in medical confidentiality and protect the benefits that follow from that public trust. This may help protect health professionals, and the health service more generally, from the kind of imputation of indiscretion feared for Dr Hawkins, and the view that they have done something wrong by disclosing confidential patient information when the law permits or requires it.

Acknowledgements

Sincere thanks to Edward (Ted) Dove, Graeme Laurie, and David Lind for their extremely helpful comments on an earlier draft of this chapter.

Notes

1 William Cobbett, Thomas Jones Howell, Thomas Bayly Howell and James Louis Petigru, *Cobbett's Complete Collection of State Trials and Proceedings for High Treason and Other Crimes and Misdemeanors from the Earliest Period to the Present Time*, vol 20 (R. Bagshaw 1771–1777) 573.

2 Ibid.

3 As noted below, there are a number of legal constraints that operate to hedge a duty of confidence: these include the courts not recognizing information confided to a health professional to be legally privileged in the way that, for example, information confided to a lawyer is legally privileged. There is no need to consider here the extent to which the justification for different kinds of limitation may be reasonably reduced to public interest justifications.

4 I recognize that such processes may result in the disclosure of a person's information without their consultation or consent. In such circumstances, it may seem odd to suggest that the person has "voluntarily relied" upon the process. However, I would suggest that reliance occurs at the point that the person voluntarily provides their information to a system that has the decision-making process as a constituent part.

5 The focus of this argument is on those who determine whether there is a public interest in disclosure: it is about public interest decision-making. I recognize as important the question of whether those who receive data, e.g. following a decision to permit use, act in the public interest, and maintain public trust. I suggest, however, careful thought would need to be given to whether the conceptual connection proposed here endures across different contexts, especially those that do not require *public interest* decision-making.

6 Cobbett, n 1, 572.

7 [1988] RPC 379.

8 Ibid., 386 [15].

9 [2004] UKHL 22.

10 (1997) 25 EHRR 371.

11 Ibid., 405 [95].

12 I am here discussing the value of medical confidentiality in the context of healthcare rather than, for example, health research. I take this to be the focal case but the central thrust of the argument I offer may be extended to other contexts: there is value in decision-makers recognizing the conceptual connection between the concept of public interest and trustworthiness. The nature or content of the interests to be traded or balanced may vary, but not the requirement that the justification for the decision meet certain common requirements. In order for the argument to translate meaningfully to other contexts there needs to be only the common environmental element that the value/interest perceived can only be realized if people *voluntarily* share confidential information with others.

13 For example, there is a widely recognized public interest in the use of data for the purposes of both health and non-health-related surveillance. For an examination of the variance in regulatory requirements associated with public interest decision-making in relation to health and non-health related surveillance, see Mark Taylor and Richard Kirkham, "Health Data, Public Interest, and Surveillance for Non-health-Related Purposes", in Ron Iphofen and Dónal O'Mathúna (eds), *Ethical Issues in Covert, Security and Surveillance Research* (Emerald Publishing 2021) 93–118.

14 [1990] 1 All ER 835.

15 *W* v *Egdell* [1990] 1 All ER 835, 848 [h].

16 [1990] 1 All ER 835.

17 [1988] 3 All ER 545.

18 Ibid., 659.

19 (1997) 25 EHRR 371 [25], [97].

20 *Source Informatics Ltd, Re An Application for Judicial Review* [1999] EWCA Civ 3011, [54]. Also, extending to include a confidential inquiry into deaths in the nuclear industry. *Lewis* v *Secretary of State for Health and Redfern* [2008] EWHC 2196 (QB).

21 Public Benefit and Privacy Panel for Health and Social Care, "Guiding Principles and Policy for Decision Making v1.0", available at: https://www. informationgovernance.scot.nhs.uk/pbpphsc/who-are-the-public-benefit-and-privacy-panel-and-what-do-they-do/.

22 G Owen Schaefer and others, "Clarifying How to Deploy the Public Interest Criterion in Consent Waivers for Health Data and Tissue Research" (2020) 21 *BMC Medical Ethics* 23 (doi: 10.1186/s12910-020-00467-5).

23 For an example of the latter, see Mark J Taylor and Tess Whitton, "Public Interest, Health Research and Data Protection Law: Establishing a Legitimate Trade-Off between Individual Control and Research Access to Health Data" (2020) 9 *Laws* (doi: 10.3390/laws9010006).

24 Public Benefit and Privacy Panel for Health and Social Care, "How to access health data in Scotland", available at: https://www.informationgovernance.scot. nhs.uk/pbpphsc/.

25 Health Research Authority, "Confidentiality Advisory Group", available at: https://www.hra.nhs.uk/about-us/committees-and-services/confidentiality-advisory-group/.

26 [1990] 95 ALR 87.

27 Ibid., 125.

28 Ibid.

29 Annie Sorbie, "Sharing Confidential Health Data for Research Purposes in the UK: Where are 'Publics' in the Public Interest?" (2020) 16 *Evidence & Policy* 249, 255.

30 Schaefer and others, n 22, 4.

31 Ibid., Table 2.

32 Ibid., 5.

33 In fact, the working definition they offer arguably only considers one side of the scale: "Contribution to the public interest: Substantial expected advancement of the health-related interests of members of a group whose interests are, or should be, or particular concern to the society in question". Schaefer and others, n 22, 4.

34 "However, these criteria cannot provide on their own a formulaic or definitive answer to which studies meet a public interest criterion and which do not. Due to the nature of the concept of public interest, such a formula is unfortunately not possible, nor indeed is it desirable". Schaefer and others, n 22, 5.

35 Schaefer and others, n 22, 6.

36 Aileen McHarg, "Reconciling Human Rights and the Public Interest: Conceptual Problems and Doctrinal Uncertainty in the Jurisprudence of the European Court of Human Rights" (1999) 62 *The Modern Law Review* 674.

37 William D Zarecor, "The Public Interest and Political Theory" (1959) 69 *Ethics* 277, 277.

38 See e.g. HLA Hart, *The Concept of Law* (Clarendon 1961) 133. Hart describes as one of the two minimum conditions of a legal system that "its rules of recognition specifying the criteria of legal validity, and its rules of change and adjudication must be effectively accepted as common public standards of official behaviour by its officials".

39 Schaefer and others, n 22, 7.

40 Taylor and Whitton, n 23.

41 Note there is a significant distinction to be drawn between what people can accept as reasonable and what they would prefer. See Mark J Taylor and Natasha Taylor, "Health Research Access to Personal Confidential Data in England and Wales: Assessing Any Gap in Public Attitude Between Preferable and Acceptable Models of Consent" (2014) 10 *Life Sciences, Society and Policy* 15 (doi: 10.1186/s40504-014-0015-6).

42 Judy Allen, Carolyn Adams, and Felicity Flack, "The Role of Data Custodians in Establishing and Maintaining Social Licence for Health Research" (2019) 33 *Bioethics* 502, 503.

43 Pam Carter, Graeme T Laurie, and Mary Dixon-Woods, "The Social Licence for Research: Why *care.data* Ran Into Trouble" (2015) 41 *Journal of Medical Ethics* 404.

44 Allen, Adams, and Flack, n 42, 503.

45 David L Deephouse and Mark Suchman, "Legitimacy in Organizational Institutionalism", in Royston Greenwood and others (eds), *The Sage Handbook of Organizational Institutionalism* (SAGE Publications Ltd 2008) 49–77.

46 Ibid., 50.

47 See e.g. Mark C Suchman, "Managing Legitimacy: Strategic and Institutional Approaches" (1995) 20 The Academy of Management Review 571, 573. For example, Suchman defines social legitimacy as "a generalized perception or assumption that the actions of an entity are desirable, proper, or appropriate within some socially constructed system of norms, values, beliefs, and definitions", 574.

48 Seymour Martin Lipset, *Political Man: The Social Bases of Politics* (Johns Hopkins University Press 1981).

49 Deryck Beyleveld, *The Dialectical Necessity of Morality* (University of Chicago Press 1992); Alan Gewirth, *Reason and Morality* (University of Chicago Press 1980); Immanuel Kant, *The Groundwork of the Metaphysics of Morals* (Christine M Korsgaard, Jens Timmermann and Mary Gregor, eds, 2nd edn, Cambridge Texts in the History of Philosophy 2012).

50 Roger Brownsword, "Law and Technology: Two Modes of Disruption, Three Legal Mind-Sets, and the Big Picture of Regulatory Responsibilities" (2018) 14 *Indian Journal of Law and Technology* 30, 54–58.

51 Beyleveld, n 49; Kant, 49.

52 Mark J Taylor, "Health Research, Data Protection, and the Public Interest in Notification" (2011) 19 *Medical Law Review* 267.

53 Taylor and Whitton, n 23.

54 For an overview, see Jonathan Quong, "Public Reason", *The Stanford Encyclopedia of Philosophy* (Summer edn, 2022), available at: https://plato.stanford.edu/archives/sum2022/entries/public-reason/. Even those unpersuaded by rationalist moral philosophy may still agree there to be an obligation on those with coercive power to provide a justification for its exercise, or else represent no more than the rules of the powerful.

55 Exceptional circumstance to be assessed here in accordance with the normative commitments of western liberal democracy and something akin to Mill's "harm principle": "the only purpose for which power can be rightfully exercised over any member of a civilised community, against his will, is to prevent harm to others". See John Stuart Mill, *The Collected Works of John Stuart Mill, Volume XVIII— Essays on Politics and Society Part I* (University of Toronto Press 1977) 223.

56 Public Benefit and Privacy Panel for Health and Social Care, "Guiding Principles and Policy for Decision Making", n 21.

57 Sorbie, n 29.

58 Taylor and Taylor (n 41).

59 Rebecca M Bratspies, "Regulatory Trust" (2009) 51 *Arizona Law Review* 575, 589.

60 It may not be enough to say that you trust something or someone, or even to believe that you trust it or them, if you never actually rely upon that belief in a way that exposes you to a vulnerability you may never *actually* trust them: short of acting upon the belief you may only ever be said to be willing to trust and not actually to trust them.

61 Roger C Mayer, James H Davis and F David Schoorman, "An Integrative Model of Organisational Trust" (1995) 20 *Academy of Management Review* 709, 717–720.
62 Onora O'Neill, *Autonomy and Trust in Bioethics* (Cambridge University Press 2009), especially Chapter 1: "Gaining autonomy and losing trust?".
63 Ibid.
64 Sorbie, n 29.
65 Ibid., 256.
66 Mayer, Davis, and Schoorman, n 62, 719.
67 Ibid.
68 "Good reason" here is a reason that conforms with general and social norms.
69 Onora O'Neill is one of those who has doubted Annette Baier's suggestion that "reasonable trust will require grounds for … confidence in another's good will, or at least the absence of grounds for expecting their ill will or indifference". See Annette Baier, "Trust and Antitrust" (1986) 96 *Ethics* 231, cited in O'Neill, n 62, 13–14.
70 O'Neill, n 62, 25.
71 Office of the National Data Commissioner, "Introducing the DATA Scheme", available at: https://www.datacommissioner.gov.au/the-data-scheme.
72 Revised Explanatory Memorandum to the Data Availability and Transparency Bill 2022, para 22.
73 Noting that the DATA Scheme extends beyond health and medical data and that medical research is specifically dealt with differently from other purposes, the Scheme is nevertheless offered as an example of an approach to decision-making that relies upon the concept of "public interest" without connecting that concept to the justificatory requirements necessary to demonstrating trustworthiness.
74 Data Availability and Transparency Act 2022 (Cth) s 16(2)(a).
75 Data Availability and Transparency Code 2022 (Cth) s 6(2).
76 Ibid., s 6(3).
77 I have commented with colleagues on such waivers in another context and will not repeat concerns with lack of transparency or accountability in relation to them here. See Lisa Eckstein and others, "Reversing the 'Quasi-Tribunal' Role of Human Research Ethics Committees: A Waiver of Consent Case Study" (2023) 46 *UNSW Law Journal* 498.
78 Data Availability and Transparency Act 2022 (Cth) s 16B(3); Data Availability and Transparency Code 2022 (Cth) s 6(4).
79 Revised Explanatory Memorandum: Data Availability and Transparency Bill 2022, para 21.
80 Data Availability and Transparency Code 2022 (Cth) s 6(a)-(b).
81 Data Availability and Transparency Act 2022 (Cth) s 13(e).
82 Revised Explanatory Memorandum: Data Availability and Transparency Bill 2022, para 19; Data Availability and Transparency Act 2022 (Cth) s 130(2)(l).
83 Data Availability and Transparency Act 2022 (Cth) s 19(7)(a).
84 Data Availability and Transparency Code 2022 (Cth), s 6, Note 2.
85 This happened in the United Kingdom when, for a period, there was a practice of sharing information between the National Health Service and the Home Office for the purposes of informing decisions relating to applications for visa. The body responsible for providing the data was required to apply a public interest test to the disclosure and expressed "its consistent conclusion has been that the public interest in supporting the effective enforcement of immigration law outweighs concerns that this minimal level data sharing in relation to this very tightly defined set of individuals might genuinely impact broader public trust in a confidential health service". This was a view that the Select committee thought paid

insufficient attention to the issues of ethics and public confidence. They recommended that the balancing operation be carried out again with the benefit of input from the General Medical Council and the National Data Guardian. See House of Commons, Health and Social Care Committee, *Memorandum of understanding on data-sharing between NHS Digital and the Home Office* (Fifth report of Session 2017-19) 9.

86 Richard E Flathman, *The Public Interest: An Essay Concerning the Normative Discourse of Politics* (John Wiley & Sons, Inc. 1966), 9, cited in James Wilson and others, "Providing Ethics Advice in a Pandemic, in Theory and in Practice" (2013) 38 *Bioethics* 213.

3

BIG DATA RESEARCH

Can confidentiality and fiduciary duties fill in the gaps in privacy and data protection?

David Townend

Introduction

Health research has changed radically with advances in the opportunities of processing large datasets. Advances in data science have changed methodologies from enabling predominantly stand-alone projects with datasets gathered for a particular piece of research, perhaps with some further processing for a further project often by the same team, to "Big Data" projects where the emphasis is on the production of large data repositories and linking between large datasets held by different institutions to enable interrogation of those data by a range of researchers from different projects and perspectives. Indeed, it is seen as good stewardship of public research money that data gathered from one funded project should be made available generally to the research community for further research. The methodologies offer a greater international potential for the research, more so than the previous stand-alone projects; the projects range from "blue skies" to applied research; they are the backbone of the emerging field of "personalized medicine". The new methodologies offer the promise of solving wicked medical, health, and social problems. This is a very exciting development in medicine and health research (hereafter *health research*), but it poses challenges to the governance and regulatory framework within which the research is conducted. The governance and regulatory paradigm for health research that processes personal data is largely based on the overarching concept of privacy as articulated in human rights regimes, and in the various iterations of personal data protection laws seen internationally. Thus, Big Data research seeks to be "privacy-preserving" and "data protection compliant".[1]

This chapter seeks to address this legal situation. First, a project using the Big Data methodology is explained briefly to locate the issue in a practical situation. Thereafter two sections will ask whether first privacy and then data protection are sufficient to safeguard the needs of research participants in

DOI: 10.4324/9781003394518-5

these new methodologies. The argument is that neither privacy nor data protection meets those needs. Privacy, it will be argued, is either a subjective concept that cannot crystallize easily into objective rights and duties, or, taking Laurie's view that privacy is a space within which relationships are negotiated, does not have procedural spaces for that discourse.[2] Data protection, a space where privacy should be given its granular objectivity, or a space where the discourse of privacy is conducted, does not realize either opportunity. Further, data protection is not easily suited to the demands of Big Data as it is primarily focused in protecting personal data rather than the people to whom those data relate.

From this critique of privacy and data protection, the potential offered by confidentiality to fill the gaps in the privacy and data protection regime will be presented. Confidentiality's focus on the duty of the principal to the beneficiary will be discussed, and the nature of the duty of confidentiality seen in medical practice will be considered as a better model for the responsibility of the researcher to their participants. The question will then be asked as to whether the duty should go beyond a duty of confidentiality into a full equitable fiduciary duty.

SHERLOC: An example of the new methodology challenges

There are some cancers that are very difficult to diagnose. In their early stages, they are somewhat hidden in plain sight, in that an individual begins to feel unwell but the symptoms that present at the early stages are very similar to common, minor ailments—cold and fever symptoms, stomach upsets, and the like. Individuals visit their general practitioner (GP) increasingly regularly because the symptoms persist. Some patients are referred for further investigation; others are rather dismissed. At the same time, those patients might begin to take steps to address their concerns for themselves. This might be through internet searches about their symptoms, but it might also include purchasing over-the-counter medications or making changes in diet or lifestyle to attempt to alleviate the symptoms.

SHERLOC was a project idea (yet to be funded and realized) that sought to address this situation.[3] The hypothesis underpinning the project was that the behaviours indicated above all generate personal data. Data would be generated by the discussions with the GP, at the hospital, in internet searches, and when shopping. These data would be found in different datasets held by a variety of institutions—the GP, the hospital, the internet search provider, and through customer loyalty schemes at supermarkets and pharmacies. SHERLOC would draw on these data to create an app that would alert individuals who used the software to the potential health risk identified through the analysis of their data through an algorithm created from analysing the data of individuals who had experienced the same health (and disease) trajectory in the past, measured against an analysis of the same range of data from individuals who had not experienced the same health (and disease) trajectory. The app would produce a "nudge"—not a claim that the user had a particular illness, but an alert that their behaviour had changed such that it was similar to behaviour changes seen in individuals who displayed particular symptoms and had experienced particular health outcomes. It would be a classic personalized medicine app: it proposed the use of Big Data to take personal data about one individual, to read it in the context of the data of a large number of other individuals, and to predict from that collective experience a possible health trajectory that raised particular sorts of concerns.

In order to create the *SHERLOC* app, the data analysis would be undertaken through a federated data model. The consortium included a number of stakeholders with different datasets potentially relevant to the analysis—data from hospitals, GPs, supermarkets, internet search engines. In these datasets different data were collected for different purposes. *SHERLOC* would not be generating these data as novel data, but would be accessing the stakeholders' datasets for secondary processing of their already gathered data. These data sets would be "live" in the sense that they would contain data about individuals arranged in such a way that the data were being updated over time. Individuals would be present within the different datasets. Therefore, it would be necessary to order the datasets internally in such a way that data relating to particular individuals could be connected within *SHERLOC* so that the "history" of each individual could be seen: *SHERLOC* needed to see the medical information contained in the GP's dataset, the hospital data, the internet search history, and the shopping data relating to a particular individual to see the pattern that emerged as the disease did (or did not) develop. This was not to be able to identify the individual as an identifiable individual (in the sense of being able to contact the individual or to make judgements or decisions about the individual); rather, the interest was a technical one to link the data into one list relating to the same subject. Therefore, in the hands of the individual datasets, the data had to remain personal (so that it could be updated) for the purpose of maintaining the dataset for the original (non-*SHERLOC*) purpose (which could include the purpose of contacting the particular individual, for example, as part of the GP relationship with the patient). For *SHERLOC*, the data only had to be connectable to show the trajectory of the disease and responses to it.

The data science in *SHERLOC* was based on a federated data processing method called "the Personal Health Train".[4] Each data provider creates a "station" for the train to visit. At each station the train interrogates the dataset with a set of questions to which only answers are taken. In order to ensure the answers can be connected to the same person at the next station, the data in all the datasets (at all the stations) have to be ordered such that each person appears in the same place on the list of participants in each dataset. This is achieved by ordering the data in each dataset according to a common code.[5] The data that are received are only answers to the questions asked in the order of the code. To this, further data are added ("salting" the data) so that in the hands of a third party, the dataset is incomprehensible; the data are only connectable within the operation of the algorithm, and the algorithm only produces mathematical patterns. Taking data of individuals known to have experienced the particular disease or health problems in question and plotting their data from the different data-sets against the data of individuals known not to have experienced the same issues produces formulae that allow individuals who so choose to map their own data against those formulae. The development of the algorithm is the first stage of the project. The second phase of the project is building the interface that enables individuals to compare their own data and produce a personalized nudge.

This is a typical Big Data, data science methodology, engaging machine learning and questions of either gathering data together from a number of sources, or interrogating the data in situ (a federated data approach). The datasets can be in one jurisdiction or many, and can be created and owned by various types of institutions (for-profit, charitable, healthcare, research, public, private, etc.). These new methodologies are far removed from stand-alone projects where data are gathered solely for the purposes of that research, relying on achievable anonymization and specific informed consent as the governance mechanisms. The new methodologies certainly pose a number of data science research challenges, but my concern in this chapter is the challenges they pose to the law and how those might be resolved.

The next parts of the chapter consider the two main elements of the current regulatory regime in relation to Big Data health research: privacy and data protection. Privacy, it will be argued, is conceptually weak. Privacy, in its current conceptual state, does not offer objective normative standards that resonate with different individuals in different communities; more radical conceptualizations of privacy have yet to gain traction in the regulatory process. Data protection, it will be argued, is a regime that is primarily based in creating rights over personal data, and lacks fundamental duties to bind the ongoing relationship between the data controller and their data subjects.

The problem of the privacy paradigm

Big Data science is very much created within a narrative of the privacy rights of the individual: processing must be "privacy preserving". This should give a conceptual, paradigmatic framework to resolve the conflicts between different interests in data sharing and the issues raised by *SHERLOC*. Taking Anita Allen's typology of genetic privacy,[6] we can see that *SHERLOC* certainly engages two of Allen's four areas of privacy: informational privacy (information about identifiable individuals are processed); decisional privacy (the question of who determines whether or not the datasets are engaged in the project, and how individuals are engaged in the project—the determination of the direction of the project). Proprietary privacy could be engaged if the question is resolved as to whether personal information or data are owned by either the person to whom they relate or the person who has gathered data and added the value of interpretation to create information from the data. Physical privacy is not engaged in the secondary processing of already gathered personal data, but could be brought into play by the novel gathering of, for example, blood samples if the project required data from analysis of blood to add to the information about the patient in the second phase of the project (the implementation of the project with particular patient-users of the developed app). Broad conceptual pillars of privacy are therefore engaged. However, the argument in this section of the chapter is that privacy does not have enough granularity and has not developed sufficiently as a concept to be able to give strong normative answers. There is no conceptually necessary next sentence giving the detail of privacy after the first sentence, "research must be privacy-preserving and data science must respect the privacy of the participants". The void has been filled to some extent with the idea that privacy must mean "individual privacy" as a respect for the autonomy of the individual, leaving aside concepts such as "group privacy". These moves, first, do not reflect the definition we do have of privacy within the human rights instruments, and, second, they create privacy as a presumption of exclusion from interference in (in this instance) the use of personal data.

Within human rights legislation, the right to privacy or private life is not an absolute right; it is tempered by the public interest. Article 12 of the Universal Declaration of Human Rights frames the right thusly:

> No one shall be subjected to arbitrary interference with his privacy, family, home or correspondence, nor to attacks upon his honour and reputation. Everyone has the right to the protection of the law against such interference or attacks.

The two key words are "privacy" and "arbitrary". There can be warranted interference with one's privacy. The same concept is seen in Article 8 of the European Convention on Human Rights:

> 1. Everyone has the right to respect for his private and family life, his home and his correspondence.

2. There shall be no interference by a public authority with the exercise of this right except such as is in accordance with the law and is necessary in a democratic society in the interests of national security, public safety or the economic well-being of the country, for the prevention of disorder or crime, for the protection of health or morals, or for the protection of the rights and freedoms of others.

Again, the right is conceptualized around a right to private life within the context of the rights of others protected in the public interest. The case law of the European Court of Human Rights has built up jurisprudence to define the meaning of both privacy and the public interest, but on a case-by-case basis that makes it very difficult to see a normative definitional thread of what one can expect one's private life to be.[7] Arguably that is the very heart of the right—that one should have a space where one can define one's own private life—but jurisdictions wish to place limits upon that space to create a community of private individuals. Beyond that, there cannot be absolute independence from others in a consumer, wage-labour economy; our economies, our means of production and wealth generation, demand interpersonal interaction, which in turn demands a collective culture.

An alternative understanding of privacy

Conceptually, privacy as it appears in legal theory and other academic disciplines creates typologies of areas where privacy is recognized, but arguably it does not have the internal power to create a definition of the private space that one can expect.[8] It is, at best, a patchwork of the different laws and manners that operate in societies to define the interaction of individuals in a community. And in that sense, the articulation of the privacy right is perhaps the affirmation of Hannah Arendt's caution against the separation of the legal and physical person.[9] The recognition of the individual's right to their individuality within a local culture operating within the general, internationally agreed human rights and the rule of law prevents individual States from losing sight of the personhood of its citizens. There is value in affirming a privacy right, but it is at the level of recognizing a general right to personhood. The right to a particular definition of individual private life (or privacy) is defined only loosely by the general legal culture of the particular country. Constitution and human rights courts can weigh a balance between specific competing interests when a particular case is brought for adjudication, operating within the margin of appreciation of the particular legal culture within which the dispute is set; the privacy of a particular moment can be observed. However, to create a definition of privacy, one would have to describe the whole of a legal and social culture. Yet even that would only produce a description rather than an agreed normative statement of privacy. Therefore, while the purpose of data protection can be described as seeking to safeguard the private space of individuals in relation to the information that is processed within a particular culture, an appeal to "privacy" as a basis for data protection law will not of itself unlock definitions. The appeal to "privacy" is one that connects the definition to the culture of the place and time. Hence, in a largely individualistic, consumer society, the dominant expression of privacy, and the public interest, reflect the values of that society. And the seemingly uncomfortable conundrum that personal data can have de facto commercial property value for the creator of datasets, but not for the data subject about whom the data relate, reflects the confusion of values in the particular society where the issue is raised. And again, in a society that struggles with the welfare basis of its healthcare system in a largely market-driven individualist society, an appeal to altruistic use of personal health data can appear equally confused. Privacy at this level is not a definer of norms but is merely a reflection of social values in all their complexity and confusion.

This is a claim about privacy as a legal value. Privacy, one's private life, is also an expression of an individual expectation about one's place in society. It is, essentially, a microcosm of the concept described above. An individual, defined by their culture, education, and psychology, creates a private explanation of, and set of explanations about, their place in the world. In that way, the right to privacy and to a private life is about a right to construct that free expression of how one wishes the world to be. It is at once a freedom from unjustified interference from the State (and others) that allows the individual a free expression of who they believe themselves to be. It is a political freedom. However, it is one that is tempered by the liberal view that one only has a right of self-expression and self-determination to the point where one does not harm others.[10] And that is where the internal discourse about how one wishes to be and to imagine the world becomes an external discourse; privacy and the public interest are about the right, and duty, of the individual to participate in a public discourse about the definition of the culture within which they live (and the right that such a public discourse be facilitated in their culture). This is very much the concept of privacy that Laurie develops—the "sphere of separateness".[11] Laurie sees this as a space for the negotiation. This would be a very different approach from the more negative exclusionary expressions of privacy.[12] And in that sense, privacy is the right and duty of individuals in a community to fine-tune their culture to enable as great an inclusion of diverse opinions as possible both about how individuals wish to live and the impact of one's life on others.[13] Under these conceptualizations, privacy is a dynamic paradigm of social discourse. However, this is not operationalized (yet), and Big Data projects' references to privacy, while showing an earnest intent to respect rights of individual citizens, are not able to connect to or realize clear normative standards. Put more optimistically, the enthusiasm of the data science research community to locate its work in respect for individuals' privacy can make the projects themselves spaces where the negotiation of privacy expectations can be undertaken.[14]

The data protection gaps underlined by Big Data

Data protection law can, at one level, be seen as an opportunity for regulatory flesh to be put on the conceptual bones of privacy.[15] The EU General Data Protection Regulation (GDPR) represents an iteration of a democratic expression of informational privacy.[16] Researchers in *SHERLOC* and other Big Data projects should be able to find guidance about the balance of different interests in relation to their processing of personal data; they should find clear definition of their rights and duties.

However, such clarity is not found in the GDPR. Further, even on its face, the concept underpinning the GDPR is one based on limited duties owed to the data subject by the data controller with rights afforded to the data subject to ensure that the data subjects' interests are safeguarded.[17] It is arguably much more about the protection of the data in personal data rather than the individuals to whom the data relate.

This is problematic. There is arguably a structural imbalance of power between the data subject and the data controller (in the latter's favour). The rights of the data subject depend first upon a stark choice of either accepting the controller's terms for the processing or not being included, or, where the controller is processing one's personal data without a need for consent, to object to the processing and be removed from the dataset or the particular processing activity. These actions on the part of the data subject depend upon a power relationship where the data subject feels capable of declining the data controller. To click "reject all" on a pop-up consent in accessing a website might require a low level of confidence; to refuse a medical practitioner's request to participate in a research study, or to challenge a company's standard terms about participating in a research project from one's shopping data, could be quite another matter.

This becomes important when considered against the importance of trust and confidence in health research, and, perhaps more importantly, the recent decline in such trust and confidence.[18] There is a strong argument that the data protection balance is one that favours commercial interests, perhaps unsurprisingly as the legal basis for the creation of the GDPR under the EU Treaties is in seeking harmonization of Member States' laws to create a single market.[19] It is a *General* Data Protection Regulation, and not a sector-specific Regulation to balance competing interest in health research. While the Regulation is concerned to safeguard citizens' fundamental rights and freedoms, it is designed to do so within the context of the social market.[20] The next part of the chapter will defend these claims.

The data protection principles do not create strong duties for the data controller

Article 5 of the GDPR creates a series of principles that govern the processing of personal data. The principles themselves are written in an abstract, rather passive voice: "Personal data shall be [...] processed lawfully, fairly and in a transparent manner in relation to the data subject" (Article 5(1)(a)). The principles continue to explain "purpose limitation" (that the processing must be for "specified, explicit and legitimate purposes" with the possibility of further compatible processing) (Article 5(1)(b)); "data minimisation", limiting the amount of data processed to that which is necessary for the stated purpose (Article 5(1)(c)); "accuracy" of the data (Article 5(1)(d)); "storage limitation", requiring that data only be kept in a form that can identify individuals for as long as is necessary for the stated purpose (Article 5(1)(e)); and, "integrity and confidentiality", which in the GDPR is defined as relating to ensuring "appropriate security of the personal data, including protection against unauthorised or unlawful processing and against accidental loss, destruction or damage, using appropriate technical or organisational measures" (Article 5(1)(f)). Article 5(2) indicates that "[t]he controller shall be responsible for, and be able to demonstrate compliance with, paragraph 1 ('accountability')."

There are weaknesses in the principles. The concepts of fairness and transparency are not further defined in the Regulation. Lawfulness is defined in as much as lawfulness must first require conformity to the legal obligations set out in the GDPR, and in conformity to national rules that bite on the processing of personal data (insofar as Member States have discretion to regulate beyond the requirements of the GDPR). Thus, in a jurisdiction with confidentiality, lawfulness would suggest conformity with that law (in so far as it conforms with the requirements of the GDPR), but that does not produce a harmonized environment for the regulation of the processing of personal data across the EU. Data minimization and storage limitation appear strong, but the limitation is determined by what is required for the purpose of the processing. This is, of course, sensible, and prevents abuse of the opportunity, but as in many of the issues about definition, it is not clear who will be the de facto arbiter of many of the data controller's choices. There are, however, more fundamental concerns about the regime.

The data subject's rights seem to create an almost "self-help" protection regime for the data subject

Articles 13 and 14 require the data controller to notify the data subject of the identity of who is processing their data and for what purpose. Articles 15 to 22 give the data subject a series of rights upon which they can act to protect themselves. They have a "right of access" (Article 15). This is the right to further information about the nature of the processing of data relating to them from the data controller, including a copy of the data being processed (for a fee). There is a "right to rectification" (Article 16) whereby the data subject can require the correction of inaccuracy in the data.[21] The GDPR reframes the "right to erasure" as the "right to be forgotten" (Article 17). This is limited. The data controller must erase data where they are no longer required for the purpose of processing, where the data subject withdraws consent to the processing where that is the legal basis for processing, or in response to an Article 21 ("right to object") request from the data subject where the objection is a legitimate objection to processing on the legal basis of the data controller's legitimate interest to process the data or that the data are processed in the public interest (Articles 6.1.e and 6.1.f), or where the processing is for direct marketing purposes. The "right to be forgotten" was designed to be a response to the difficulty of personal data remaining as a shadow on the internet and electronic media. However, Article 17(2) concedes a reality that once published, it is very difficult to remove the data, limiting the duty of data controllers to going as far as is reasonable "taking account of available technology and the cost of implementation", including notifying other controllers who are processing the personal data. Under Article 18, the data subject has a "right to restriction of processing" available during the period that the data are being corrected under Article 16, where the processing is unlawful as an alternative to the erasure of the data, where the purpose is exhausted but the data are required by the data subject in legal claims, or while establishing the legitimacy of an objection to processing of the data under Article 21(1). Article 19 establishes a right to be notified of any changes made in relation to Articles 16, 17(1), and 18.

Article 20 gives the data subject, further to the right of access in Article 16, a "right to data portability". This is commonly spoken of as a right to a copy of the data held by the data controller about the data subject "in a structured, commonly used and machine-readable format" that the data subject can transfer to another controller. However, what is not discussed is the wording of the data that are available under data portability: "the personal data concerning him or her, *which he or she has provided to a controller*" (emphasis added). This makes strong commercial sense. A data controller will add value to gathered personal data—convert the personal data to personal information through processing the original raw data—and it would be improper to allow a data subject make that work available to a third party, but this is a limit on the access a data subject has to data that relate to them in the hands of the data controller.

The rights are outlined above in some detail to show two things: they are limited in their scope, but also the data subject must initiate the rights. The data subject must know, or suspect, a problem with the processing of their personal data, and this places the emphasis strongly upon the data subject for the protection of their interests. However, is this sufficient to sustain a claim that the GDPR creates a largely "self-help" regime for the data subject?

Under Article 24, the data controller owes a duty to assess the nature of the potential impact on the data subject and to mitigate those risks through "appropriate technical and organisational measures" to ensure compliance with the GDPR and any sector-specific codes created under Article 40 of the same. Under Article 25, the data controller must ensure that processing is designed to be compliant with the requirements of the GDPR (rather than designing the processing and then attempting to ensure that it is complaint), and in this the data controller can balance the severity of the risk with "the state of the art [and] the cost of implementation". Under Article 30, the data controller must maintain a "record of processing activities". This record ties back to the requirements of the data protection principles (Article 5) and the information given to the data subject under Articles 13 and 14. It includes a requirement to consider the time period for the processing, and to describe the "technical and organisational security measures" used. This does not apply to all organizations, but it would, arguably, apply to research institutions (Article 30(5)). This sits with the Article 35 requirement to make a data protection impact assessment in advance of processing, and to seek a "prior consultation" with the Supervisory Authority where the data controller identifies the processing as potentially of high risk and without measures to mitigate that risk. Article 37 requires the appointment of a "data protection officer" (DPO) where the data controller or processor is a public body, engaged in the "systematic monitoring the data subject on a large scale", or is engaged in the large-scale processing of sensitive personal data. In other cases, a DPO may be appointed. The DPO is employed by the company, as an independent guardian of GDPR observance in the enterprise. Article 32 creates an obligation on the data controller to ensure the "security of processing". This is a strong duty to ensure the security of the data, and this goes a long way to ensuring the protection of the data subject. The data controller, under Article 33, is under a duty to notify the supervisory authority in the event of a breach in relation to personal data, with a strict timeframe and procedures to follow. The fines that can be imposed for a breach are very high.

Is it then fair to say that the GDPR creates a largely self-help regime for the data subject?

This is a step too far, but the analysis shows that the data protection regime is exactly that: it is a regime that protects the personal data. The focus is, on the one side, on the duties owed by the data controller in relation to the personal data, and, on the other, on the rights of the data subject to act in response to notifications of the processing of their personal data. As seen above, the data protection regime does not create a strong duty of care between the data controller and the data subject. This claim is supported by two further elements: the GDPR does not place the data subject in a position to negotiate the terms of their interaction with the data controller; the data controller is likely to be an institution rather than an individual.

That the data subject has very limited opportunities, if any, to negotiate the terms of the use of their data reflects the EU single market environment that the GDPR is largely created to serve. The data controller must safeguard personal data they are processing in line with the GDPR. However, the duty extends only for such time as the data are "personal data" within the scope of the GDPR. The duty ends once the data in the possession of the data controller cease to be capable of identifying an individual (either within the data themselves or when linked to other data reasonably likely to come into the possession of the data controller) (Article 4(1)) and Recital 26). There is the technical difficulty in finding a clear definition of "reasonably likely" to be used to identify an individual. However, the larger issue is that this limits the protection of the integrity of the data subject. The data subject is offered no protection against a use of data that relate to them without identifying them; the data subject has no recourse if, for example, their anonymized medical data were used for the development of a chemical weapon (assuming that such a use would be repellant to the data subject). Once identifiers and the reasonable possibility of identification are removed, the data protection regime is predicated on the idea that data subject can have no further interest in the data.[22] There is a similar lack of engagement with the data subject in relation to the legal basis upon which the data are processed. A data controller must have a legal basis under Article 6 (and a basis for lifting the moratorium against processing special, sensitive personal data under Article 9). The data subject must be informed of that legal basis, and from that the data subject can choose to exercise the rights outlined above. Where informed consent is used as the legal basis, the data subject's choice is stark; where the data subject wants or needs the processing to be undertaken, there is a theoretical space for negotiation of the terms, but practically this must only happen very rarely, perhaps again mirroring the essentially commercial setting of the GDPR. Even in health research, where an information sheet and informed consent protocol has been agreed with a research ethics committee, it is unlikely that a research participant will be able to negotiate the terms of the use of their data.

The definition of the "data controller" is perhaps the most interesting indicator of the underpinning nature of the GDPR. Article 4(7) states: "'controller' means the natural or legal person, public authority, agency or other body which, alone or jointly with others, determines the purposes and means of the processing of personal data". This would seem very clearly to envisage that the controller, in the case of a research project, would be at least the

Principal Investigator (PI) of the project—the person determining the scientific choices in relation to the project. This person might be a joint controller with their employer, but the key element of the *data protection* definition of data controller is the control of the purposes and processes of the enterprise. One can see that where an employee simply carries out the data protection policies of an employer, then they do not exercise such control. However, it is argued widely, that, for instance, in a university or research institution, there should be only one data controller, and that should be the institution or the figurehead of the institution. This could be said to be an *employment law* definition of data controller. This would sit with a general reading of the GDPR as an essentially economic instrument; the ability to compensate the data subject in the event of a breach of the personal data would be the key and sufficient purpose of the definition of a data controller. However, this approach underlines a lack of sufficient connection between the data subject and the individuals dealing with their personal data. It is argued that employment law makes that connection; the researcher could be given all the data protection duties through their contract of employment. However, this is arguably not in the plain meaning of Article 4(7). Further, a data subject may not want mere compensation in the face of a breach of their personal data; private information cannot be un-known in the mind of the recipient, and the function of data protection law arguably should be to create an environment of trust and confidence between the data subject and the person choosing what to do with their data and who is processing it. In analysing the definition of data controller, Lee Bygrave and Luca Tosoni indicate that the intention of the legislators and the "Article 29 Working Party" (and since the GDPR, the European Data Protection Board) is to locate the responsibility of controllership with the decision-maker.[23] However, they suggest that the role of controller will not usually sit with an individual within a corporation, to increase stability for the data subject, although (and this is very much in line with vicarious liability law) where the individual employee exceeds their authority, then that individual is seen as the data controller. This they support with analysis of judgments of the Court of Justice of the European Union.[24] Therefore, and concluding this point, how far in practice a research PI will be held accountable as a data controller is somewhat moot; there is certainly disagreement within the data protection community around this point. And yet, this is a crucial point in relation to building trust and confidence between the data subject and the processing of their personal data.

Confidentiality: A way of addressing the regulatory difficulties of privacy and data protection

A sustainable conclusion from the previous sections is that privacy and data protection do not serve *SHERLOC* and Big Data research well. The new data science methodologies need members of the public to trust researchers who process their data at a very large, macro scale searching for both normal and unexpected results that can then be used as an index against which the situations of individuals with particular conditions can be read. Data science can go some way to create tools that assist in building that trust,[25] but the regulatory environment must address the need to build trust between researchers, participants, and general publics. A case has been made above that privacy lacks normative authority to set robust boundaries that resonate with citizens, or provide discourse opportunities for them to create those normative boundaries for themselves; data protection is designed primarily to protect personal data as the means of protecting data subjects without creating trust between data subjects and data controllers (or the individuals processing personal data). There is a need to find a way of making the individual researcher (in our health research example) accountable to the data subject for the protection of their personal data and their broader interests. Confidentiality, well known in the clinical health setting, offers those connecting duties. It can meet some of the gaps visible in data protection law.

At this point, it is worth focusing on medical confidentiality,[26] as this operates in many different jurisdictions.[27] The duty of confidentiality is owed by the individual health practitioner, and not primarily by the institution. This is so well established that it is part of the professional character of health professionals.[28] A healthcare professional has a duty of confidentiality to those in their care that binds them almost against the world. And the duty is such that any healthcare professional coming into contact with the information of a patient is bound by the duty. Confidence exists between the immediate professional and the patient, and then with anyone with whom they discuss the case, and anyone who comes into contact with the patient's information. This is a fundamental of healthcare professionalism. It is not agreed by contract; it simply applies.[29]

Medical confidentiality is a well-established case, but it is an application of a more general duty. Confidentiality operates, for example, in English equity, in situations where the relationship and information has a quality of confidence.[30] The duty of confidence has been established independent of a contract in English law since at least the mid-1800s.[31] In the commercial setting, employees owe a duty of confidentiality to their employer beyond the terms of their contract.[32] Paparazzi potentiality owe a duty of confidentiality to celebrities they seek to photograph unless a public interest or freedom of expression argument can be established to justify a breach of that duty.[33] There is a link to the human right to privacy and a breach of a tort in relation to that right,[34] but a duty of confidence has a particular quality in equity in that it exists because of the situation in which the information was found; an individual, once aware of the information, owes a duty of confidence regardless of whether it is negotiated or implied in a contract. Throughout the case law, the duty extends over information that has a quality of confidential information.

Based in equity, confidentiality has a strong element of discretion—it is found according to the situation and is not rule-bound. It is a concept of duty towards the individual to whom information relates rather than simply to the information itself. It is a fine distinction to draw with data protection: confidentiality is fundamentally, in data protection language, about the relationship between the data controller (or data processor) and the data subject, where the data controller is the natural person actually determining the purpose of processing and processing the information. Perhaps it is better expressed that it is not simply processing the information, but it is concerned with the processing of the person behind the data. Equitable remedies in relation to breach, as in the case of data protection, cannot create an unknowing of published information, but they extend and enforce a duty to anyone into whose hands the information falls in breach of the duty of confidence.

In the case of health research, the conditions are visible for the application of a duty of confidence. Researchers receive information that has a quality of confidence—the participants from whom it is gathered can have a "reasonable expectation" that the information is confidential.[35] The recognition of this duty by the courts in equity would require litigation, which is costly; researchers do not have a professional body to issue a guideline embracing the duty. There is an argument for the express acceptance of the duty of confidentiality in data protection law, for example as a data protection principle under Article 5 of the GDPR, although, as argued above, it would take further amendments to move the focus of data protection law from the protection of data to the primary protection of the data subject. And yet the acknowledgement of such a duty of confidence in the research community might not be a great imposition. In the empirical work of the project *DataTerms*, one of the concerns expressed by the data scientists and other researchers who participated in focus groups or were surveyed by questionnaire in the work was around the protection of the rights of research participants over their personal information and the provenance of the information and its integrity for ensuring high-quality science.[36] Confidentiality could meet some of the concerns expressed in *DataTerms*, but also those expressed around ensuring and strengthening trust in research.

Would embracing equity's fiduciary duty be a step too far in developing the research governance landscape?

The express inclusion of the duty of confidence in health research would address some of the concerns raised about the application and focus of data protection. It could also go some way to addressing the normative shortfall in the concept of privacy. Confidentiality creates a duty of respect between individuals. It does not go as far in that regard as the equitable principle of the fiduciary duty, and confidentiality does not depend upon or create of itself a fiduciary duty. The final question of this chapter is whether acknowledging a fiduciary duty between the researcher and the research participant would create a stronger environment for the development of trust and confidence in the public towards Big Data research.

The fiduciary duty at the heart of modern equity can be seen as an extreme expression of duty.[37] Cases such as *Keech* v *Sandford*[38] and *Boardman* v *Phipps*[39] hold that where a fiduciary duty is established a principal owes a supervening duty of care to the beneficiary. This operates such that the principal must subordinate all their interests to protect the interests of the beneficiary. *Keech* v *Sandford* concerned the renewal of a lease over a market. Despite the landlord expressly stating that he did not wish to renew the lease in favour of the beneficiary, a minor, the principal of the beneficiary (and the original legal owner of the lease) had to hold the new lease he had negotiated for himself on constructive trust for the original beneficiary because of the fiduciary duty he owed to that beneficiary. There was no sense of dishonesty; simply the necessary rigidity of the fiduciary duty had to be maintained. Likewise, in *Boardman* v *Phipps*, a constructive trust was imposed in favour of beneficiaries of a family trust over profits made by principals who invested their own money and skill in a complex commercial takeover of an underperforming company in which a family trust had shares. Again, there was no dishonesty in the dealings, but the principle of the strength of the fiduciary duty was of paramount importance. In *Boardman*, remuneration for the skill of the principals was recommended on a generous scale, but the supervening nature of the duty was upheld.

In both *Keech* and *Boardman*, the fiduciary relationship was concerned with the use of information that was made available to the principal by virtue of the relationship they had to the beneficiary (being the legal owner of the lease to the minor's beneficial interest in the former; gaining knowledge of the situation of the underperforming firm in the latter). Many of the situations where a fiduciary duty of care is imposed in English equity are commercial situations, and there is case law that indicates that in English equity the doctor–patient relationship is not a fiduciary relationship.[40] However, this is not the case in other jurisdictions, where the doctor–patient relationship is established as a fiduciary duty.[41] Would taking this step add to the trust environment for health research?

SHERLOC and similar Big Data projects require the processing of large datasets. The potential for health research using the new methodologies depend on the ability to use large, if not whole, population datasets. This is not to identify individual people because of an interest in them as individuals or to seek to contact them or interact in their lives. However, there is a necessity to be able to identify individuals at the level of connecting data relating to that individual across datasets; the value of the data is increasingly in the information that it gives by the connection of different dimensions of the individual life that it discloses. The information is about a particular individual, but the interest is not in the individual but in the abstract information that the connections yield.[42] Accepting that the relationship between the researcher and the participant creates a fiduciary duty would send a strong message establishing a high professional standard among researchers that is currently missing. Indeed, it would address some of the distrust around the use of Big Data seen in, for example, "care.data".[43] It would place researchers on a level with commercial professionals (and in some jurisdictions, medical professionals) and their beneficiaries. Crucially, it would accept that there is an imbalance of power: researchers have conflicts of interest with their participants that must be managed, and the fiduciary duty is a particularly strong way of acknowledging and managing the relative weakness of the research participant in the relationship. Modern fiduciary relationships acknowledge that there are legitimate benefits that a fiduciary can take (e.g. remuneration for work done, benefits from the use of information under the relationship) where those benefits are articulated and agreed. Crucially, for Big Data research, it would require those developing projects to articulate and negotiate the terms of the relationship with their immediate participants (where novel information is gathered), and would impose a visible, strong duty of care in the situation of secondary processing of already gathered data. The duty of care is towards the individual; the fiduciary duty requires the principal (the person interacting with information from another person) to consider the integrity of the person. It creates a moral compass recognized by the law that neither privacy nor data protection offers in their current forms.

Conclusion

Big Data projects have the potential to change the lives of citizens for good. *SHERLOC*, if the hypotheses are correct, could enable the use of different silos of data, gathered for different purposes, including commercial interests, to benefit individuals in relation to their health. Currently, for many people the regulatory and governance framework for the processing of personal data is not strong enough to allay fears that, instead of being used for the benefit of them as individuals, the risk of it being used to harm them is too great. After forty years of data protection legislation crafted on the basis of a privacy narrative, a root and branch reimagining of the paradigm must be considered, as it still does not function coherently to provide a sufficiently robust framework to enable citizens to explore the future potentials in healthcare and data science without fear of regulatory and governance failure. Privacy, it can be argued, serves a very different function in society from that needed for the underpinning of data protection. Privacy should be about ensuring a conversation about the relationships of individuals within society and the extent of free expression and the exploration of personhood in democracy. Undoubtedly, the regulatory and governance landscape for Big Data research—for all medical research—will continue to be dominated by privacy and data protection. The next stage in creating that landscape is to refine those concepts and laws so the participants in research (and that is increasingly whole populations) have trust in the researchers and research governance structures to safeguard their interests. The duty of confidentiality and the fiduciary duty provide both a narrative upon which to address the meanings of the duties expressed in data protection and a set of enforceable values to establish a relationship between the data subject and data controllers and data processors that reimagines those relationships in a more complete and coherent way. The next part of the privacy and data protection story should be a reimagining of the regulatory and governance landscape through the duties offered in equity, in confidentiality, and in the fiduciary duty.

Notes

1 See Johan van Soest and others, "Using the Personal Health Train for Automated and Privacy-Preserving Analytics on Vertically Partitioned Data" (2018) 247 *Studies in Health Technology and Informatics* 581.
2 Graeme Laurie, *Genetic Privacy: A Challenge to Medico-Legal Norms* (Cambridge University Press 2002), Chapter 5.
3 *SHERLOC* (Signs of Health and Risks Looking Out for Cancer) was a proposal originally developed for Cancer Research UK's Global Grand Challenge 2018. It was selected for the final ten proposals and given funds to develop the bid. It was not selected as one of the winning proposals. Since 2018, the consortium has continued to develop the proposal and apply for funding (as yet, unsuccessfully) for elements of the proposal.
4 van Soest and others, n 1.
5 A national health number or citizen identity number would be a good candidate for this. However, it only operates within the particularly jurisdiction, and in some jurisdictions the use of such numbers for research is prohibited. This is the case in the Netherlands, where the BSN (national citizen number) is unique to the individual citizen, but research using the BSN is banned under Dutch law. Therefore, one of the tasks in creating the Personal Health Train is to identify a set of data within the different datasets that allow the data to be coded in such a way that, effectively, a unique identification number is created for each person so that their data within each dataset is connectable across the datasets. It should be noted that the EU development of and ambition for the European Digital Identity, if available for researchers, would allow an enormous step forward in working with personal data across differently structured datasets. See Regulation (EU) No 910/2014 of the European Parliament and of the Council of 23 July 2014 on electronic identification and trust services for electronic transactions in the internal market and repealing Directive 1999/93/EC, and the proposed amendments to it: 2021/0136(COD).
6 Anita Allen, "Genetic Privacy: Emerging Concepts and Values", in Mark Rothstein (ed), *Genetic Secrets: Protecting Privacy and Confidentiality in the Genetic Era* (Yale University Press 1997), 31–59, 33.

7 European Court of Human Rights, "Guide on Article 8 of the European Convention on Human Rights Council of Europe" (2022), available at: https://www.echr.coe.int/documents/d/echr/guide_art_8_eng.

8 Beate Roessler and Judith DeCew, "Privacy", *The Stanford Encyclopedia of Philosophy* (Winter 2023 Edition), Edward N Zalta & Uri Nodelman (eds.), available at: https://plato.stanford.edu/archives/win2023/entries/privacy/); Alan F Westin, "Social and Political Dimensions of Privacy" (2003) 59 *Journal of Social Issues* 431; Alan F Westin, *Privacy and Freedom* (Atheneum 1967); Samuel D Warren and Louis D Brandeis, "The Right to Privacy" (1890) 4 *Harvard Law Review* 193.

9 Hannah Arendt, *The Human Condition* (University of Chicago Press 1958).

10 See e.g. John Stuart Mill, *On Liberty* (John W Parker and Son 1859).

11 Laurie, n 2.

12 See e.g. Warren and Brandeis, n 8.

13 See Mark J Taylor and David Townend, "Towards a New Privacy: Informed Consent as an Encumbrance to Group Interests?", in Edward S Dove and Niamh Nic Shuibhne (eds), *Law and Legacy in Medical Jurisprudence: Essays in Honour of Graeme Laurie* (Cambridge University Press 2022), 367–390.

14 See e.g. the *CARRIER* project, funded by the Dutch NWO research council, which includes such public engagement work, available at: https://www.nwo.nl/en/projects/628011212.

15 Data protection is not only about privacy, but at one level it concerns a granular expression of privacy in relation to the processing of personal data. The forerunner of the EU's GDPR, Directive 95/46/EC, indicated that the Directive concerned the protection of the fundamental rights and freedoms of natural persons, "and in particular their right to privacy with respect to the processing of personal data" (Article 1.1). However, there are more bases for data protection than privacy. See e.g. Lee A Bygrave, *Data Privacy Law: An International Perspective* (Oxford University Press 2014).

16 Regulation (EU) 2016/679 of the European Parliament and of the Council of 27 April 2016 on the protection of natural persons with regard to the processing of personal data and on the free movement of such data, and repealing Directive 95/46/EC (General Data Protection Regulation). The EU has, arguably, managed to establish the GDPR as a template that other jurisdictions have followed, by requiring that any data generated within the EU and processed elsewhere have to be processed in a compatible manner to the processing in the EU, and that data generated outside the EU but processed within it are processed in compliance with the GDPR. Therefore, it will be used as the basis of the discussion of data protection law in this chapter.

17 This structure of the GDPR can be seen in the EU's 1995 Directive, which, in turn, had its roots in the Council of Europe's Convention 108 of 1981 and the OECD Privacy Guidelines of 1980. The framework of the GDPR is that there are basic definitions of key concepts in the Regulation (Article 4), data protection principles (Article 5), legal bases for processing (Article 6) and for the lifting of the moratorium on the processing of sensitive personal data (Article 9), information requirements to ensure the notification of processing to the data subject (Article 13 and 14), and a series of rights given to the data subject (Articles 15–21).

18 Vincenzo Carrieri, Sophie Guthmuller, Ansgar Wübker, "Trust and COVID-19 Vaccine Hesitancy" (2023) 13 *Scientific Reports* 9245; Angeliki Kerasidou and Charalampia (Xaroula) Kerasidou, "Data-driven Research and Healthcare: Public Trust, Data Governance and the NHS" (2023) 24 *BMC Medical Ethics* 51 (doi: 10.1186/s12910-023-00922-z); NHS England, "NHS England sets out the next steps of public awareness about care.data", available at: https://www.england.nhs.uk/2013/10/care-data/; Sigrid Sterckx and others, "'You Hoped We Would Sleep

Walk Into Accepting the Collection of Our Data': Controversies Surrounding the UK care.data Scheme and Their Wider Relevance for Biomedical Research" (2016) 19 *Medicine, Health Care, and Philosophy* 177; Denis Campbell, "Patients May Shun New NHS Data Store Over Privacy Fears, Doctors Warn" (10 November 2023) *The Guardian*, available at: https://www.theguardian.com/society/2023/nov/10/patients-may-shun-new-nhs-data-store-over-privacy-fears-doctors-warn.

19 Treaty on the Functioning of the European Union, Article 114.
20 Treaty of European Union, Article 24.
21 Member States may derogate from Articles 15, 16, 18, and 21 under Article 89, where the safeguard of de-identification or pseudonymization is applied.
22 This fits with the historical "gold standard" in research ethics that protection is found in informed consent and anonymization.
23 Lee A Bygrave and Luca Tosoni, "Article 4(7). Controller", in Christopher Kuner and others (eds), *The EU General Data Protection Regulation (GDPR): A Commentary* (Oxford University Press 2020) 145–156.
24 They point to, inter alia, C-101/1 *Lindqvist*, and C-25/17 *Jehovan todistajat*.
25 Huma Saeed and others, "Blockchain Technology in Healthcare: A Systematic Review" (2022) 17 *PLoS One* e0266462.
26 See Shaun D Pattinson, *Medical Law and Ethics* (6th edn, Sweet & Maxwell 2020) Chapter 6. For discussion of confidentiality in equity, see "Breach of Confidence", in John McGhee and others, *Snell's Equity* (34th edn, Sweet & Maxwell 2020), Chapter 9.
27 See e.g. Article 7:457 on patient confidentiality of the Dutch Civil Code, Book 7 Medical Treatment Agreement Act (Wet geneeskundige behandelingsovereen-komst—WGBO), available at: https://wetten.overheid.nl/BWBR0005290/2012-06-13/#Boek7.
28 See generally General Medical Council, *Good Medical Practice* (2024), available at: https://www.gmc-uk.org/professional-standards/professional-standards-for-doctors/good-medical-practice, and specific guidance on confidentiality, available at: https://www.gmc-uk.org/professional-standards/professional-standards-for-doctors#confidentiality.
29 See e.g. *NHS Constitution for England* and *Handbook to the NHS Constitution* (2023), available at: https://www.gov.uk/government/publications/the-nhs-constitution-for-england, created under the Health Act 2009.
30 *Coco v A N Clark (Engineers) Ltd* [1969] RPC 41.
31 *HRH Prince Albert v Strange* (1849) 1 Mac. & G. 25, 41 ER 1171; *Saltman Engineering Co v Campbell Engineering Co* [1948] 1 WLUK 12; *Argyll v Argyll* [1967] Ch 302.
32 *Faccenda Chicken Ltd v Fowler and Others* [1987] Ch 117; see also *Attorney General v Guardian Newspapers No. 2* [1990] AC 109.
33 *Campbell v Mirror Group Newspapers* [2004] UKHL 22, [2004] 2 AC 457; *Douglas v Hello! Ltd No 3* [2005] EWCA Civ 595, [2006] QB 125.
34 *PJS v News Group Newspapers* [2016] UKSC 26, [2016] AC 108.
35 For a full discussion of the reasonable expectation of confidentiality, see *Snell's Equity*, n 26, 9-013 *et seq.*, and particularly the discussion therein of *AB v Sunday Newspapers (t/a The Sunday World)* [2014] NICA 58.
36 Annie Sorbie and others, "Examining the Power of the Social Imaginary through Competing Narratives of Data Ownership in Health Research" (2021) 8 *Journal of Law and the Biosciences* lsaa068 (doi: 10.1093/jlb/lsaa068).
37 See *Snell's Equity*, n 26, Chapter 7.
38 [1726] EWHC Ch J76, (1726) 2 Eq Cas Abr 741; 25 ER 223.
39 [1967] 2 AC 46.

40 *Sidaway* v *Bethlem Royal Hospital and the Maudesley Hospital Health Authority and Others* [1985] 1 All ER 643 (HL).

41 *Meinhard* v *Salmon*, 164 NE 545, 546, (NY 1928); *Witherell* v *Weimer*, 421 NE2d 869 (1981); Sophie Ludewigs and others, "Ethics of the Fiduciary Relationship Between Patient and Physician: The Case of Informed Consent" (forthcoming) *Journal of Medical Ethics* (doi: 10.1136/jme-2022-108539).

42 There is a question about the duties that are then owed to the individual where connections that are useful to the individual are revealed—incidental findings from the research—but this is beyond the scope of this chapter.

43 N 18.

PART II

Country and region-specific issues

4

MANAGING ACCESS TO HEALTH DATA FOR RESEARCH AND INNOVATION IN THE EU

Is a better regulatory approach possible?

*Aisling McMahon and Ciara Staunton** *

Introduction

The digital era has led to an unprecedented proliferation of information by and about individual people: we are generating vast amounts of data through our everyday online interactions (from emails to social media activities to our browsing histories) and consumer transactions. Such activities can reveal information about our individual behaviours and preferences, and from this, in some instances, inferences can be drawn about society, or certain groups within a society. Alongside this, third parties (including professional service providers) may need to collect, generate, and store significant digital information about individuals, including sensitive personal data. More specifically, in the health context, data are being generated in a range of digital interactions, including in the context of people's electronic health records, public health prevention, treatment programmes, and as part of health research. Such health data can be used for research into human behaviours as well as to uncover insights around the genetic basis of disease. This research has the potential to develop predictive models that improve healthcare decision-making, to develop and improve treatment interventions, as

* Both authors contributed equally to this chapter. Author names are listed in alphabetical order. The discussion of intellectual property rights in the chapter, and in particular, the section entitled "Limited oversight around how other legal protections may impact sharing of data: The competing interests at stake?", is based on research conducted by Aisling McMahon as part of the ERC-funded PatentsInHumans Project. That research is funded by the European Union (ERC, PatentsInHumans, Project No. 101042147). Views and opinions expressed are, however, those of the authors only and do not necessarily reflect those of the European Union or the European Research Council Executive Agency. Neither the European Union nor the granting authority can be held responsible for them.

DOI: 10.4324/9781003394518-7

well as drive innovation around developing new health-technologies, such as medicines, diagnostics, medical devices, and other health interventions.[1]

Such research involves significant levels of processing (i.e. collection and various uses) of health data. The collection, use, and sharing of health data is, however, fraught with ethical and legal issues.[2] This includes issues related to the protection of: individual data subjects' human rights, including their right to privacy, private family life, and confidentiality, as protected under Article 8 of European Convention on Human Rights (hereafter ECHR), which entails the need for data subjects to be informed about how such data are used and for what purpose to vindicate their broader autonomy interests, and in turn links with concerns related to data protection; and issues of transparency around data use.[3] Moreover, and relatedly, there are risks of data harms for individual health research participants and third parties arising from such research. Such risks have been discussed in detail elsewhere, but include risks of data breaches, data leaks (raising issues under Article 8 ECHR), and individual and group discrimination which also engages rights to non-discrimination under Article 14 ECHR.[4]

Accordingly, new mechanisms have been adopted which seek to deter data uses which could lead to harms and to protect data subjects' rights and interests at stake. This includes oversight bodies such as data access committees (DACs),[5] proposed data trusts,[6] and legal frameworks on the use of data.[7] In the health context, health data that are not anonymous are not only personal data, as defined under the European Union's General Data Protection Regulation (GDPR); they are also considered to be special category (i.e. sensitive) personal data under the law. As such, processing of health data is subject to stricter rules and extra protections must be met.[8] Moreover, since coming into force in 2018, the GDPR has strengthened the protection of personal data in the European Union (EU) and provided rules and procedures that must be followed in the processing of personal data, including the rights of data subjects that must be respected.[9] Like other data protection regulations, the GDPR is a general legal framework and not sector specific (i.e. it is not tailored to the health context). However, due to the importance of research in society, and the concerns that new data protection requirements could have adverse impacts on research, certain exceptions to some of the strict processing requirements were put in place for research contexts. The exceptions and derogations contained in the GDPR have been considered elsewhere in detail,[10] but what is also important to note in the health research context is that there has been a fragmented application to the GDPR in the context of health research across EU Member States. Thus, accessing personal data often requires a complex navigation of differing national approaches.[11] Furthermore, uncertainty in the application of some of the provisions in the health research context, and concerns about potential fines, has resulted in (some instances) an overly cautious approach to data protection, leading to claims that it is hindering the sharing of personal data for health research purposes.[12] Herein lies a key tension around data within the health research context: although individual rights and interests can be implicated by data breaches and data harms, health research may be hindered by lack of access to relevant health data. Moreover, a lack of data can impact diversity in available datasets,[13] our understanding of health, and the types of health technologies (including medicines, vaccines, etc.) that may be developed, with knock-on effects for individual people's health which can also impact individual human rights, up to and including, in some cases the right to life (Article 2 ECHR), and collective societal interests in maximizing health benefits and understandings.

To address some of the problems with the GDPR and to improve the European digital environment, including to balance interests of individual data subjects with collective interests of society in making relevant data available for health research, a number of legislative initiatives have been introduced as part of the European Strategy for Data. This is a strategy that is aiming to make Europe a leading player in the data economy.[14] This includes the Data Governance Act, which seeks to increase trust in data sharing, increase data availability, and overcome technical obstacles to data sharing.[15] The Data Governance Act is focused on facilitating the reuse of data held by the public sector, but it is not just public sector data that can be accessed for research and innovation, with the European Parliament estimating that 80% of industrial data is not used, due to low trust in data sharing, conflicting economic incentives, and technological obstacles.[16]

To encourage data sharing in the health space, a draft Regulation for a European Health Data Space (EHDS) was introduced by the European Commission in May 2022. The EHDS is part of the Commission's ambition to build a strong European Health Union through realizing the potential that electronic health data holds for the economy and for the realization of healthcare benefits.[17] In part to address some of the problems that have arisen from the fragmented application of the GDPR at a national level in the context of research and innovation, the EHDS proposes to introduce one legal framework across the EU to enable access to electronic health data for eight specified purposes. These are purposes that have been identified as benefiting society: "such as research, innovation, policy-making, patient safety, personalised medicine, official statistics or regulatory activities" (Recital 1). The ambition of the EHDS is that by introducing one legal framework applicable to all Member States, it will address some of the elements of the GDPR that were perceived as hampering data sharing.

A framework that provides a harmonized approach to accessing personal data is undoubtedly needed, and depending on its final form, should improve Europe's competitiveness in data-driven research and innovation. However, the evolving regulatory landscape requires frameworks that enable research and innovation in a manner that adequately protects personal data, while also considering some of the other important individual and collective rights and interests at stake. This includes the rights to privacy, autonomy, and non-discrimination, and the collective/individual interests in the right to health, and societal interests in enabling access to any downstream benefits of the research developed. As we argue in this chapter, data governance in the health research context should be grounded in processes that consider and balance all the relevant rights and interests at stake. This requires a careful balance to be struck between individual and collective interests, and consideration of the interests of a range of different stakeholders.

Given the emerging nature of the EHDS at the time of writing,[18] and ongoing advances within the digital health space in Europe, it is useful at this juncture to assess the GDPR and the proposed EHDS to determine whether and to what extent they are adequately engaging with and balancing the competing rights and interests that are at stake in the collection, use, and sharing of data for health research and innovation purposes. This chapter focuses on these issues, examining specifically whether and to what extent the current and proposed data regulatory frameworks in Europe for the use of health data for research and innovation adequately engages with and balances the range of key rights and interests at stake.

In what follows, we set the scene by providing an overview of the key rights and interests in health research with reference to five key (in some instances overlapping) actors or stakeholders involved bearing rights and interests, namely research participants, patients, researchers, national governments, and industry. We argue that there are a range of competing interests at stake which will impact parties' views and interests in how data are accessed, shared, and used downstream. Following this, we provide an overview of the current GDPR framework and the key elements of the proposed EHDS. Although the Data Governance Act will impact access to data, due to constraints of space, and due to their more specific impact on the use of data in the health space, we confine our focus here to the GDPR and the proposed EHDS. We then critique the current and proposed framework under the GDPR and proposed EHDS, arguing that the current risk-based approach to data sharing underpinning the GDPR and EHDS fails to fully engage with the range of interests at stake that have been outlined in the chapter, and in particular, with the broader collective interests at stake. We then conclude by arguing that a new data sharing framework is needed, but there needs to be greater engagement with the breadth of competing rights and interests at stake in this context if we are to deliver a sustainable and functional landscape for health research in the digital age.

Rights and interests relevant to personal data uses in health research contexts

Health research is critical in society. It can offer insights which improve diagnosis, treatment, and prevention of illness. It can also contribute to and improve health innovation around the development of new health technologies. Relatedly, fostering health research sectors can play a key role in contributing to employment, industry, and the broader economy. Thus, health research and research-enabling processes can be an important feature of a bioeconomy. As such, there are a considerable number of stakeholders involved in health research, including: patients, research participants, researchers, academic institutions, research centres, healthcare professionals, regulators, policymakers, industry, employees, and the wider public. These stakeholders have a range of (often) competing rights, interests, and motivations around data access, use, and sharing. For example, research participants may make their data available for research due to altruism and the desire for health technologies to be developed that will improve health outcomes for all;[19] patients may be motivated so that therapies can be developed to benefit their individual health or others; researchers can be motivated by a range of factors, including with the aim of contributing to science and public good, contributing to the improvement of health, and also to advance their own career via published research, patents or funding, etc.[20] For industry, employees, and government, alongside potential public interest motivations in terms of generating better health outcomes, they may also have commercially orientated motivations, including leveraging health research in particular areas as a means to maximize profitable activities, for example via its use in the development of new health technologies, which in turn can result in patents and other intellectual property rights (IPRs), generating increased profits, increased tax revenues, and new industries, and contributing to a lower unemployment rate.

Considered in this light, it is thus unsurprising that it is often claimed that health research is needed to facilitate the "public interest" given the range of health benefits, societal benefits, and private sectors benefits that can arise. However, "public interest" as a concept is undefined and arguably confuses the discourse in discussions of health data, as "public interest" is a legal basis on which to process personal data within the European data protection frameworks. Nonetheless, while not advocating for the use of the term, if we take public interest—in terms of its broader general conception—as something that could improve individual and public health while also improving the overall economy, it quickly becomes clear that there are a range of competing interests and aims at stake in the health research context that may be in tension with each other. Indeed, broad claims that research is in general in "the public interest" is contested and fraught with challenges, no less in defining what is meant by the "public" or what the "public" interest is.[21] Not only are there are different groups within society at a national and regional level that we have pointed out, but also at a global level who have different (at times competing) interests or priorities in the development of, and downstream access to, health data, health research, and/or new technologies developed via health research.[22] Given such issues, there has been a shift away from considering "the public" as a separate entity to an understanding that "the public" is composed of many "publics".[23] Knowing "the public" to whom the research pertains to is critical, as it is a key factor to determine the risk and benefits of potential health research activities.[24] In short, differing publics have diverse needs and interests, and these needs and interests can compete against those of other publics.[25] We further expand on some of the publics in health research to demonstrate our point.[26]

In the health research context, at least five key "publics" can be identified with their own rights and interests which need to be carefully considered and balanced in any effective system for the regulation of health data for health research purposes. This section takes each of these five categories in turn in order to highlight the key rights and interests at stake which must be balanced. In doing so, we also see the ongoing tension between parties who may favour data sharing and openness in use of data, and those who may not favour data sharing (for a range of reasons) or secondary uses, and differing considerations which may apply depending on the context for individual and societal interests.

First, there are the research participants who may provide data and/or biospecimens for health research and whose Article 8 ECHR rights are engaged by providing health data and in participating in health research.[27] By participating in health research, a range of individual participant rights are implicated, including participants' right to autonomy in being provided with adequate information about the research and their ability to give informed consent, right to privacy around use of their data and biospecimens, and right to data protection around use of data collected or derived related to their health and person can be engaged—rights that as noted are protected under Article 8 ECHR. Such participants will likely be concerned with the mitigation of any potential data harms in the use of their health data in research, which in some instances may lean in favour of restrictive uses of data, but also that their contribution is given maximum effect via the use and sharing of such data (within the confines of the permission they give) in the health research context.[28] Second, and relatedly, patients may have an interest in the development of new health technologies arising from health research (whether they participate in this research or not), but they will also have an interest in ensuring such technologies, once developed, are accessible and available to them and others.[29] Research participants may in some cases also be patients or may have family members who are patients. Thus, such participants may have an interest in both how their personal data are used (Article 8 rights), and in how any downstream knowledge or technologies, if developed via such research, are accessed and made accessible.[30] Patient interests in access to health-technologies may also engage the right to health, and right to life (Article 2 ECHR), such as where a patient is suffering from a terminal condition and requires access to life-sustained or curative health-care. Again, for such patients, their interests will be around supporting the maximization of data use (in a safe manner) within the health research context, while ensuring accessibility of the downstream benefits such as technology and scientific knowledge developed.

Third, national governments have an interest in supporting health research that improves the public health of its population, thereby improving overall societal well-being and reducing economic burdens on the national state. Governments also have an interest in supporting strong health research systems by encouraging innovation with potential knock-on benefits for the national economy, employment, and so on. The realization of these aims will require crafting policies that provide for data openness and incentives for industry involvement in research and development. However, governments also have an interest and duty to protect individual citizens and to mitigate against individual and group data harms which may arise in the health research context,[31] and which can impact trust in the health data sharing landscape with knock-on effects for societal trust and participation in health research more generally. Thus, governments must take a nuanced and balanced approach to data sharing and data use and ensure that regulatory frameworks embed systems that manage risks of data harms when promoting data sharing as far as possible while also enabling the system to be workable for health researchers, and alongside this maintaining equity of benefits.

Fourth, researchers have an interest in research to develop healthcare benefits which many scientists may be intrinsically motivated by. Successful health research outcomes may also further their career, either for example, via publications or being named as an inventor on patent applications, which may arise from technologies developed and contributed to by such research. Being awarded and attaining patents (or being named as inventor on such patents) and publications are key facets within many academic promotion systems and can enable better employment prospects in industry contexts. Moreover, depending on the context where new technologies from health research are developed—and the applicable IPRs and employment policy in place (see below)—researchers may in some instances share the potential IPRs over technologies developed, and profits arising. In such cases, researchers will often have an interest in obtaining access to secondary data to further develop their own research. However, the originality of insights for academic publishing and the "novelty" of an invention is a requirement for patent applications; hence, researchers may also in some instances have an interest in not openly sharing data until the point of publication or prior to patent grant/application. If they share data with other researchers for a secondary use or otherwise for other projects, they may be concerned that others could achieve the outcome they are working on first. Hence, a range of competing interests around data sharing and openness are at stake and must be carefully mediated.

Fifth, in terms of the role of industry, currently health research is often conducted within a private industry context or within public–private partnership settings. Industry has an important role to play in research in the current health innovation landscape, particularly in the translation of research to therapies. In many cases the early-stage research may be conducted within a university context or a university-company partnership, while the translational stage, given in part the high costs and resources needed, often takes place within industry settings. In such cases, generally companies will hold IPRs over health technologies developed, as employment contracts usually provide—unless modified by prior negotiation—that any IPRs created in the course of employment will be held by the employer (e.g. the relevant company or university). Such IPRs allow the rightsholders to exclude others from use of an IP-protected technology, unless that third party obtains a licence from the rightsholders. Hence, rightsholders (including companies and industry more generally) can use IPRs to develop an income stream from technologies developed and have a strong financial interest in investing in health research where it is likely to lead to a new health technology. Such entities may also have a preference to gain access to data under secondary uses where this would assist their researchers to develop new technologies, but they may prefer not to share data with other groups where to do so would enable such groups to achieve outcomes they may also be working on. For such reasons, again within the industry context, a complex picture emerges and there are likely a range of competing interests or concerns around secondary use of data, around data sharing, and around sharing or openness in the knowledge produced via such health research.

All the forgoing rights and interests are important and in vibrant bioeconomy, but it is critical that they are balanced with each other so that one does that supersede another. As research evolves, so regulations must evolve, ensuring balance between these competing rights and interests must be maintained. Changes to regulatory structures are necessary at times. For example, the emergence of biobanks, genomics, and data-driven medicine has resulted in changes to consent models and oversight mechanisms, such as DACs.[32] Artificial intelligence (AI) and its application to health are now requiring ethical and legal reflection, and the EU's recently enacted Artificial Intelligence Act will impact this space.

The advent of other new technologies will likely lead to a continued need for our research regulatory processes to adapt and evolve. Indeed, it is critical that the regulation of research is dynamic, evolving in line with developments in science and technology, and aims to balance the competing interests that arise in research. With this in mind, and the impact of the GDPR and likely impact of the EHDS on the regulation of research, we now consider the GDPR and the EHDS in the context of health research, prior to critiquing these regulatory initiatives in light of the foregoing observations below to assess the extent to which the current and proposed frameworks adequately balance the range of stakeholders interests and rights we have observed in this section.

The GDPR and EHDS: Key principles and processes

The GDPR sets out the six principles that must be met in the processing of personal data: lawfulness, fairness, and transparency; purpose limitation; data minimization; accuracy; and storage limitation. It sets out the rights of data subjects in the processing of personal data and other procedures that must be followed in the processing. Overall, the GDPR takes a risk-based approach to the processing of personal data with tools contained within it to mitigate against that risk.[33] The purpose of the GDPR was to provide a harmonized framework to the processing of personal data. Due to concerns about the impact some of these strict processing requirements would have on research, certain derogations and exemptions are provided for either by directing invoking the provisions of the GDPR, or through Member State law.[34]

These derogations for research are critical, particularly in data-driven research that is reliant on accessing and using vast quantities of data and data sharing. Despite this, we share the concerns expressed by many others about the potential impact that the derogations have had on research participants' rights and on research. These issues have been covered in depth elsewhere,[35] but the main concerns are worth summarizing here.

First, the provisions enabling Member States to provide for derogations to research has resulted in well-documented criticisms of the fragmented application of the GDPR for research. This has resulted in a multitude of differing approaches to the protection of personal data for research across the EU Member States, a situation that is making data sharing even more challenging.[36]

Second, the GDPR provides considerable rights for data subjects, which includes rights to being informed when their data are processed, having a right to object, or a right to restrict the processing of their personal data. These rights are essential for a participant to exercise their autonomous choices on how their data are used (and fulfil their Article 8 ECHR rights), particularly when consent is not the lawful basis for processing. Without these rights, a data subject will be left in the dark as to when and for what purpose their data are being used. The GDPR provides that a data controller can exempt themselves from upholding these rights if the processing is for research purposes.[37] Importantly, if the personal data are not being collected from the data subject directly, a data controller can be exempted from the right to information (Article 14(5)(b)). As a result, in such instances, a data subject will be unaware that their data have been collected and are being used for research, irrespective of whether the personal data were collected for research or some other purpose at the time of initial collection. Without knowing that their personal data are being processed, a data subject cannot exercise any of their rights under the GDPR. This right to information is thus essential to the exercise of their other rights.[38]

Third, although the GDPR is not a research regulatory framework, it is de facto treated as such. It has come to be a key framework and shaped how data are processed, used, and shared not only for research within the EU, but also for researchers outside the EU who work with the EU framework and EU-based data.

EHDS—Proposals on secondary use of data

Alongside these existing criticisms of the GDPR, significant changes have been proposed to the secondary use of electronic health data under Chapter IV of the EHDS, which also give rise to concerns. If the EHDS is passed in the form currently proposed, it will create a legal obligation to share electronic health data if certain conditions have been met. Slokenberga has comprehensively critiqued the proposed legal framework,[39] and Staunton and others have critiqued the proposed framework from a bioethical perspective,[40] but certain key points are worth mentioning here. Under the proposed new framework, any natural or legal person can apply for access to the electronic health data (called a "data user") from a data holder ("any natural or legal person, which is an entity or a body in the health or care sector or performing research in relation to these sectors"). Electronic health data is broadly defined and includes electronic health records, genetic data, and population-based health data. This electronic health data may be personal data (and thus fall under the GDPR) or anonymous data (and thus outside of the GDPR). Interestingly, considering that governance mechanisms that have been adopted by biobanks and databanks (such as DACs discussed above to decide on access) have been *communicated* to their participants, the proposal takes the decision on assessment and access to the electronic health data from the data controller (as would likely be the case under the GDPR) or data holder, and places it in a new independent body called a Health Data Access Body (HDAB), with a HDAB to be established in each Member State.

The draft EHDS sets out the criteria to be met in an access request to the HDAB: an application must detail the purpose of the data use; description of the requested data; a justification if pseudonymized data are requested; (undefined) safeguards to prevent unauthorized use and the rights and interests of the data holder and natural persons; an estimated time period the data are required; and details on a secure processing environment. If the application requires access to personal data, applicants must provide details on how the processing complies with the GDPR. Article 44 of the draft EHDS also makes it clear the importance of data minimization and purpose limitation in the HDAB's assessment. Finally, an applicant should also provide information on any applicable ethical aspects. These ethical aspects are undefined but most likely relate to national ethical requirements.

The draft EHDS requires the HDAB must make an assessment within two months of receiving an application, a time limit that can be extended by two months for complex applications. Once an application is approved by a HDAB, a data permit is issued specifying the terms and conditions of the data use. The data holder must make the data available to the data user within two months through a secure processing environment.

The draft EHDS aims to streamline access to electronic health data for many purposes by introducing one legal framework with the same rules and processes to be followed in accessing electronic health data. As discussed, under the GDPR the right to information (and the resulting impact on other rights) can be derogated from if the processing is for research purposes. Under the EHDS the derogation of this right to information has been extended to the other purposes for which electronic health data can be accessed for the secondary use of data. The extension of this derogation (and other issues) has been criticized by the European Data Protection Board (EDPB) and the European Data Protection Supervisor (EDPS). Their joint opinion on the EHDS states that the extension is unjustified, and this and many proposals under the draft EHDS do not conform with the GDPR.[41] More recently, the European Parliament in its report on the draft EHDS recommends the introduction of an opt-out for natural persons so that they can decide to opt out of the use of their electronic health data for any secondary purpose that they did not want their data processed.

Balancing rights and interests: A critique

Having briefly set up the legal framework for the GDPR and the proposed EHDS, we now turn to consider these frameworks, examining the extent to which they adequately balance the risks of data harms and individual privacy interests with collective and individual interests in data sharing for health research. For a range of reasons discussed above, data sharing is critical for data-driven research methods and for the provision of healthcare. Data sharing promotes transparency and reproducibility, optimizes the use of a valuable resources, and enables meta-analyses.[42] Moreover, it is well recognized that there are biases in datasets.[43] It is critical that data from unrepresented populations are shared to begin to correct bias in our current datasets, to enhance the generalizability of research findings across populations, and to begin to address health disparities. If we do not have regulatory frameworks in place that enable data sharing, downstream products may only be applicable to populations coming from research regulatory environments that provide for data sharing. It is not, however, enough for regulatory frameworks to enable data sharing; instead, such frameworks must embed ethical, legal, equitable, and socially and culturally appropriate data sharing. By this we mean data sharing that responds to ethical concerns, is appropriate to the specific cultural contexts, and that there is equitable access to the data, and to the use of the data, and reasonable and appropriate equitable access to downstream technologies arising from uses of data.

However, a key concern in this context is that as the GDPR and the EHDS were developed distinct from research regulatory frameworks, they do not necessarily engage with or appropriately balance the competing rights and interests between the individuals and collective rights and interests in the health research context. This is particularly problematic as the GDPR (and likely that the same will arise for the EHDS) has become a de facto research regulatory framework. In particular, we highlight three key concerns in relation to how the GDPR and proposed EHDS frameworks will impact the rights or interests of stakeholders in health research: (i) there is a focus on data protection and risk-based protections for individual data subjects against data harms, but limited consideration of other rights such as individual's right to autonomy over how their data are used, and individual interests and rights in data sharing to secure health benefits; (ii) there is limited focus on the rights or interests of the *collective*, such as groups within society, around how data may be used or risks of discrimination to such groups; (iii) there is also a limited engagement in relation to how industry or other data users may use or share data, and relatedly, limited focus on how resulting knowledge or findings generated may be accessible and shared with the public, due to the competing interests at stake in these contexts.

A risk-based legal framework primarily concerned with data protection: Need to consider data subjects' broader rights and interests

The GDPR, and indeed data protection regulations generally, take a risk-based approach to the protection of personal data that are framed around anticipating and seeking to minimize data harms for the individual data subject.[44] Individual data subjects, as distinct from groups or communities, are provided with legal protection. The EHDS continues with this approach in that the focus is on the protection of the individual, and the individuals' data protection rights. They do not consider data harms that can occur beyond data protection, nor do they account for the data harms to groups and communities. The GDPR and the EHDS also do not account for the context in which data are used. In other words, who is using the data, for what purpose, the application of AI to the data use, or the linking of data. Frameworks that seek to provide protection from data harms must consider potential data harms broadly, the potential for harm beyond the individual, and the fact that data harms are often context dependent.

This chapter is not seeking to diminish or detract from the important rights and processes introduced by the GDPR, but in the health research context, this individualistic risk-based framing is problematic, particularly considering the GDPR's (and other data protection regulations') influence on the regulation of health research. The focus within the GDPR is on the protection of personal data and not the other rights and interests at stake. Under the GDPR, the further processing of personal data can be permitted without informing the data subject, under the derogations provided by the GDPR, if personal data are not collected directly from the data subject and they are to be used for scientific research and subject to appropriate safeguards. This is justified due to the important value of research in society and that the use of personal data for research is subject to safeguards under Article 89 GDPR.[45] A data subject's right to autonomy is limited in this context, but it is considered justified, proportionate, and subject to safeguards.

Similarly, under the proposed EHDS, the focus is on ensuring that electronic health data are accessed in a manner that ensures that they meet data protection standards. The proposed opt-out of data uses is critical for providing natural persons with some control over the use of their electronic health data, particularly as electronic health data may be used for a purpose and by an entity beyond which they have provided their consent.[46] For example, would a patient in a public health system expect that their data be accessed and used by a commercial for-profit company to develop and train AI? Without an opt-out, the balance of interests in the proposed legislative framework is arguably too heavily weighted towards providing access to the data, without due consideration of the individual autonomy rights (including those under Article 8 ECHR) and interests around how their data will be used and by whom. An opt-out would go towards rebalancing these competing interests.

This is important as attitudes towards data sharing vary according to the context in which the data takes place: the purpose for which data are being used and who is using the data.[47] For example, there is evidence that members of the public can be wary of commercial involvement in health research.[48] We cannot simply ignore these differing perspectives and seek to address it by introducing a legal framework that creates an obligation to share data. Experience elsewhere has shown us that legal legitimacy alone is never enough.[49] Legal legitimacy does not equate to trusted governance. Thus, in addition to legal frameworks, there must be mechanisms, such as accountable and transparent procedures on data use, public and community engagement, and other initiatives that can promote the integrity of the data lifecycle and strengthen the social licence for the use of the data.

Yet in making this point, we acknowledge that if all individuals who provide health data for research purposes are given a right to autonomy over how data are used, depending on scope of such rights, and how they choose to exercise these, this could hinder health research. For example, if following the collection of personal data from a person which is subsequently included within and processed as part of a larger dataset, and that individual at a later stage requests removal of all data: (a) depending on the context removal of data may be impracticable; and/or (b) may impact the usability of the other data in the dataset (which may affect other data subjects' autonomy and other interests over how their data are used). Hence, a balanced approach must be adopted, with proportionate restrictions which may need to provide for derogations on the right to autonomy, for the benefit of collective interests. A narrow individualistic view could be to the detriment of the collective interests, as if too many individuals refuse to share their data, this could introduce bias into the dataset, or the data may lose its value. On the other hand, if we require the sharing of the data due to the public value or collective interests in sharing the data, without respecting the autonomous decision of an individual, this could damage trust in the governance. A nuanced consideration of such issues is needed to adopt an appropriate balance of the rights and interests at stake here.

Need to consider collective risks of discrimination of certain groups which may arise due to secondary use and data sharing

Beyond the right to autonomy, data use also brings the risk of discrimination and stigmatization of certain groups. Such risks can pertain to the individual but are also a risk for the collective community from which the data comes. However, under the GDPR and proposed EHDS, there is no focus on the collective interests at stake. Data access oversight mechanisms, such as DACs, do often take these collective rights and interests into account as they can consider the importance of the research to the community, and the risk to discrimination and stigmatization. But what future do they have under the proposed EHDS? It is the HDAB that sets out the rules for data access, determines access, processes applications, issues data permits, and makes the data available to a data user in a secure processing environment. The HDAB will make available the results or outcomes of projects that arise from the secondary use of electronic health data under the EHDS (Article 38(1)). Should the HDAB be made aware by a data user of a finding that may impact the health of an individual, they *may* (but are not obliged to) inform the natural person. The HDAB are also required to publish an annual report under Article 39, and this will include the "number of digital health products and services, including AI applications, developed using data accessed via EHDS". Thus, many of the responsibilities of a DAC now fall under the HDAB. More importantly, there seems no scope for a DAC to be involved in decisions on access. If a HDAB will soon have this power, it is critical that interests other than the individual data subject's data protection rights are considered and at a minimum, we need to consider the risk of discrimination and stigmatization. Staunton and others have previously called for an integrated bioethics approach to data protection.[50] Considering the potential power of the HDAB on data access, it is a call that we would reiterate and apply to the EHDS as well.

Limited oversight around how other legal protections may impact sharing of data: The competing interests at stake?

Moreover, as noted, one of the rationales around the proposed EHDS is to enable increased ease of data sharing to maximize health research benefits that may arise from this. For instance, the EHDS imposes obligations around secondary use and access to data; however, it is not clear how this will interact with other legal protections in place, including with various IPRs which may be applicable over relevant datasets or compilations developed from individuals' data. For instance, in some cases, the value of data will be the knowledge or insights gained by the collation of datasets gathered together. Moreover, while there is no IP in data per se,[51] compilations or collections of data, knowledge generated using data from multiple participants, or certain aspects of findings resulting from the processing of people's data may be protected by IPRs. It is plausible that IPRs could be in tension with current discussions around mandating obligations for entities to share data under secondary uses of data provisions within the proposed EHDS. Accordingly, it is questionable how the EHDS's right to information will apply to this area, or whether entities will be able to exert their IPRs to refuse to share this data and in what contexts. The role of IPRs in this and related contexts may also have a very real impact on individuals' autonomy interests over how data they provide, or which relate to them are used and for what purposes, and over downstream access they (and others) may have over knowledge and other benefits that may arise from health research.

For example, a sui generis database right exists in Europe which offers certain protections to collections of data collated from multiple sources in a database (such as potentially in the genetic database context); the exercise of this right may potentially conflict with requests to share certain data to third parties.[52] Other IP rights may also apply; for example, trade secrets may be applicable over insights or knowledge gleaned via use of data which are kept confidential by the entity processing the data. It is not clear how potential tensions between entities holding IPRs over such knowledge or related aspects to such data, and the discussions around secondary uses of data, will be resolved under the EHDS. There is already criticism from industry around proposals for the general right to information for third parties and how this may impact their IPRs and other commercial interests related to data.[53]

Indeed, Article 33(4) of the EHDS anticipates such tensions and currently states that

> **Electronic health data** entailing protected intellectual property and trade secrets from private enterprises shall be made available for secondary use. Where such data is made available for secondary use, all measures necessary **to preserve the confidentiality of IP rights** and trade secrets shall be taken.
>
> *(emphasis added)*

The first line of this article appears to suggest that even where IPRs apply, companies will have an obligation to disclose such health data for secondary uses. However, it is not clear how this provision would operate in practice. Moreover, if the intention is that IPRs could not impede sharing of data, there is potential that the last sentence could undermine this aim as it suggests confidentiality will be preserved. In practice, depending on how a provision like this were to be adopted or interpreted, it could water down the potential benefit of the provision in terms of open sharing of information for secondary uses in the health research context. For example, it could lead to data being shared but only when redacted in some contexts, and this could limit the usefulness of secondary use provisions.

Moreover, a related but separate issue in terms of IPRs and use of data for health research is that IPRs, including patents, will often arise over health technologies such as new medicines which may be contributed to by data provided for health research purposes. Such IPRs over medicines (and other health technologies) give rightsholders the ability to exclude third parties from use of the technology under patent (e.g. medicines) for the duration of the patent term, which is generally 20 years. Patents allow rightsholders to decide how patented technologies can be used and by whom during this term, and this in turn can impact how the publics can access and use such technologies,[54] with implications for the rights to life and health in some cases.

Moreover, the role of IPRs over technologies contributed to by health research can create tensions. For example, as one of us has discussed elsewhere, even where individuals provide data and biospecimens for use for health research purposes in an altruistic manner to publicly funded biobanks, where their motivation in providing such samples or data may be to contribution to public health, there are no binding European legal obligations mandating that downstream technologies that may be developed are publicly accessible, or that such individuals be informed of the potential impacts IPRs could have on access to technologies that may be developed downstream. This can give rise to a range of bioethical implications.[55] Within such data governance frameworks, there is often a lack of engagement with how benefits generated via research using participants' data (or contributed to by such data) will be accessed by such participants and the broader publics. The result can be that although current data protection frameworks seek to ensure that individuals are protected from data harms that may arise at an individual level, there is limited consideration of the interests and rights individuals have in being able to share in the technological benefits generated by the knowledge gleaned from use of their (and other publics') data. This warrants deeper consideration in terms of how we can best balance private and public interests in such contexts. Such issues also impact broader collective interests, including various publics' right to access the benefits from scientific knowledge, with knock-on effects on population health needs, and for public health systems more generally. Moreover, while a balance must be delivered which engages with various publics interests, needs, or rights and commercial incentives to participate in and conduct health research in such contexts, the lack of engagement with such issues in the health research context, including in the current EHDS discussions around data use and sharing and secondary use of data, should be revisited.

Concluding thoughts: A pathway towards a European Health Data Framework to balance the competing interests at stake?

A new data sharing framework approach is needed for health research in the digital data-driven age. It is essential for the promotion of science, but also to meet individual and public health needs. A new regulatory framework, however, must strive to balance the competing rights and interests of the range of different stakeholders within the health innovation and research landscape. This is a complex task given the range of stakeholders and publics implicated in such contexts, and requires a nuanced approach. The draft EHDS is attempting to push the data sharing agenda forward. However, the current proposal is doing so with a focus primarily on data protection and re-identification as the key concerns. Similar to the GDPR, it is primarily a risk-based approach which focuses on privacy and data protection concerns—one that does not sufficiently account for the need to ensure we also engage with other interests at stake, including the right to autonomy of data subjects in how data may be used for secondary purposes, within what contexts, and by whom. This also connects with the collective interests in ensuring and maintaining trust within the data governance context. Moreover, the current GDPR and proposed EHDS frameworks also do not sufficiently engage with the equity of benefit in downstream access to therapies and knowledge generated or contributed to by health research and participants' data.

A more holistic approach is needed—one that is underpinned by transparency and by respect for individuals and a broader range of communities and publics involved—which seeks to maximize the benefits from health research that may arise, without disproportionately affecting or harming individuals and the collective interests at stake.

Notes

1 For an overview of some of the potential benefits that data has in the health context, see Charles Auffray and others, "Making Sense of Big Data in Health Research: Towards an EU Action Plan" (2016) 71 *Genomic Medicine* 1, 3; Javier Andreu-Perez and others, "Big Data for Health" (2015) 19 *IEEE Journal of Biomedical and Health Informatics* 1193, section II; Aisling McMahon, Alena Buyx, and Barbara Prainsack, "Big Data Governance Needs More Collective Responsibility: The Role of Harm Mitigation in the Governance of Data Use in Medicine and Beyond" (2020) 28 *Medical Law Review* 155, 158–159; Roberta Pastorino and others, "Benefits and Challenges of Big Data in Healthcare: An Overview of the European Initiatives" (2019) 29 *European Journal of Public Health* 23; Israel Júnior Borges do Nascimento, "Impact of Big Data Analytics on People's Health: Overview of Systematic Reviews and Recommendations for Future Studies" (2021) 23 *Journal of Medical Internet Research* e27275; Xiaoming Wang and others, "Big Data Management Challenges in Health Research—A Literature Review" (2019) 20 *Briefings in Bioinformatics* 156; Mark Walport and Paul Brest, "Sharing Research Data to Improve Public Health" (2011) 377 *The Lancet* 537.
2 Evelyn Anane-Sarpong and others, "Application of Ethical Principles to Research Using Public Health Data in The Global South: Perspectives from Africa" (2018) 18 *Developing World Bioethics* 98; Angela Ballantyne and G Owen Schaefer, "Consent and the Ethical Duty to Participate in Health Data Research" (2018) 44 *Journal of Medical Ethics* 392; Mark Sheehan, "Can Broad Consent Be Informed Consent?" (2011) 4 *Public Health Ethics* 226; Phaik Yeong Cheah and Jan Piasecki, "Data Access Committees" (2020) 21 *BMC Medical Ethics* 12; Sara Gerke, Timo Minssen and Glenn Cohen, "Ethical and Legal Challenges of Artificial Intelligence-Driven Healthcare" (2020) *Artificial Intelligence in Healthcare* 295; Signe Mezinska and others, "Ethical Issues in Genomics Research on Neurodevelopmental Disorders: A Critical Interpretive Review" (2021) 15 *Human Genomics* 16; Ciara Staunton and others, "Ethical and Social Reflections on the Proposed European Health Data Space" (2024) 32 *European Journal of Human Genetics* 498; Francesca Forzano, Maurizio Genuardi, and Yves Moreau, "ESHG Warns against Misuses of Genetic Tests and Biobanks for Discrimination Purposes" (2021) 29 *European Journal of Human Genetics* 894.
3 Laura J Damschroder and others, "Patients, Privacy and Trust: Patients' Willingness to Allow Researchers to Access Their Medical Records" (2007) 64 *Social Science & Medicine* 223.

4 Forzano and others, n 3; Yann Joly and others, "The Genetic Discrimination Observatory: Confronting Novel Issues in Genetic Discrimination" (2021) 37 *Trends in Genetics* 951. For a discussion of potential harms that may arise via uses of data within algorithmic systems, see Joanna Reddan and Jessica Brand, "Data Harm Record" available at: https://datajusticelab.org/data-harm-record/; McMahon and others, n 2, 158–160.

5 Cheah and Piasecki, n 3.

6 Sylvie Delacroix and Neil D Lawrence, "Bottom-up Data Trusts: Disturbing the 'One Size Fits All' Approach to Data Governance" (2019) 9 *International Data Privacy Law* 236.

7 Santa Slokenberga, "Scientific Research Regime 2.0? Transformations of the Research Regime and the Protection of the Data Subject That the Proposed EHDS Regulation Promises to Bring Along" (2022) 2022 *Technology and Regulation* 135; Staunton and others, n 3.

8 Ciara Staunton, "Individual Rights in Biobank Research Under the GDPR", in Santa Slokenberga, Olga Tzortzatou, and Jane Reichel (eds), *GDPR and Biobanking: Individual Rights, Public Interest and Research Regulation across Europe* (Springer 2021), 91–104.

9 Ibid.

10 Santa Slokenberga, Olga Tzortzatou, and Jane Reichel (eds), *GDPR and Biobanking: Individual Rights, Public Interest and Research Regulation across Europe* (Springer 2021); Luca Marelli, Elisa Lievevrouw, and Ine Van Hoyweghen, "Fit for Purpose? The GDPR and the Governance of European Digital Health" (2020) 41 *Policy Studies* 447; Kärt Pormeister, "Genetic Data and the Research Exemption: Is the GDPR Going Too Far?" (2017) 7 *International Data Privacy Law* 137; David Peloquin and others, "Disruptive and Avoidable: GDPR Challenges to Secondary Research Uses of Data" (2020) 28 *European Journal of Human Genetics* 697; Ciara Staunton, Santa Slokenberga, and Deborah Mascalzoni, "The GDPR and the Research Exemption: Considerations on the Necessary Safeguards for Research Biobanks" (2019) 27 *European Journal of Human Genetics* 1159.

11 Slokenberga and others, n 11.

12 Peloquin and others, n 11; Marelli and others, n 11.

13 Segun Fatumo and others, "A Roadmap to Increase Diversity in Genomic Studies" (2022) 28 *Nature Medicine* 243.

14 Communication from the Commission to the European Parliament, the Council, the European Economic and Social Committee and the Committee of the Regions—A European strategy for data' (COM(2020) 66 final), available at: https://eur-lex.europa.eu/legal-content/EN/TXT/?uri=CELEX%3A5202 0DC0066.

15 Regulation (EU) 2022/868 of the European Parliament and of the Council of 30 May 2022 on European data governance and amending Regulation (EU) 2018/1724 (Data Governance Act) (Text with EEA relevance), available at: https://eur-lex.europa.eu/legal-content/EN/TXT/?uri=CELEX%3A32022R0868.

16 European Parliament, "Boosting data sharing in the EU: what are the benefits?" (6 April 2022), available at: https://www.europarl.europa.eu/topics/en/article/20220331STO26411/boosting-data-sharing-in-the-eu-what-are-the-benefits.

17 The explanatory memorandum to the EHDS states:

> The EHDS will create a legal and technical environment that will support the development of innovative medicinal products and vaccines, and of medical devices and in vitro diagnostics. This will help to prevent, detect, and rapidly respond to health emergencies. In addition, the EHDS will help

> to improve understanding, prevention, early detection, diagnosis, treatment and monitoring of cancer, through the EU cross-border secure access and sharing between healthcare providers of health, including cancer related data of natural persons. Therefore, by providing secure access to a wide range of electronic health data, the EHDS will open new opportunities for diseases prevention and treatment of natural persons.

18 February 2024.

19 By "health technologies", we are referring to a wide range of technologies, including medicines, diagnostics, medical devices, and vaccines.

20 David Carr and Katherine Littler, "Sharing Research Data to Improve Public Health: A Funder Perspective" (2015) 10 *Journal of Empirical Research on Human Research Ethics* 314; Winner Dominic Chawinga and Sandy Zinn, "Global Perspectives of Research Data Sharing: A Systematic Literature Review" (2019) 41 *Library & Information Science Research* 109; Anna Middleton and others, "Global Public Perceptions of Genomic Data Sharing: What Shapes the Willingness to Donate DNA and Health Data?" (2020) 107 *The American Journal of Human Genetics* 743; Roberta Biasiotto and others, "Public Preferences for Digital Health Data Sharing: Discrete Choice Experiment Study in 12 European Countries" (2023) 25 *Journal of Medical Internet Research* e47066.

21 See discussion of the contested nature of the "public interest" as a concept in Annie Sorbie, "The Public Interest", in Graeme Laurie and others (eds), *The Cambridge Handbook of Health Research Regulation* (Cambridge University Press 2021), 65–72. See also John Bell, "Public Interest: Policy or Principle?" in Roger Brownsword (ed), *Law and the Public Interest: Proceedings of the 1992 ALSP Conference* (Stuttgart: Franz Steiner Verlag 1993), 27–36; Annie Sorbie, "Sharing Confidential Health Data for Research Purposes in the UK: Where Are 'Publics' in the Public Interest?" (2020) 16 *Evidence & Policy* 249.

22 For example, in the COVID-19 context, in early stages of the pandemic there were limited global supplies of COVID-19 vaccines available—and given the way the applicable intellectual property and technology transfer issues played out in practice—national States and regions competed with each other for first access to such vaccines. See discussion in Aisling McMahon, "*Global equitable access to vaccines, medicines and diagnostics for COVID-19: The role of patents as private governance*" (2021) 47 *Journal of Medical Ethics* 142.

23 Ulrike Felt and Maximilian Fochler, "Machineries for Making Publics: Inscribing and De-Scribing Publics in Public Engagement" (2010) 48 *Minerva* 219; Sara Chandros Hull and David R Wilson (Diné), "Beyond Belmont: Ensuring Respect for AI/AN Communities Through Tribal IRBs, Laws, and Policies" (2017) 17 *The American Journal of Bioethics* 60.

24 Sonja Erikainen and others, "Public Involvement in the Governance of Population-Level Biomedical Research: Unresolved Questions and Future Directions" (2021) 47 *Journal of Medical Ethics* 522.

25 The public interest as set out in data protection law does not take such a granular approach to considering the differing publics and their differing interests. In considering the public under the GDPR and its interests, the public is seen as a monolithic entity, thus not reflecting the reality that what is in the interest of one public is not necessarily in the others.

26 Acknowledging that there are differing publics with competing interests should cause us to re-consider the legal concept of public interest, but this is beyond the scope of this chapter.

27 Article 8(1) of the European Convention on Human Rights stipulates that "Everyone has the right to respect for his private and family life, his home and his correspondence".

28 Biasiotto and others (n 21).
29 In the context sharing of benefits in the biobank context based on donors contribution of biomaterials/data, see discussion in Aisling McMahon, "Patents, Human Biobanks and Access to Health Benefits: Bridging The Public–Private Divide", in Jessica Lai and Antoinette Maget Dominicé (eds) *Intellectual Property and Access to Im/material Goods* (Edward Elgar 2016), 176–203; Aisling McMahon and Opeyemi Kolawole, "Biobank Donation in Search of Public Benefits and the Potential Impact of Intellectual Property Rights Over Access to Health-Technologies Developed: A Focus on the Bioethical Implications" (2024) 32 *Medical Law Review* 205.
30 Ibid.
31 On the role of "harm mitigation" bodies, see McMahon and others, n 2; Barbara Prainsack and Alena Buyx, "A Solidarity-Based Approach to the Governance of Research Biobanks" (2013) 21 *Medical Law Review* 71; Barbara Prainsack and Alena Buyx, *Solidarity in Biomedicine and Beyond* (Cambridge University Press 2017).
32 Victoria Nembaware and others, "A Framework for Tiered Informed Consent for Health Genomic Research in Africa" (2019) 51 *Nature Genetics* 1566; Nicki Tiffin, "Tiered Informed Consent: Respecting Autonomy, Agency and Individuality in Africa" (2018) 3 *BMJ Global Health* e001249; Sheehan, n 3; Isabelle Budin-Ljøsne and others, "Dynamic Consent: A Potential Solution to Some of the Challenges of Modern Biomedical Research" (2017) 18 *BMC Medical Ethics* 4; Roberta Biasiotto, Peter Pramstaller, and Deborah Mascalzoni, "The Dynamic Consent of the Cooperative Health Research in South Tyrol (CHRIS) Study: Broad Aim within Specific Oversight and Communication" (2021) 21 *BioLaw Journal—Rivista di BioDiritto* 277; Deborah Mascalzoni and others, "Ten Years of Dynamic Consent in the CHRIS Study: Informed Consent as a Dynamic Process" (2022) 30 *European Journal of Human Genetics* 1391; Jane Kaye and others, "Dynamic Consent: A Patient Interface for Twenty-First Century Research Networks" (2015) 23 *European Journal of Human Genetics* 141.
33 Raphaël Gellert, "Understanding the Notion of Risk in the General Data Protection Regulation" (2018) 34 *Computer Law & Security Review* 279.
34 Staunton and others, n 11.
35 Staunton, n 9; Ciara Staunton and others, "Appropriate Safeguards and Article 89 of the GDPR: Considerations for Biobank, Databank and Genetic Research" (2022) 13 *Frontiers in Genetics* 719317 (doi: 10.3389/fgene.2022.719317); Marelli and others, n 11; Peloquin and others, n 11; Pormeister, n 11; Anne-Marie Duguet and Jean Herveg, "Safeguards and Derogations Relating to Processing for Scientific Purposes: Article 89 Analysis for Biobank Research", in Santa Slokenberga, Olga Tzortzatou, and Jane Reichel (eds), *GDPR and Biobanking: Individual Rights, Public Interest and Research Regulation across Europe* (Springer 2021), 105–120; Dara Hallinan, "Broad Consent under the GDPR: An Optimistic Perspective on a Bright Future" (2020) 16 *Life Sciences, Society and Policy* 1.
36 Slokenberga and others, n 11; Peloquin and others, n 11; Marelli, n 11; Pormeister, n 11.
37 Staunton, n 9.
38 Ibid.
39 Slokenberga, n 8.
40 Staunton and others, n 3.
41 EDPB-EDPS, *EDPB-EDPS Joint Opinion 03/2022 on the Proposal for a Regulation on the European Health Data Space* (adopted 12 July 2022), available at: https://edpb.europa.eu/system/files/2022-07/edpb_edps_jointopinion_202203_europeanhealthdataspace_en.pdf.
42 Walport and Brest, n 2.
43 Fatumo and others, n 14.

44 On the limitations of risk-based frameworks to data within the digital and big data contexts, see McMahon and others, n 2, 160–161.

45 Staunton and others, n 11.

46 Staunton and others, n 3.

47 Biasiotto and others, n 20.

48 Christine Critchley, Dianne Nicol, and Margaret Otlowski, "The Impact of Commercialisation and Genetic Data Sharing Arrangements on Public Trust and the Intention to Participate in Biobank Research" (2015) 18 *Public Health Genomics* 160; Dianne Nicol and others, "Understanding Public Reactions to Commercialization of Biobanks and Use of Biobank Resources" (2016) 162 *Social Science & Medicine* 79; Gill Haddow and others, "Tackling Community Concerns About Commercialization and Genetic Research: A Modest Interdisciplinary Proposal" (2007) 64 *Social Science & Medicine* 272, 277.

49 Pam Carter, Graeme Laurie and Mary Dixon-Woods, "The Social Licence for Research: Why Care.Data Ran into Trouble" (2015) 41 *Journal of Medical Ethics* 404. See also discussion in Graeme Laurie and others, "A Review of Evidence Relating to Harm Resulting from Uses of Health and Biomedical Data" (Report for Nuffield Council on Bioethics Working Party on Biological and Health Data and the Wellcome Trust's Expert Advisory Group on Data Access) (June 2014), 161, available at: https://www.nuffieldbioethics.org/wp-content/uploads/FINAL-Report-on-Harms-Arising-from-Use-of-Health-and-Biomedical-Data-30-JUNE-2014.pdf.

50 Staunton and others, n 32.

51 See also discussion in: Guido Noto La Diega, "Ending Smart Data Enclosures: The European Approach to the Regulation of the Internet of Things between Access and Intellectual Property", in Stacy-Ann Elvy and Nancy Kim (eds), *The Cambridge Handbook on Emerging Issues at the Intersection of Commercial Law and Technology* (Cambridge University Press, forthcoming).

52 The tensions between IPRs and data sharing in the digital age are discussed in detail in Timo Minssen and Justin Pierce, "Big Data and Intellectual Property Rights in the Health and Life Sciences", in I Glenn Cohen and others (eds), *Big Data, Health Law, and Bioethics* (Cambridge University Press 2018) 311–323. See also Noto La Diega, n 51. On the database right more generally, see Jasper A Bovenberg, "Should companies set up databases in Europe?" (2000) 18 *Nature Biotechnology* 907.

53 For a discussion of some of the industry objections, including a framing of IP as a human right, see MedTech Europe, "MedTech Europe's position on the proposed European Health Data Space Regulation" (22 February 2023), available at: https://www.medtecheurope.org/wp-content/uploads/2023/02/230222-ehds-position-paper-final.pdf; European Federation of Pharmaceutical Industries and Associations, "European Health Data Space: Key Aspects to be Considered in the Trilogue Discussions" (31 January 2024), available at: https://www.efpia.eu/news-events/the-efpia-view/statements-press-releases/european-health-data-space-key-aspects-to-be-considered-in-the-trilogue-discussions/; DigitalEurope, "Position Paper on the European Health Data Space proposal" (January 2023), available at: https://cdn.digitaleurope.org/uploads/2023/01/DIGITALEUROPEs-Position-Paper-on-the-European-Health-Data-Space-proposal-1.pdf.

54 The nature and role of IPRs in the health context, focusing on the COVID-19 context, are discussed in Aisling McMahon, "Global Equitable Access to Vaccines, Medicines and Diagnostics for COVID-19: The Role of Patents as Private Governance" (2021) 47 *Journal of Medical Ethics* 142.

55 For a discussion of IPRs in biobank context and tension that can arise, see McMahon, n 30. For a discussion of the broader bioethical issues posed in such contexts, see McMahon and Kolawole, n 30.

5

SECONDARY USES OF PATIENTS' DATA IN THE EUROPEAN HEALTH DATA SPACE

A UK-German comparison

Miranda Mourby and Fruzsina Molnar-Gabor

Introduction

What "secondary uses"[1] of health data should patients reasonably expect? Particularly when our healthcare increasingly depends on the re-use of our records for research and innovation?[2] The European Union (EU) is proposing, via Regulation, a statutory "European Health Data Space"[3] (hereafter, the EHDS Proposal) to develop new infrastructure for secondary uses of patient information across national boundaries. The definition of "electronic health data" in the EHDS Proposal is very broad; consequently, we will also refer to "health data" throughout this chapter as information which identifies patients, could identify patients, or is otherwise derived from their healthcare records. These types of information can only be made available throughout the EU on the basis of interoperable standards, and some common understanding of the value of secondary uses of health data. These secondary uses (for purposes beyond the patient's care) have proved one of the more difficult issues within the negotiation of the Regulation,[4] with the current Proposal condemned by some interest groups as a violation of patients' reasonable expectations of privacy.[5]

Common agreement on the appropriate scope of patients' rights appears elusive. In its mandate for negotiations with the European Parliament, the Council of the EU suggests leaving the question of patient autonomy up to individual EU Member States:

> Member States may introduce a specific right to object from the processing of personal electronic health data for secondary use which complements the right to object set out by article 21 of Regulation (EU) 2016/679 [i.e. the General Data Protection Regulation, or "GDPR"]. It is appropriate to leave Member States free to decide to introduce and

DOI: 10.4324/9781003394518-8

modulate such a right as it involves a balance between individual autonomy and the availability of health data for secondary use purposes,
which is best made at national level, taking into account Member States'
specific situations and historical experiences. Should a Member State
choose to provide for such a right, it should also define how and where
to exercise it and facilitate its exercise.[6]

As such, whether patients should have a right to opt out of the EHDS may
well be left as a question of national policy. This is particularly problematic,
considering that (as we will show) there are no guarantees that the right to
object under Article 21 GDPR[7] will apply in the context of further processing
of health data for scientific research. There appears to be a risk that the
EHDS will not cure the issue of regulatory fragmentation across the EU that
currently affects health research under the GDPR, and data subjects will have
different rights, depending on which Member State they live in (or where
their health insurance provider is based).

Given the apparent difficulty in achieving pan-EU consensus in this area, this
chapter compares two European countries with different regulatory approaches
to (and legal traditions of) secondary uses of health data: Germany and the
United Kingdom (UK). The UK can be seen as less insistent on individual autonomy, as (for example) its regulators do not recommend consent as a legal basis
when processing health data for research.[8] It will be a "third country" for the
purpose of the EHDS, but it may still be able to exchange health data due to its
adequacy status under data protection law.[9] Indeed, it appears that the national
health services in England, Wales, and Northern Ireland (NHS) are keen to participate in the EHDS. NHS Confederation (which represents healthcare providers in these nations) has contributed to the relevant scoping work with an
account of UK-style "opt-out" models to legitimate secondary uses of health
data. Under the NHS "opt-outs"[10] for England, for example, health data are
routinely collected for secondary purposes unless individuals actively object
(albeit in a pseudonymised form, and subject to safeguards).[11]

In Germany, the Data Protection Conference has accepted "broad consent" for the processing of health data for scientific research purposes. This
was done in recognition of the privileged status of research guaranteed by
Article 13 of the Charter of the Fundamental Rights of the EU and Article 5(3)
of the Basic Law, as well as in the GDPR, in particular Article (5)(1)(b).[12]
Albeit, the consent in question is one that broadly encompasses research,
rather than permitting specific tailoring to individual preferences.[13] Federal
data protection law takes a cautious approach to the non-consented use of
personal data for scientific research; it permits this only when the controller's
interest in processing "substantially outweighs" the data subject's interest in
not processing the data.[14] It remains to be seen how these different regulatory
approaches to the secondary use of health data will affect the introduction of

the EHDS infrastructure. It is likely, however, that the EHDS Regulation itself will provide the "basis in Union law" for processing personal data under Article 6(1)(e) of the GDPR, as an alternative to affirmative consent under Article 6(1)(a).[15] It can also provide the necessary basis in EU law for Article 9(2)(j) GDPR—an additional condition which should be satisfied when health-related personal data are processed for research. By providing an EU law basis for these justifications within the GDPR, which are alternatives to consent, the EHDS Proposal can integrate into German data protection law. National implementation has also been implemented by the federal Health Data Use Act, which introduces an opt-out procedure for processing of data from the electronic health record for secondary purposes.[16] At most the EHDS Proposal only seems likely to allow Member States the possibility to introduce an option to opt out (as in England's NHS): no draft published to date has required active, opt-in consent for secondary uses of health data.[17]

Despite the difference in UK and German legal cultures—and their respective implementations of the GDPR—we suggest that a right to object to secondary uses within the EHDS would be compatible with both German *and* UK law. Whether a right to object to secondary purposes in the EHDS could be implemented in other EU jurisdictions, to create a more consistent framework of rights across the EHDS, merits further investigation. We would support further research on this point, to encourage Member States to implement opt-outs in a consistent way across the EU. This approach to the EHDS—based on the availability of patient opt-outs, rather than consent, will need to be integrated not just with EU and Member State data protection laws, but also with the European Convention on Human Rights (ECHR). Ultimately, we argue that an EHDS based on opt-outs (as opposed to opt-in consent) *can* be compatible with the net effect of these privacy and data protection rights. However, it is important that these opt-outs are as consistent as possible in their scope and availability across the EU (and authorized participant States). At the time of writing, Member States have discretion as to whether they should introduce opt-outs. Our comparison of Germany and the UK supports the hypothesis that opt-outs from secondary use of health data can be consistently implemented across the EHDS. We would therefore encourage further work on the development of a "best practice" opt-out model for the EHDS.

Policy background

As a (non-EU) outsider to the forthcoming EHDS, the UK has a track record of ambitious schemes for secondary uses of patient data from its NHS—i.e. for research and for other purposes beyond providing care to the data subject.[18] In England, the main central repository of health data for secondary uses is NHS Digital, which has since merged with NHS England.[19] NHS

England has since entered into a number of contracts with the US public company Palantir Technologies Ltd, to set up a "Federated Data Platform" for the integration and secondary use of patient data. Media suspicion has been entrenched by litigation brought by openDemocracy to make the terms of these contracts public.[20]

Commentators within the UK can imply that NHS patient data are a "unique resource",[21] unavailable in multi-payer systems with dispersed healthcare data. However, controversy regarding control and benefit within secondary uses of health data is not uniquely British—and neither is the claim to a valuable informatics resource. Of the roughly 62 million patients registered with a GP practice in England,[22] some 3.37 million people have exercised the national data opt-out to prevent NHS England for sharing their health information for secondary uses,[23] putting the remaining pool at around 59 million data subjects (although this could change as adult patients opt in/out). But Germany—although a multi-payer system—supports approximately 90% of its population (i.e. roughly 75 million people) through statutory, state-funded health insurance.[24] The 2019 Digitale-Versorgung-Gesetz (DVG 2019 or Digital Healthcare Act) has legislated for greater integration of these data for secondary uses, creating an estimated pool of 73 million recipients of statutory health insurance who may have their data pooled into a federal Research Data Centre.[25] In December 2023, a draft Health Data Use Act was published, which will make pseudonymised electronic patient data available for research on an opt-out basis.[26]

As with the UK's Federated Data Platform, the German Research Data Centre has met with objection. Although the DVG did indeed become law, its centralization of 73 million patients' records has been challenged in the domestic courts, with proceedings stayed in 2023 while it is established how the Research Data Centre will operate within the framework of emerging European and national legislation.[27]

Given the controversies which have arisen at the national level, it is perhaps unsurprising that the EHDS has not been met with universal approval.[28] But the EHDS will constitute an even bigger step for secondary uses of health data. At the EU level, Commissioners have discussed the EHDS as an opportunity to bring together the health data of 450 million patients, which could make the EU a global leader in science, medicine, and analytics driven by Big Health Data.[29] Echoing the UK's experience of building infrastructure for secondary data uses, early investigation of citizens' expectations of the EHDS suggests greater ambivalence on the part of the patient population towards the involvement of the private sector, particularly when compared to other stakeholders.[30] The EHDS Proposal has (thus far) defined the scope of secondary uses for which health data may be made available, but has kept the definition of a health data "user" broad, e.g. per the Council's draft:

"health data user" means a natural or legal person who has lawful access to personal non-personal electronic health data for secondary use based on a data permit or a data request pursuant to this Regulation.[31]

As such, there appears to be no bar in the private sector accessing health data for a broad range of secondary purposes under the EHDS, albeit there is a proposed requirement to publish the results of their processing within 18 months,[32] so that any insights beneficial for the provision of healthcare can be shared more widely.

Where EHDS data are made available voluntarily under the data altruism provisions of the EU's Data Governance Act,[33] patients may be offered a range of options to exercise a degree of control over their medical information: from UK style opt-outs[34] to the broad consent model accepted by the German data protection supervisory authorities' conference,[35] or the opt-out model due to be introduced under the German Health Data Use Act.[36] Where health data are collected through the mandatory provisions of the EHDS Regulation under Article 33 of the EHDS Proposal, however, patients will not have an equal opportunity to withdraw or withhold their information, unless their Member State passes legislation to enable them to do so. Under the Article 35F of the EHDS Proposal, the right to opt out (above and beyond the GDPR right to object, with its public interest exemptions) is left to individual Member States to grant or withhold from patients. As such, it becomes all the more important that patients' expectations are understood and respected within the EHDS. This is considered further in the next section.

Secondary uses in the EHDS

The European Commission adopted its "European strategy for data" in February 2020.[37] This document acknowledged the ongoing challenge of sharing data across Member State boundaries under the GDPR, in part because of differing national interpretations of its requirements, and also derogations under Articles 6(4) and 9(4) which allowed countries to introduce their own bases for processing health data.[38] These discrepancies were explored more fully by the Commission the following year, when it released an assessment of Member States' rules on health data in light of the GDPR.[39] Having conducted workshops and surveys of stakeholders, the Commission concluded:

> variation in interpretation of the law and national level legislation linked to its implementation have led to a fragmented approach which makes cross-border cooperation for care provision, healthcare system administration or research difficult.[40]

The EHDS is an explicit response to these lingering points of disjuncture in national data protection laws, by providing a common framework across Member States for the integration of health data. The original Proposal was published in May 2022, and its text was debated and amended for the best part of 18 months. In December 2023, the Commission and European Parliament agreed their political positions on the proposed Regulation, meaning that three-way "trilogue" negotiations with the Council of the EU will take place over 2024 (or beyond) to finalize the text of the Regulation.[41]

A key sticking point in the negotiations has been the degree of control data subjects should have over the secondary use of their health data in the EHDS—above and beyond the rights they have in health data which can be linked to them—i.e. which constitutes "personal data" under the GDPR.

A key respect in which individuals will clearly *not* enjoy strengthened control their electronic health data is within the mandatory cross-border data infrastructure for secondary uses of health data. Article 33 of the EHDS Proposal sets out an extensive list of types of health data which must be made available across the data "space" for such secondary purposes. The drafters evidently envisaged that this mandatory sharing of data could conflict with the laws of Member States which have interpreted the GDPR as requiring consent for the further use of health data. Article 33(5) therefore states:

> Where the consent of the natural person is required by national law, health data access bodies shall rely on the obligations laid down in this Chapter to provide access to electronic health data.

This provision is telling. Whether the data subject's consent is needed for research, as opposed to a specific national legislative basis for research, is one of the key discrepancies in the implementation of the GDPR across the EU.[42] This can cause difficulties when researchers in a consent-focused Member State attempt to integrate data with a team in a country which either permits, or even encourages, reliance on other bases.[43]

Regardless of the basis for processing, it is evident that patients in the EHDS are intended to have the opportunity to exercise their data subject rights under the GDPR.[44] Indeed, it is clear that the "health data access bodies"— the key data custodians of the EHDS—are obliged to provide information on how data subjects can access their GDPR rights.[45]

However, there are two important limitations on individuals' control over their data under the EHDS. First, Article 38(2) makes it clear that "health data access bodies" do not need to provide information about their processing directly to the data subjects involved under Article 14 GDPR. The EDPB and the EDPS have strongly objected to this derogation from the GDPR, stating in their joint opinion:

Such exemption undermines the possibility for data subjects to exercise an effective control over their personal data rather than strengthen it and thus appears to be at odds with the objective laid down in Article 1(2)(a) of the Proposal.[46]

Second, even where patients are aware of the processing of their data within the EHDS, and are able to exercise their data subject rights, these rights are already subject to significant research exemptions under the GDPR. The rights of erasure,[47] objection,[48] and restriction[49] are all subject to derogations for scientific research and statistical purposes under the Regulation. This means that these rights can be disapplied where their exercise would be contrary to the prevailing public interest of the research processing. For example, Article 21(6) GDPR provides:

> Where personal data are processed for scientific or historical research purposes or statistical purposes pursuant to Article 89(1), the data subject, on grounds relating to his or her particular situation, shall have the right to object to processing of personal data concerning him or her, unless the processing is necessary for the performance of a task carried out for reasons of public interest.

This "task in the public interest" could well cover many of the secondary uses of health data under the EHDS that patients might otherwise wish to "opt out" of. The uncertain availability of these GDPR rights is thus problematic for patients wishing to know the extent of their rights under the EHDS. These three GDPR data subject rights would, where they do apply, provide a mechanism with the closest conceptual and practical resemblance to an "opt-out" for patients, in the absence of reliance on their consent.[50] Given the contingent nature of data subject rights, therefore, it is not clear that a higher standard of transparency would give individuals enough control over their information to opt out of the EHDS entirely. Even if data subjects did receive, read, and understand the information Articles 13–14 GDPR require, and were thus made aware of their rights in relation to the processing, these rights could still be disapplied through the research exemptions. This makes it all the more concerning that the most recent compromise draft of the EHDS Proposal has left it to Member States to decide whether to provide an additional right to opt out of secondary uses of health data, which would otherwise be more certain than the GDPR.[51]

This is not to suggest that there may not be genuine "public interest" reasons to prioritize comprehensiveness of data in the EHDS. Rather, the concern is more that the legitimate scope of "public interest" uses is also a contentious issue, which adds to the uncertainty lurking within the current Proposal. In his analysis of the EHDS Proposal, Terzis suggests the text transforms the conventional informed consent requirement in biomedical research into a transparency requirement, but that this is "not by itself a bad idea as the complexity of medical research often justifies flexible arrangements at place for the use and reuse of health data".[52] However, like other commentators,[53] he points to the variety of actors who could potentially access data for (equally various) secondary purposes under the EHDS—contrasting a "wholly legitimate claim of a medical research group" to use data from a clinical trial with a technology company developing of an experimental AI system.[54]

Whether there is, in fact, a bright ethical line to be drawn between AI development and a clinical trial is debatable. The capacity of machine learning to yield clinically significant insights within health data platforms has (in general terms) been defended as a "reasonable" use of health information, at least by some UK ethicists.[55] The societal benefit of developing and translating AI into healthcare is not necessarily lesser than the promise of a clinical trial, and both forms of experiment will carry their own risks. Likewise, the fact that research is conducted by a company—as opposed to medical researchers based only in a university or hospital—does not necessarily undermine its potential public benefit. This is a contested issue that precedes the EHDS, with some expressing concern that the GDPR is too broad in including the private sector within its definition of scientific research.[56]

The GDPR thus does not provide certainty as to when data subjects will be able to successfully object to the secondary use of their health data. The Regulation contains broad public interest exemptions to data subject rights, and in the absence of national legislation enabling a *lex specialis* EHDS opt-out, the scope of informational self-determination remains unhelpfully unclear for EU patients. EU Member States are also signatories of the ECHR[57] and thus must observe the right to respect for private life under Article 8 ECHR. We will consider, in the next section, the additional importance of opt-outs for this right.

Secondary uses and Article 8 ECHR

The successful development of the EHDS requires the alignment of its infrastructure with three broad sources of law: national law, EU law, and the ECHR. The relationship between these laws varies within our national case studies. In the UK, EU law no longer applies but the ECHR has (at least limited) direct effect through the Human Rights Act 1998. This means that UK public authorities (including public hospitals and other public controllers of NHS patient data) must perform their functions in a way which is compatible with the Convention rights of natural persons. The national Courts must also interpret UK law in a way which is compatible with the ECHR (even when a dispute is litigated between private citizens).[58] This includes the right to respect for private and family life under Article 8 ECHR. The Convention right thus has vertical and horizontal direct effect in the UK: that is, individuals can bring claims against the state, and (via civil law cause of action, interpreted compatibly) against other citizens or companies who infringe their privacy.

In Germany, primary EU law (such as the Treaties) is directly applicable, with most secondary legislation (including the EHDS Regulation) also having direct effect, insofar as its requirements are framed with sufficient clarity.[59] The horizontal direct effect of EU law rights (i.e. between citizens) is a more contested area, although aspects of the EU Charter of Fundamental Rights[60] have been found to have direct horizontal effect.[61] Germany is also signatory to the ECHR. The ECHR does not have constitutional status in German law, and cannot be directly enforced in national courts; however, the German Constitutional Court also interprets national laws in accordance with the ECHR.[62]

Germany and the UK are thus both signatories to the ECHR even if they have absorbed its requirements differently. Article 8 ECHR expresses the fundamental right to privacy. The article has two key elements, which can be summarized as relating to "scope" and "justification":

1. Everyone has the right to respect for his private and family life, his home and his correspondence.
2. There shall be no interference by a public authority with the exercise of this right except such as is in accordance with the law and is necessary in a democratic society in the interests of national security, public safety or the economic well-being of the country, for the prevention of disorder or crime, for the protection of health or morals, or for the protection of the rights and freedoms of others.

Article 8(2), the "justification" half of the provision, considers the lawfulness, necessity, and proportionality of any intervention with privacy rights (such as using, disclosing or collecting patients' data). Article 8(1), however, outlines the scope of the right to privacy. The word "reasonable" does not appear within its text, but it has come to be associated with the application of Article 8 through discussion in European Court of Human Rights (ECtHR) case law, set out below.

Article 8 ECHR in the UK

As we have outlined above, the NHSs in the various nations in the UK make data available for secondary uses on an "opt-out" basis. It is therefore, perhaps, unsurprising to suggest that this status quo is generally considered compatible with the Article 8 right to respect for private life, as available in a "domestic" version under the Human Rights Act 1998.

Although the Human Rights Act 1998 applies across the UK, there are subtle discrepancies in case law (as well as NHS practices) across the UK's four constituent nations. For ease of reference, this section will focus specifically on Article 8 as it has been interpreted in English law. Mark Taylor and James Wilson have argued that the Article 8 (as it applies within English confidentiality law) requires both sufficient notice of the use of identifiable information, and the opportunity to object—the latter being an expression of the value of individual autonomy within Article 8.[63] The importance of the opportunity to object does not, however, seem to stem from English law, but rather from the jurisprudence of the European Court of Human Rights—particularly *Avilkina and Others* v *Russia*,[64] where a prosecutor's order requiring doctors to disclose medical records was deemed oppressive in the absence of (inter alia) the patients' opportunity to object or agree to the disclosure.

The opportunity to object has not been robustly required by the English Courts, however. In the Court of Appeal's judgment in *R (W, X, Y & Z)*[65] (which has been criticized by some UK commentators[66]), the disclosure of NHS patient information to the Home Office for immigration purposes was held not to interfere with the patients' rights under Article 8 ECHR. This was because the Court found that the applicants lacked a "reasonable expectation of privacy",[67] as they were overseas visitors who had not paid for their NHS care and a patient liable to such charges would reasonably expect that, in the event of default, steps would be taken to enforce payment, which may include informing others of the fact, duration, and cost of their stay at the hospital concerned. The "reasonable expectation" of privacy appears central to the English interpretation of Article 8 ECHR, and represents a lower bar even than an "opt-out" scheme based on the opportunity to object (which is, in turn, a lower bar than active "opt-in" consent, conventionally required under the principle of informational self-determination).

This leaves open the question of whether other national interpretations of Article 8 ECHR set the bar any higher. It is evidently possible to interpret the scope and requirements of Article 8 more robustly than the UK Government. The ECtHR places less emphasis on "reasonable expectations" as a qualifying factor, and takes a more expansive approach to the application of Article 8. It is notable that the Strasbourg Court has repeatedly rejected the UK Government's submission that Article 8 was not engaged because the applicants did not have a reasonable expectation of privacy.[68] Within ECtHR jurisprudence, it has long been established that use and retention of information relating to a person's health engages the right to respect for private life under Article 8 ECHR, even when the intended use of the information by the State is entirely benign.[69] This strongly implies the engagement of Article 8 ECHR by the processing of patient data in the EHDS.

Given the potential for a more stringent approach to Article 8, the next section will explore whether the German interpretation of the right to privacy could be satisfied with an "opt-out" scheme.

Secondary uses in Germany[70]

The German constitution commits to inviolable and inalienable human rights, particularly through Article 1 II of the German Basic Law,[71] which states:

> The German people therefore acknowledge inviolable and inalienable human rights as the basis of every community, of peace and of justice in the world.

This provides domestic support for human treaties such as the ECHR, which in Germany has the status of an international treaty. The organs of the Federal Republic of Germany are thus bound by the ECHR, and all legal acts must be interpreted in its light. Although in the hierarchy of norms it remains on the level of ordinary (non-constitutional) law, due to the international law-friendly nature of German Basic Law, it can take precedence.[72] The judgments and interpretation of the ECtHR are also binding for German courts.[73] In individual cases, court decisions or laws may even become inapplicable due to a violation of the ECHR.[74] Both non-compliance with an ECtHR decision by German authorities and its schematic "enforcement" in violation of higher-ranking law can violate fundamental rights in conjunction with the rule of law principle of Article 20(3) of the German Basic Law.[75]

The ECHR, as the fundamental basis for human rights, binds German government bodies universally, regardless of whether they are applying national, EU, or international law. Although the German Basic Law has the "last word" with regard to fundamental rights, this rests on a co-operative relationship between the Basic Law and the ECHR.[76]

Against this backdrop, Germany has interpreted ECHR rights through its own legal culture of privacy.[77] The wider-ranging scope of the ECHR (requiring cohesion with multiple sources of national law) means it is more susceptible to interpretation through each national socio-legal culture.[78] The German Constitution (or "Basic Law") prioritizes human dignity as a value at stake in private information.[79] It is the first value enshrined in the Basic Law, which took on constitutional status in 1949. Since then, the inviolable dignity of the individual has guided the German Constitutional Court into shaping rights to control one's own personal data, most notably in the form of the right to informational self-determination,[80] as a subset of the general right to personality under Article 2(1) and the corresponding importance of individuals' consent to the use of their information.

This is understood in sympathy with the emphasis on autonomy developed by the ECtHR in its interpretation of Article 8 ECHR.[81] Cases citing Article 8 ECHR have emphasized the importance of consent as an aspect of informational self-determination, particularly in the context of health and genetic data.[82]

Where consent is required, this prioritizes data subjects' control over the completeness of health data available for secondary use. The tension between comprehensive datasets and individual control is at the heart of the concerns around the development of the EHDS. In the context of "primary" uses of data (i.e. for the patient's healthcare), greater systemic interoperability supports the patient's right to data portability, which in turn can give them more control over their information.[83] Within secondary uses of data, however, the systemic capacity to connect and transfer health records does not necessarily empower individual patients. Rather, the interoperability of these more comprehensive and longitudinal health datasets comes with privacy compromises for the patients involved, as more information can be ascertained about them, and by a greater range of actors.[84]

Like the UK, Germany has attempted to define an appropriate and feasible level of control for patients within systems for secondary data use. At a federal level, the Medical Informatics Initiative has used a "Consent" working group to explore the various models of patient consent.[85] In the UK, however, it is made clear that secondary uses of health data are not normally conducted on the basis of consent. The absence of an opt-out is not taken as consent to the sharing of health data.[86]

The EHDS poses a greater integrative challenge to the German legal culture than it would for a country such as the UK. This does not mean, however, that Germany cannot accommodate the EHDS into its national law. Even when the GDPR was in its early stages, there was recognition in German scholarship that consent could not be a "philosopher's stone" within data protection law, as individuals can easily become overwhelmed by trying to exercise their personal will to regulate complex systems within multiple forms and purposes of processing.[87] Given these limitations, control of these information channels should—it has been argued—be exercised by legislative requirements.[88]

The EHDS Proposal represents exactly such a set of legislative requirements for informational control. If combined with adequate transparency, and accessible opportunities for opt-out, the systemic safeguards within the EHDS Proposal could be enough to prevent any dignitary harm from the partial loss of informational self-determination. But there is one significant caveat before we can consider the matter concluded. Some high-level interpretations of the GDPR have left open the possibility that scientific research can be conducted on personal data without the need for a corresponding legal basis.[89] If this were the case, "health data access bodies" in the EHDS could make personal data available without complying with the legislative safeguards provided for in the EHDS Proposal—or even under national law. This would be a bold—and problematic—interpretation of the GDPR, which would undermine the protections for individual rights afforded by the EHDS Proposal. However, as this interpretation has some authoritative support within the EU, we will consider it in our final section below.

Secondary uses under the GDPR

As an initial point, the GDPR does not use the term "secondary use". Instead, it discusses "further processing" of personal data—a phrase which is not explicitly defined, and thus has an ambiguous overlap with the idea of "secondary uses" of health data.[90] For the purposes of this section, however, the GDPR's concept of "further processing" overlaps with the secondary uses we discuss here: data collected for one purpose (e.g. providing healthcare) are then made available for further uses under the EHDS.

The UK and Germany alike are bound by versions of the GDPR which may (or may not) widen the scope for scientific research using health data which are compatible with patients' reasonable expectations.[91] Whether or not the GDPR can be legitimately interpreted in this way has significant implications for the EHDS, which must be shaped in accordance with a nationally harmonized understanding of data protection requirements.

Recital 50 GDPR makes reasonable expectations a more important benchmark in the secondary processing of health data, stating:

> In order to ascertain whether a purpose of further processing is compatible with the purpose for which the personal data are initially collected, the controller, after having met all the requirements for the lawfulness of the original processing, should take into account, inter alia: any link between those purposes and the purposes of the intended further processing; the context in which the personal data have been collected, in particular the reasonable expectations of data subjects based on their relationship with the controller as to their further use.

While a version of this recital did exist under the previous EC Data Protection Directive,[92] the reference to the reasonable expectations of the data subjects as a benchmark is new. Also new within Recital 50 is the potentially cryptic statement when personal data are used for secondary compatible purposes:

> [...] no legal basis separate from that which allowed the collection of the personal data is required [and] ... (f)urther processing for archiving purposes in the public interest, scientific or historical research purposes or statistical purposes should be considered to be compatible lawful processing operations.

This has sparked a controversy as to whether personal data can be re-used for research without satisfying the original legal basis for collection, or indeed a new legal basis. The European Commission suggested this would not be the case when they advised (in the context of the Clinical Trials Regulation):[93]

[…] even when the presumption of compatibility is found to apply, the scientific research making use of the data outside the protocol of the clinical trial must be conducted in compliance with the relevant legal basis and all other relevant applicable provisions of data protection law as stated under Article 28(2) CTR.

However, this position has since been unsettled by provisional comments from the European Data Protection Board in 2019:[94]

[…] the controller could be able, under certain conditions, to further process the data without the need for a new legal basis. These conditions, due to their horizontal and complex nature, will require specific attention and guidance from the EDPB in the future. For the time being, the presumption of compatibility, subject to the conditions set forth in Article 89, should not be excluded, in all circumstances, for the secondary use of clinical trial data outside the clinical trial protocol for other scientific purposes.

The European Data Protection Supervisor has made the most recent contribution to this debate, and has taken a relatively cautious approach to the presumption of compatibility. In a 2020 preliminary opinion on scientific research, they note:

The recital thus appears to assimilate purpose specification and lawfulness in the case of reuse for the purposes of scientific research. As the recital is not accompanied by a specific provision in the main body of the GDPR, this appears not so much a blanket exemption to the separate steps set out in the Charter Article 8(2)—applicable to all circumstances—but rather advisory (hence "should be considered to be compatible"). We would therefore argue that, in order to ensure respect for the rights of the data subject, the compatibility test under Article 6(4) should still be considered prior to the reuse of data for the purposes of scientific research, particularly where the data was originally collected for very different purposes or outside the area of scientific research.[95]

Indeed, according to one analysis from a medical research perspective, applying this test should be straightforward.[96]

The EDPS position is less problematic for our current purposes. If the "further processing" requirements simply involve additional—advisory—consideration of compatibility with the original purpose of data collection, this only adds a safeguard without taking any protections away. By way of hypothesis, two simple examples would be a research or innovation use of data that might undermine the original purpose of the collection, such as:

- a German participant in a clinical trial makes their information available a help find a treatment for their disease. A subsequent use of this data to create intellectual property (IP) unavailable within the German market would thus undermine the original purpose of the collection, and present an incompatible purpose for processing;
- a Welsh patient receives healthcare for a rare condition: a study challenging the health economic case for this care, which could ultimately lead to its withdrawal, could also be an incompatible use of personal data stemming from their care.

In other words, the GDPR principle of purpose limitation can introduce helpful consideration of the patient's interests and aspirations. But if, contrary to our arguments here, it is treated as a replacement for the lawfulness principle, and eliminates the need for a legal basis for research, these considerations are not enough. A lawful basis based on legislation—including EU legislation such as the EHDS Proposal itself—should contain carefully negotiated rules about purposes, actors, and information security, providing clarity upstream as to who can access health data, and on what terms. Ad hoc consideration of "compatible purposes", even when coupled with the GDPR's requirements for research safeguards under Article 89, is no substitute. An infrastructure setting out the scope and aim of secondary uses—and not negotiating them piecemeal—will have the necessary requirements of clarity and accessibility for more systemic forms of oversight.

In short, the GDPR should not be interpreted in such a way to disapply the EHDS Proposal as a necessary legal basis for processing. Although, as the time of writing, definitive guidance from the European Data Protection Board on this point is still forthcoming, we would support a clear requirement for research to be governed by a legal basis for processing under the GDPR. Otherwise, all the negotiated safeguards and careful balancing of interests that go into the EHDS (and the national implementing legislation which will integrate it into Member State law) can effectively be bypassed through a loophole in the GDPR.

The EHDS Proposal itself (or said national implementing legislation[97]) should provide an appropriate legal basis under Article 6(1)(e) (a task in the public interest, which must have some basis in EU or Member State law) for processing personal data. This may not address all concerns which have been raised by data rights groups to date—for example, if these instruments do not rule out commercial access to health data through HealthData@EU.[98] But uses of data founded in these pieces of legislation will at least have to comply with the concessions to data subjects' interests that *have* been built into the EHDS Proposal: the duty to make findings public within 18 months,[99] the transparent purpose limitation set by the "data permit" system,[100] and the confinement of health data analysis to secure processing environments.[101] The proposed text of the EHDS Regulation introduced by the Council in December 2023 requires "health data access bodies" to ensure that health data processing complies with Article 6 GDPR,[102] meaning that personal health data re-used in the EHDS should have a basis for processing.

At the time of writing, the main question which appears only partially resolved is the question of patients' ability to opt out. We suggest this is a sufficiently important question to require resolution at EU level. To leave the question to individual Member States may seem a politically expedient compromise if the question of opt-outs has proved intractable within negotiations.[103] However, on a practical level, this risks recreating we have already seen in the implementation of the GDPR,[104] which itself allows scope for multiple derogations at the Member State level, resulting in (in the Commission's own assessment) obstacles to sharing health data across national boundaries.

Member States will need to bear in mind the "principle of coherence" when they implement the EHDS. This doctrine derives from the EU Treaties,[105] and requires the Union to ensure consistency in the application of its laws. This requires both harmonization of measures between the EU and its Member States, and between the Member States themselves within the scope of application of EU law.[106] An important aspect of this is the coherence of fundamental rights, which is understood as the seamless interlocking of the protection of fundamental rights in the multi-level system, in which duplications and contradictory decisions are avoided or resolved through clear rules of priority.[107]

The principle of coherence requires consistency of fundamental rights at a European and national level. In this case, the rights at stake are those relating to privacy and data protection. Where interference with these rights is permitted, it is essential that Member States' discretion be as narrow as possible to avoid diverging legal standards. Narrowly defined options for derogations, subject to specific conditions, can help maintain a minimum degree of coherence between national measures. At the time of writing, however, Article 35F of the Council's draft EHDS Proposal contains areas of potential incoherence in its "right to object": most significantly, in the discretion whether to implement the right in the first place,[108] but also in the potential to restrict this right (if implemented) for broadly defined public interest purposes.[109]

The principle of coherence is not simply a question of bureaucratic alignment: it goes to the heart of the vision of the EU as a union of free and equal citizens. It therefore seems unfair to allow the same health data infrastructure to be compulsory for some, but voluntary for others, depending on decisions of their respective governments. Leaving the proposed opt-out mechanism in Article 35F as a derogation, rather than a broadly available right, suggests informational privacy is a question of national politics, and undermines the principle of solidarity in biomedical research,[110] which should underscore the moral authority of the Proposal in the first place.

Conclusion

In conclusion, we are broadly supportive of an EHDS Proposal based on an "opt-out" system for secondary uses, but have expressed concern at the European Commission's suggestion that the question of individual autonomy versus secondary uses is best left to Member States. We have considered two legal cultures within Europe—the UK and Germany—which have distinct historical and contemporary differences in their implementation of privacy rights. Despite these differences, however, we have concluded that both legal frameworks would be compatible with an "opt-out" system for the EHDS. We would welcome further research on other European jurisdictions to test the generalizability of these findings.

The EHDS poses a challenge to the legal-bioethical paradigm in countries such as Germany, where broad consent has conventionally been seen as a minimum requirement to preserve informational self-determination in research. However, this challenge is apparently surmountable, with the Health Data Use Act introducing secondary uses of patient data on an opt-out basis.[111] As such, it should be possible to integrate the EHDS infrastructure into German law without infringement of patients' constitutional rights, even without introducing an "opt-in" system of objection. However, this should be balanced with careful attention to patient feedback while the EHDS Proposal can still be amended. Any evidence that patients are unhappy with certain uses—e.g. commercial uses generating exclusive IP—should be taken seriously. If control and co-design are not offered upstream through public engagement, it may be exercised downstream through the imperfect tool of individuals opting out of all secondary uses, including those uses they would otherwise support.

Ultimately, if the EU does not include a right to opt out of secondary uses within the EHDS Proposal itself, we can only call for consistent exercise of the derogation among Member States (and third country-authorized participants)[112] to avoid regulatory fragmentation and unfair national discrepancies.

Acknowledgements

The authors would like to acknowledge Anna Lina Gummersbach and Noemi Aguirre Chan for their work on the Bundesministerium für Bildung und Forschung project awarded to Fruzsina Molnar-Gabor: Datenschutzrechtliches Reallabor für eine Datentreuhand in der Netzwerkmedizin—TrustDNA (16DTM108A). This work was a valuable part of the background to this chapter. The authors would also like to thank Adam Dampc for his input related to constitutional law. Miranda Mourby is also grateful to Elisabetta Biaisin for her thoughts on the EHDS Proposal.

Notes

1 This is a very broad term but, in essence, it means any purpose other than using an individual's data to provide their healthcare. See EHDS Proposal Article 2.
2 See, for example, UK Department for Health and Social Care, "Data Saves Lives: Reshaping Health and Social Care with Data" (Policy Paper, 15 June 2022), available at: https://www.gov.uk/government/publications/data-saves-lives-reshaping-health-and-social-care-with-data/data-saves-lives-reshaping-health-and-social-care-with-data.
3 European Commission, "Proposal for a Regulation of the European Parliament and of the Council on the European Health Data Space" COM (2022) 197 final, hereafter referred to as the "EHDS Proposal". Unless specified otherwise, references will be to the text of the original proposal, as at the time of writing the status of proposed amendments is unresolved.
4 Giedre Peseckyte, "EU Parliament Solving Riddle of Secondary Use of Data in Health Data Space", Euractive (3 July 2023), available at: https://www.euractiv.com/section/health-consumers/news/eu-parliament-solving-riddle-of-secondary-use-of-data-in-health-data-space/.
5 European Digital Rights, "EU's Proposed Health Data Regulation Ignores Patients' Privacy Rights" and Position Paper (6 March 2023), available at: https://edri.org/our-work/eu-proposed-health-data-regulation-ignores-patients-privacy-rights/; European Digital Rights, "Joint Public Letter to EU Lawmakers on Patients' Rights in the European Health Data Space" (13 April 2023), available at: https://edri.org/wp-content/uploads/2023/04/Joint-public-letter-on-consent-in-EHDS-2.pdf.
6 Council of the European Union, "Proposal for a Regulation on the European Health Data Space—Mandate for negotiations with the European Parliament" (2023, December 7), available at: https://data.consilium.europa.eu/doc/document/ST-16048-2023-REV-1/en/pdf, Recital 37a (hereafter referenced as "EHDS Proposal: Council Version").
7 Regulation (EU) 2016/679 of the European Parliament and of the Council on the protection of natural persons with regard to the processing of personal data and on the free movement of such data (General Data Protection Regulation) 2016 (hereafter cited as "the GDPR"). When the UK domestic version of the GDPR is referenced, it will be termed "the UK GDPR".
8 Health Research Authority, "Consent in Research" (19 April 2018), available at: https://www.hra.nhs.uk/planning-and-improving-research/policies-standards-legislation/data-protection-and-information-governance/gdpr-guidance/what-law-says/consent-research/. "Legal basis" is used here the sense of a lawful basis under Article 6 of the GDPR (as discussed later in this chapter). However, there

are parallels with the de-emphasis on consent through the "reasonable expectations of privacy" test in English common law, also discussed later in this chapter.

9 Elizabeth Redrup Hill, "The European Health Data Space", PHG Foundation (5 October 2023), available at: https://www.phgfoundation.org/briefing/ehds.

10 Patients can choose between type 1 opt-outs, which prevent General Practitioners from sharing information with NHS England (which holds the central repository for secondary uses of health data), whereas the "national data opt-out" prevents NHS England sharing information with other organizations. See: https://www.nhs.uk/using-the-nhs/about-the-nhs/opt-out-of-sharing-your-health-records/.

11 Towards the European Health Data Space ("TEHDAS"), "TEHDAS' Proposals for Promoting Data Altruism in the EHDS" (29 September 2023) 34, available at: https://tehdas.eu/results/tehdas-proposals-for-promoting-data-altruism-in-the-ehds/.

12 Cf. the resolution of the Datenschutzkonferenz, the conference of all supervisory authorities, Decision of the 97th Conference of the Independent Data Protection Supervisory Authorities of the Federation and the Länder on the interpretation of the term "certain areas of scientific research" in Recital 33 of the GDPR (3 April 2019), available at: https://www.datenschutzkonferenz-online.de/media/dskb/20190405_auslegung_bestimmte_bereiche_wiss_forschung.pdf.

13 TEHDAS, n 11, 43.

14 Federal Data Protection Act: Act to Adapt Data Protection Law to Regulation (EU) 2016/679 and to Implement Directive (EU) 2016/680, s 27(1), as cited in Mette Hartlev and others, "EU-STANDS4PM Report: Legal and Ethical Review of In Silico Modelling" (Deliverable 3.1) (March 2020), available at: https://www.eu-stands4pm.eu/publications.

15 Recital 32 GDPR clarifies that consent under Article 6 should be given "by a clear affirmative act", meaning that this legal basis requires "opt-in" consent.

16 Bundesministerium für Gesundheit, "Health Data Use Act (GDNG): Better Research in Healthcare", available at: https://www.bundesgesundheitsministerium.de/ministerium/gesetze-und-verordnungen/guv-20-lp/gesundheitsdatennutzungsgesetz.html.

17 See section on "Secondary Uses in the EHDS" below.

18 The EHDS Proposal defines secondary uses of electronic health data with reference to a list of eight purposes in Article 34, including (e) scientific research related to health or care sectors, (f) the development of healthcare and medicinal products, and (g) the training, testing and evaluation of algorithms to be used in healthcare. We use the term "secondary uses" in this chapter with corresponding breadth.

19 NHS Digital, "Health Education England, NHS Digital and NHS England merger", available at: https://digital.nhs.uk/about-nhs-digital/nhs-digital-merger-with-nhs-england.

20 openDemocracy, "We've Won Our Lawsuit Over Matt Hancock's £23m NHS Data Deal With Palantir" (30 March 2021), available at: https://www.opendemocracy.net/en/ournhs/weve-won-our-lawsuit-over-matt-hancocks-23m-nhs-data-deal-with-palantir/.

21 See e.g. Sir John Bell, "Life Sciences Industrial Strategy: A Report to the Government from the Life Sciences Sector" (30 August 2017), available at: https://www.gov.uk/government/publications/life-sciences-industrial-strategy.

22 As at 10 January 2024: https://digital.nhs.uk/data-and-information/publications/statistical/patients-registered-at-a-gp-practice/october-2023.

23 As at 25 October 2023: https://digital.nhs.uk/dashboards/national-data-opt-out-open-data.

24 GKV Spitzenverband, "The Statutory Health Insurance Companies", available at: https://www.gkv-spitzenverband.de/krankenversicherung/kv_grundprinzipien/alle_gesetzlichen_krankenkassen/alle_gesetzlichen_krankenkassen.jsp.

25 Social Code—Book V—Statutory Health Insurance, § 303a et seq., as amended by the Act for Better Care through Digitization and Innovation (Digital Care Act—DVG) of December 9, 2019, Federal Law Gazette Volume 2019 Part I No. 49, issued at Bonn on December 18, 2019, 2562 et seq., No. 39.

26 N 16. As part of the model (pilot) project for comprehensive diagnostics and therapy finding using genome sequencing for rare and oncological diseases, Section 64e (6) SGB V obliges the platform provider to ensure a data protection-compliant, barrier-free and uniform design of the declaration of consent of the insured persons. This assumes an "additional" consent requirement for the subsequent use of the data for case identification and scientific research, which must be obtained by the service providers participating in the pilot project. To this end and to the extent possible, existing and nationally used sample texts should be used, such as the information and consent documents drawn up as part of the Medical Informatics Initiative, which would include the templates developed for broad consent, which would also contain the templates developed for broad consent. See Cabinet draft of 30 August 2023, available at: https://www.bundesgesundheitsministerium.de/service/gesetze-und-verordnungen/detail/gesundheitsdatennutzungsgesetz.html, at 71.

27 Bijan Moini, "Preventing Data Leaks: Health Data Database of 73 Million People with Statutory Health Insurance", available at: https://freiheitsrechte.org/themen/freiheit-im-digitalen/gesundheitsdaten.

28 See e.g. concerns raised in European Digital Rights, n 5.

29 European Commission, "Remarks by Commissioner Stella Kyriakides at the Press Conference on the European Health Data Space" (3 May 2022), available at: https://ec.europa.eu/commission/presscorner/detail/en/speech_22_2790.

30 TEHDAS Project, n 11.

31 EHDS Proposal: Council's Draft, Article 2(2)(z).

32 Ibid., Article 35C(3).

33 Regulation (EU) 2022/868 of the European Parliament and of the Council of 30 May 2022 on European data governance and amending Regulation (EU) 2018/1724 (Data Governance Act) [2022] OJ L 152/1.

34 See TEHDAS, n 11, 34.

35 Decision of the 97th Conference of the Independent Data Protection Supervisory Authorities of the Federation and the Länder on the interpretation of the term "certain areas of scientific research" in Recital 33 of the GDPR (3 April 2019), available at: https://www.datenschutzkonferenz-online.de/media/dskb/20190405_auslegung_bestimmte_bereiche_wiss_forschung.pdf.

36 N 16.

37 European Commission, "Communication 2020/66 of 19 February 2020 from the Commission to the European Parliament, the Council, the European Economic and Social Committee and the Committee of the Regions: A European strategy for data", available at: https://eur-lex.europa.eu/legal-content/EN/TXT/?uri=CELEX%3A52020DC0066.

38 Ibid., para 4.

39 European Commission, DG Health and Food Safety, "Assessment of the EU Member States' Rules on Health Data in the Light of the GDPR" (12 February 2021), available at: https://health.ec.europa.eu/system/files/2021-02/ms_rules_health-data_en_0.pdf.

40 Ibid., 9.

41 European Parliament, "Legislative Train Schedule: Proposal for a Regulation on the European Health Data Space", available at: https://www.europarl.europa.

eu/legislative-train/theme-promoting-our-european-way-of-life/file-european-health-data-space.

42 European Commission, DG Health and Food Safety, "Assessment", n 39, 26.
43 See EU-STANDS4PM report, n 14, 37–40.
44 To the extent that the UK contributes patient data as a third country, UK patients will have the possibility of exercising at least as many GDPR rights to control their data as are available (subject to research exemptions).
45 EHDS Proposal, Article 38(1)(d).
46 European Data Protection Board and European Data Protection Supervisor, "EDPB-EDPS Joint Opinion 03/2022 on the Proposal for a Regulation on the European Health Data Space" (12 July 2022) para 23, available at: https://edpb.europa.eu/system/files/2022-07/edpb_edps_jointopinion_202203_european healthdataspace_en.pdf.
47 GDPR, Article 17(3)(d).
48 GDPR, Article 21(6).
49 GDPR, Article 18(2).
50 Per EHDS Proposal, Article 33(5).
51 EHDS Proposal: Council Version, Article 35F.
52 Petros Terzis, "Compromises and Asymmetries in the European Health Data Space" (2022) 30 *European Journal of Health Law* 345.
53 See EDRI position paper, n 5, 4. See also J Scott Marcus and others, "The European Health Data Space" (2022) *IPOL | Policy Department for Economic, Scientific and Quality of Life Policies, European Parliament Policy Department Studies*, 48, available at: http://dx.doi.org/10.2139/ssrn.4300393.
54 Terzis, n 52, 360.
55 Alex McKeown and others, "Ethical Issues in Consent for the Reuse of Data in Health Data Platforms" (2021) 27 *Science and Engineering Ethics* 9 (doi: 10.1007/s11948-021-00282-0).
56 Kärt Pormeister, "Genetic Data and the Research Exemption: Is the GDPR Going Too Far?" (2017) 7 *International Data Privacy Law* 137.
57 Convention for the Protection of Human Rights and Fundamental Freedoms, Rome, 1950 Council of Europe European Treaty Series 5.
58 Human Rights Act 1998, ss 3 and 6.
59 European Parliament, "60 years of Van Gend & Loos Direct Effect of EU Law and a 'New Legal Order'", available at: https://www.europarl.europa.eu/RegData/etudes/BRIE/2023/739326/EPRS_BRI(2023)739326_EN.pdf.
60 Charter of Fundamental Rights of the European Union [2000] OJ C364/1.
61 Aurelia Colombi Ciacchi, "The Direct Horizontal Effect of EU Fundamental Rights: ECJ 17 April 2018, Case C-414/16, Vera Egenberger v Evangelisches Werk Für Diakonie Und Entwicklung E.V. and ECJ 11 September 2018, Case C-68/17, IR v JQ" (2019) 15 European Constitutional Law Review 294.
62 Giuseppe Martinico, "Is the European Convention Going to Be 'Supreme'? A Comparative-Constitutional Overview of ECHR and EU Law Before National Courts" (2012) 23 *European Journal of International Law* 401.
63 Mark Taylor and James Wilson, "Reasonable Expectations of Privacy and Disclosure of Health Data" (2019) 27 *Medical Law Review* 432.
64 (2013) (application no. 1585/09).
65 *R (on the application of W, X, Y and Z) v Secretary of State for Health and Secretary of State for the Home Department, the British Medical Association* [2015] EWCA Civ 1034.
66 Taylor and Wilson, n 63, 450.
67 N 65, [43–44].
68 Specifically *Peck v United Kingdom* (2003) App. No(s). 44647/98; *Perry v United Kingdom* App. No(s). 63737/00. In *Pay v United Kingdom* (2009) 48

EHRR SE2, the ECtHR decided to "proceed on the assumption, without finally deciding, that Article 8 [was] applicable", casting some doubt on the UK Government's assertion that the applicant lacked a reasonable expectation of privacy, but not fully resolving the matter. In any event, the ECtHR found the complaint under Article 8 to be "manifestly ill-founded", placing it in comparative sympathy with the UK government overall.

69 *Chave nee Jullien v France* (1991) App. No(s).14461/88; *Z v Finland* (1997) App. No(s). 22009/93.
70 The authors would like to thank Dr Adam Dampc for his assistance in drafting this sub-section of the chapter.
71 BVerfG, Judgment of the Second Senate of 4 May 2011—2 BvR 2365/09, 740/10, 2333/08, 1152/10, 571/10, EuGRZ 2011, 297.
72 BVerfG, Order of the Second Senate of 18 March 2013—1 BvR 2436/11, 1 BvR 3155/11, BVerfGK 20, 234–249.
73 Grabenwarter/Pabel, Europäische Menschenrechtskonvention, § 3 Die EMRK im Recht der Mitgliedsstaaten, para 8–12.
74 Sauer, Die Umsetzung von EGMR-Urteilen in Deutschland—Verpflichtungen der Rechtspraxis, NJW 2023, 2073.
75 BVerfG, Order of the Second Senate of 14 Octobre 2004—2 BvR 1481/04, BVerfGE 111, 307.
76 BVerfG, Judgement of the Second Senate of 4 May 2011—2 BvR 2365/09, 740/10, 2333/08, 1152/10, 571/10, EuGRZ 2011, 297.
77 James Q Whitman, "The Two Western Cultures of Privacy: Dignity versus Liberty" (2004) 113 *Yale Law Journal* 1151.
78 BVerfG, Order of the First Senate of 6 November 2019—1 BvR 16/13 -, paras. 1–157 (Recht auf Vergessen I/"Right to be forgotten I"), para 66.
79 Basic Law, Article 1(1).
80 BVerfG, Order of the First Senate of 15 December 1983—1 BvR 209/83 -, paras. 1–214 ("Census" Judgment), BVerfGE 65, 1–71.
81 BVerfG, Order of the First Senate of 24 January 2012—1 BvR 1299/05 -, paras. 1–192, BVerfGE 130, 151–212.
82 BVerfG, Judgment of the First Senate of 13 February 2007—1 BvR 421/05 -, paras. 1–101, BVerfGE 117, 202–244.
83 Teodora Lalova-Spinks and Daniela Brešić, "The Broadening of the Right to Data Portability for Internet-of-Things Products in the Data Act: Who Does the Act Actually Empower? (Part I)" (Blogpost, KU Leuven Centre for IT & IP Law, 22 June 2023), available at: https://www.law.kuleuven.be/citip/blog/the-broadening-of-the-right-to-data-portability-for-internet-of-things-products-in-the-data-act-part-i/.
84 Petros Terzis and Enrique Santamaria Echeverria, "Interoperability and Governance in the European Health Data Space Regulation" (2023) 23 *Medical Law International* 368.
85 Sven Zenker and others, "Data Protection-Compliant Broad Consent for Secondary Use of Health Care Data and Human Biosamples for (Bio)medical Research: Towards a New German National Standard" (2022) 131 *Journal of Biomedical Informatics* 104096 (doi: 10.1016/j.jbi.2022.104096).
86 For example, the NHS Digital website refers to consent and opt-outs as separate mechanisms. See "When does a national data opt-out not apply?", available at: https://digital.nhs.uk/services/national-data-opt-out/operational-policy-guidance-document/when-does-a-national-data-opt-out-not-apply.
87 See Johannes Masing, "Data Protection Challenges" (2012) 32 *Neue Juristische Wochenschrift* 2305.
88 Ibid., 2309.

89 See e.g. European Data Protection Board, "Opinion 3/2019 concerning the Questions and Answers on the interplay between the Clinical Trials Regulation (CTR) and the General Data Protection Regulation (GDPR) (art. 70.1.b)" adopted 23 January 2019, available at: https://edpb.europa.eu/sites/default/files/files/file1/edpb_opinionctrq_a_final_en.pdf.

90 Regina Becker and others, "Secondary Use of Personal Health Data: When Is It "Further Processing" Under the GDPR, and What Are the Implications for Data Controllers?" (2022) 30 *European Journal of Health Law* 129.

91 Some commentators have argued that the GDPR inhibits the secondary use of health data. See e.g. David Peloquin and others, "Disruptive and Avoidable: GDPR Challenges to Secondary Research Uses of Data" (2020) 28 *European Journal of Human Genetics* 697.

92 Directive 95/46/EC of the European Parliament and of the Council of 24.10.1995 on the protection of individuals with regard to the processing of personal data and on the free movement of such data (OJ L 281,23.11.1995, p. 31), Recital 28.

93 European Commission Directorate-General for Health and Food Safety, "Question and Answers on the interplay between the Clinical Trials Regulation and the General Data Protection Regulation" (2019), 7, available at: https://health.ec.europa.eu/system/files/2019-04/qa_clinicaltrials_gdpr_en_0.pdf.

94 European Data Protection Board, "Opinion 3/2019", n 89, para 31.

95 European Data Protection Supervisor, "A Preliminary Opinion on Data Protection and Scientific Research" (6 January 2020), available at: https://edps.europa.eu/sites/edp/files/publication/20-01-06_opinion_research_en.pdf.

96 Marjolein Timmers and others, "Will the EU Data Protection Regulation 2016/679 Inhibit Critical Care Research?" (2019) 27 *Medical Law Review* 59.

97 Such as the German Health Data Use Act, n 16.

98 N 5, European Digital Rights' position paper on the EHDS.

99 EHDS Proposal (Council Version), Article 35C.

100 Ibid., Article 46.

101 Ibid., Article 50.

102 Ibid., Article 46(1)(c).

103 See e.g. n 4 for reports of this as a contentious issue within negotiations.

104 See n 40 for the European Commission's own assessment of the patchwork of rules created under the GDPR.

105 Specifically, Article 7 Treaty on the Functioning of the European Union, and Article 21(3) of the Treaty on the European Union.

106 Ulrike Schuster, *Das Kohärenzprinzip in der Europäischen Union* (Nomos 2017), 112.

107 Ibid., 195.

108 EHDS Proposal: Council version, Article 35F.1.

109 Ibid., Article 35F.3.

110 Barbara Prainsack and Alena Buyx, *Solidarity in Biomedicine and Beyond* (Cambridge University Press 2018).

111 N 16.

112 EHDS Proposal, Article 52.

6

THE EVOLUTION OF PRIVACY GOVERNANCE IN HEALTHCARE IN POST-APARTHEID SOUTH AFRICA

Safia Mahomed

Introduction

Prior to the advent of South Africa's democratic dispensation, the right to privacy was largely recognized at common law and not the subject of significant codification.[1] This position has significantly changed, with the right to privacy being progressively developed with specific regard to clinical practice and health research settings. With the advent of the Constitution of the Republic of South Africa, 1996, and increasing awareness of healthcare patient and research participant protections—a concept that was predominantly interpreted by ethics norms and the common law—privacy is now governed by various pieces of domestic legislation and ethical guidelines, and is also influenced by international instruments.[2]

In law, the healthcare practitioner-patient relationship is usually a contractual one, with an implied agreement that the practitioner will diagnose and treat the patient according to generally acceptable standards. A related legal concept is the fiduciary relationship where a patient places trust or confidence in the healthcare practitioner. Failure to observe and respect patient privacy strikes at the heart of this fiduciary relationship, which is critical to the optimal utilization of health services by patients for their ultimate well-being.[3] The same principles regarding protecting privacy to encourage trust apply when one considers the relationship between researcher and research participant.

This chapter explores the post-transition evolution of privacy in the healthcare context in South Africa. It showcases the legislative and ethical strides that South Africa has taken over the past 30 years in protecting patients and research participants' fundamental right to privacy, from its inception within the Bill of Rights, to its emphasis on protecting personal information under the Protection of Personal Information Act, 2013 (POPIA). It further outlines some of the challenges to privacy as a result of recent

DOI: 10.4324/9781003394518-9

statutory developments and considers ways in which privacy laws could be managed practically in an open data-driven society.

Reflections from the past

The development of privacy governance in healthcare in South Africa cannot be discussed without reflecting on the past in order to truly understand why a fundamental rights focus is critical to our context. The historical exploitation of African populations with regard to health research transgressions and health services delivery is a reality.[4] However, the gravity of some of these atrocities in the South African context was only highlighted post-democracy during the Truth and Reconciliation Commission (TRC) Hearings—a body established by the democratic government in 1995 to assist healing the country and bring about reconciliation by uncovering human rights violations which occurred under the apartheid regime. This includes the gross medical ethics and human rights abuses conducted under the guise of scientific experimentation and at the hands of the man ominously dubbed as South Africa's "Dr Death", Wouter Basson, a cardiologist and personal physician to then State President PW Botha. Ultimately, the TRC found that with the support of an extensive international network, scientists, doctors, dentists, and laboratories, among others, supported the apartheid Chemical and Biological Warfare programme, more commonly known as Project Coast. It further held that Project Coast was "evidence of science being subverted to cause disease and undermine the health of communities".[5] With such disregard to the victims' human rights, it is highly unlikely that there was any consideration towards their privacy.

Perhaps the most prominent example of medical professionalism being undermined by corrupting and morally reprehensive attitudes and actions is that of the murder of Steve Biko, an anti-apartheid activist and leader of the Black Consciousness movement, who died in 1977 while in police detention and as a result of the grossly inadequate treatment received from two doctors responsible for his care. Over five days in which they supposedly attended to Biko's care, Dr Lang and Dr Tucker failed to take his condition seriously.[6] They failed to examine Biko under proper conditions despite obvious signs of possible brain damage; no medical history was taken; simple tests regarding Biko's mental state were also not carried out; and they allowed the police to be present during the examination, which, despite influencing their diagnosis and management, clearly violated Biko's rights to privacy and confidentiality. Apart from the obvious human rights atrocities meted out against Biko at the hands of the doctors responsible for his care, who have been described as "moral monsters",[7] there was a flagrant disregard of doctor–patient confidentiality and a violation of Biko's privacy as his personal medical data was shared with the state without consent.

The fact that there have only been a handful of prosecutions[8] for the gross human rights abuses committed under the apartheid regime speaks to the need to ensure tighter regulatory measures where the dignity of the people of South Africa is at stake in order to foster trust among the population. This is even more relevant in the healthcare setting where patients are in a vulnerable position with complete trust being placed in medical professionals responsible for their care. It is with this background in mind that I turn to discuss the ethico-legal evolution of privacy governance with regard to healthcare in post-apartheid South Africa.

Current ethico-legal framework that governs the right to privacy in healthcare

As stated above, previously, the right to privacy was a right largely recognized at common law and not the subject of significant codification. Presently, the right to privacy with regard to health is protected by (1) the Constitution, 1996, (2) various pieces of legislation, and (3) the common law. Confidentiality as a concept is often discussed within the framework of privacy; however, although confidentiality and privacy are linked, there are differences between the two, as other chapters in this volume demonstrate. Privacy relates to aspects of a person's being into which no one else should intrude. Sharing private information with a healthcare practitioner results in the patient choosing to relinquish certain aspects of their privacy. However, patients have a reasonable expectation that their private information will only be shared with specific people to further their welfare. In the medical context, confidentiality will almost always invariably involve a relationship between parties, whereas privacy may not.[9] While confidentiality is often described as an ethical obligation, it is very much a legal requirement in the medical sector.[10]

Constitution of the Republic of South Africa, 1996

In South Africa, the Constitution, 1996, is the supreme law of the country. It forms the apex to our legislative framework in that no other law or government action supersedes its provisions.[11] Chapter 2 of the Constitution contains the Bill of Rights, which enumerates the fundamental rights of all persons in the country.[12] The protection and recognition of the right to privacy as a fundamental human right provides an indication of its importance. The right to privacy as outlined in section 14 of the Bill of rights of the Constitution, 1996,[13] states that:

Everyone has the right to privacy, which includes the right not to have-

(a) their person or home searched;
(b) their property searched;

(c) their possessions seized; or
(d) the privacy of their communications infringed.

In terms of section 14 of the Bill of Rights, the right to privacy includes the right not to have one's person searched. The physical examination of a person in the healthcare or health research context can then be interpreted to be an invasion of privacy. Such examination may only occur if the person waives their right to privacy for the purpose of examination in the relevant health context. Further, information related to the health status of a person is inextricably bound to issues of privacy. However, the constitutional right to privacy, like its common law counterpart,[14] is not an absolute right and may be limited in terms of law of general application to the extent that the limitation is reasonable and justifiable in an open and democratic society based on human dignity, equality, and freedom.[15] In addition to protections developed under the Constitution, 1996, the rights to confidentiality and privacy in the health context are further safeguarded in various laws and policy documents, the most relevant of which are discussed below.

National Health Act 61 of 2003

The National Health Act 61 of 2003 (NHA) provides a framework for a structured uniform health system within the Republic, taking into account the obligations imposed by the Constitution and other laws on national, provincial, and local government with regard to health services. As mentioned above, the notion of confidentiality is often discussed within the framework of privacy. The relationship between a healthcare practitioner and patient/research participant is built on trust. Confidentiality between a practitioner and patient/ research participant assists in building that trust which in turn works towards maintaining patient/participant dignity. Section 14(1) of the NHA stipulates that all information about a person receiving treatment, including information relating to their health status, treatment, or stay in a health establishment, is confidential. This is a significant guarantee under the NHA, as without an assurance of confidentiality patients may be hesitant to use health facilities and disclose necessary information for a diagnosis and treatment.

However, confidential information may be disclosed where consent is provided in writing; a court order or law requires disclosure; or where non-disclosure will represent a serious threat to public health.[16] For example, during the COVID-19 pandemic, regulations were developed for the disclosure of patients' COVID-19 status to effect quarantine or isolation and hence not infect others. The NHA creates a further exception with regard to the access of health records by allowing for a health worker or healthcare provider to disclose personal information of the person receiving treatment, if it is necessary for any legitimate purpose within the ordinary course and scope of their duties, where such disclosure is in the best interests of the person receiving treatment.[17] In addition, the NHA contains provisions for the access to and protection of health records.[18]

The NHA provides for the broad protection of patient privacy and confidentiality. But perhaps the most significant piece of legislation that was signed into law in 2013, came into effect in July 2021, and which has had an impact on privacy in the healthcare sector and challenged existing practices within the health research sector is the Protection of Personal Information Act 4 of 2013 (POPIA).

Protection of Personal Information Act 4 of 2013

Based on the European Union's General Data Protection Regulation (GDPR),[19] POPIA defines personal information broadly and covers all information related to an identifiable, living person and an identifiable, existing juristic person. POPIA aims to regulate the processing of personal information and safeguards the right to privacy. Its preamble recognizes that the constitutional right to privacy includes a right to protection against the unlawful collection, retention, dissemination, and use of personal information, and the state must respect, protect, promote, and fulfil the rights in the Bill of Rights. Unlike the GDPR, which applies to personal data of all European Union data subjects regardless of jurisdiction, POPIA only applies to personal information processed within South Africa's borders. However, it is more stringent and broader in its application in that it also applies to the personal information of juristic persons (legal entities). Any information collected about a company or other type of legal entity would enjoy the same protection as personal information of an individual—thus extending POPIA compliance to information about vendors, partners, and suppliers.

With more stringent measures in place regarding the use and transfers of personal information, one immediate tension evident from POPIA is the strain between the right to individual privacy on the one hand and data sharing in the context of open science on the other, which needs to be balanced to ensure progress on economic, social, healthcare, and educational fronts.[20] To this end, and in order to clarify the application of POPIA to research, including health research, the Academy of Science of South Africa (ASSAf) developed a draft Code of Conduct for Research (COC) which, as at the time of writing, the Information Regulator declined to accredit, citing that the formal application of the Code requires clarity. However, as the substance of the draft Code was not challenged, researchers and research institutions may continue to use the draft Code to guide their compliance with POPIA.[21]

There are eight conditions[22] which must be met when personal information is processed, and it is the responsibility of the responsible party (in the health context, this is either the practitioner or researcher) to ensure the lawful processing of personal information in a manner that does not infringe on the constitutional right of individuals to privacy. Essentially, when personal information is collected for research purposes, a participant should know what type of information is being collected, why it is being collected, what will happen to the information, for how long it will be retained, whether it will identify the participant, if and why it will be shared, and whether it will be transferred outside South Africa, and, if so, why.[23] In addition, in the health research context where transfers of personal information across international borders are commonplace, POPIA provides an added layer of regulation.

Another piece of legislation which has a bearing on personal information is the Promotion of Access to Information Act 2 of 2000 (PAIA), which, like POPIA, is currently under the ambit of the Information Regulator. PAIA attempts to balance the right to information with the right to privacy and impacts how information should be accessed. More relevant to this chapter is the processing of personal information under POPIA. Now that the privacy protections under the Constitution, 1996, the NHA, and POPIA have been briefly examined, it is prudent to canvass how the right to privacy developed with regard to healthcare under the common law.

Development of the common law position

A seminal case which recognized the independent right to privacy in South African law is O'Keeffe v Argus Printing and Publishing Co Ltd.[24] In this case, a journalist's photograph and name were published in a newspaper, without her consent, in the context of an advertisement for guns and ammunition. Watermeyer AJ concluded that: "unauthorised publication of a person's photograph and name for advertising purposes was capable of constituting an aggression upon that person's dignity where this was understood to incorporate a wide range of personality interests, including her interest in privacy".[25] Therefore, the accepted common law principle is that when a person's privacy is infringed, this results in the violation of a person's personality interests in the form of that person's dignity.[26] After the judgment in O'Keeffe, the courts began to shape the principle of privacy which now provides a remedy for the public disclosures of private facts.

In Seetal v Pravitha,[27] the court held:

> Yet a blood test on somebody without his consent is unquestionably an invasion of his privacy. And the invasion is no less such because on just about every occasion the test is otherwise innocuous.

Such information is personal and confidential and could affect a person's psychological integrity if disclosed without their permission. In addition, the wrongful disclosure of personal information may result in a breach of the affected person's privacy. A breakthrough regarding the duty of a healthcare provider to keep a patient's medical information confidential was achieved in *Jansen van Vuuren NNO v Kruger*,[28] decided before the adoption of the Bill of Rights. In this case, the HIV status of a patient was unlawfully disclosed to another doctor and dentist who knew the patient, over a game of golf. Unsuccessful in the High Court, the patient's right to medical confidentiality was upheld on appeal. Sadly, the patient succumbed to an AIDS-related illness by the time the matter was upheld on appeal.[29] The Appellate Division of the Supreme Court (now the Supreme Court of Appeal) held that a healthcare provider has both an ethical and a legal duty to respect a patient's confidentiality, and that ethical guidelines are legally enforceable providing patients with a legal remedy when guidelines are breached.[30]

In *NM v Smith*,[31] the court found that a biography about Patricia De Lille (a South African politician) invaded the right to privacy of three women whose HIV-positive status and names were disclosed in it. In addition, at least two interrelated reasons for the constitutional protection of privacy[32] were identified. The first stemmed from the constitutional idea of what it means to be a human being, implicit in which is the right to choose what personal information is released into the public arena.[33] The more intimate the information, the more important it becomes to safeguard privacy, dignity, and autonomy in that an individual makes the primary decision whether to release the information. The second reason for protecting privacy is the democratic need to reduce the power of the state and to prevent it from denying liberty and dignity by interfering with personal private space.[34] O'Regan J further highlighted in this case the interrelationship between privacy, liberty, and dignity as the key constitutional rights which construct our understanding of what it means to be a human being. Therefore, all these rights are interdependent and mutually reinforcing.[35]

As the common law principle upholds that a violation of a person's privacy results in an infringement of that person's dignity, we cannot regard these two fundamental rights as separate from each other. Additional to developments under the common law, the confidentiality requirements set out in the NHA, and provisions which regulate the protection of personal information under POPIA, healthcare providers have ethical duties, which according to *Jansen van Vuuren NNO v Kruger* are legally enforceable—thus highlighting the quasi-legal standing of national ethical guidelines. In addition, the fact that the concept of privacy is no longer limited to safeguarding discussions between a doctor and patient in clinical practice settings, and now extends to "big data" generated in the care of patients in modern healthcare,[36] means that it is prudent to outline how our ethical guidelines have been reformed to incorporate these changes.

Health Professions Council Guideline on Confidentiality, Booklet 5, revised 2021

The Health Professions Council of South Africa (HPCSA) was established by the Health Professions Act,[37] replacing the old South African and Medical Dental Council as the supreme statutory body regulating the medical profession. Being registered as a health practitioner under the Health Professions Act confers certain rights and privileges. Corresponding to these rights and privileges are the ethical duties a health practitioner or researcher owes to individuals and society. These duties are outlined in various Guidelines of Good Practice, issued by the Health Professions Council of South Africa. Apart from setting out requirements to maintain and retain patient or participant confidentiality, the importance of protecting personal information against improper disclosure is emphasized within the HPCSA Guideline on Confidentiality.[38] A healthcare practitioner may only provide information about a patient with consent (where possible), even in circumstances where the patient will not be identified by the disclosure; must anonymize data where unidentifiable data will serve the purpose; and must keep disclosures to a minimum.[39] With regard to the disclosure of information to others providing care, the Guideline indicates that any practitioner receiving personal information is bound by confidentiality, even where there is no contractual or professional obligation to protect it.[40] This statement affirms that confidentiality of medical information not only promotes a relationship of trust between patients and healthcare providers, but also contributes towards better health outcomes.[41] Where a patient cannot be informed about the sharing of personal information (for example in a medical emergency), the healthcare practitioner should disclose the information and explain the situation to the patient or an available third-party nominee after the emergency has passed.[42] In terms of disclosures other than the treatment of a patient,[43] the Guideline draws from the exceptions to confidentiality under section 14(1) of the NHA.[44]

In addition, there is a duty placed on a healthcare practitioner to ensure appropriate arrangements for the security of personal information when it is stored, sent, or received by electronic means. This extends to a healthcare practitioner taking professional advice on how to keep information secure before connecting to a network and recording the fact that such advice was obtained. The Guideline also cautions healthcare practitioners that information sent through the internet may be intercepted, and this should be a deciding factor whether and in what form to transmit personal information.[45] Therefore, the responsibilities on healthcare providers to ensure the safety of their patients' personal information have increased. Another ethical guideline which recognizes the privacy risks that come with the advent of new technologies which have driven a cultural transformation in the delivery of healthcare and more particularly for health research is the new national Ethics in Health Research Guidelines.

South African ethics in the Health Research Guidelines—Principles, structures, and processes[46]

The National Health Research Ethics Committee (NHREC) was established in accordance with section 69(1) of the NHA. One of the responsibilities of the NHREC is to determine guidelines for the functioning of health research ethics committees (RECs) to facilitate best practice.[47] Accordingly, the first edition of the Department of Health, National Ethics Guidelines was published in 2004, the second edition was published in 2015, and the third edition of the Guidelines, Principles, Structures and Processes, was published in 2024 (new Guidelines). The new Guidelines broadly recognize research participants' rights to privacy and confidentiality and that researchers have a duty to protect these rights through the course of the research process, including when disseminating research results or findings.[48] They also rely heavily on POPIA and reiterate the newly legislated stipulations in place for the processing of personal information, including cross-border transfers of information. In South Africa, the regulation of human biological materials should be set out in a Material Transfer Agreement (MTA). The new Guidelines acknowledge that although some MTAs may include clauses regulating the transfers of data, it is advisable to enter into separate Data Transfer Agreements (DTAs) for one or more data sets from the owner/provider to a third party.[49] Further guidance to RECs is outlined for consideration during the protocol review process when data transfers are envisaged.

Importantly, the new Guidelines recognize that data sharing raises specific ethical concerns in relation to privacy and that data sharing decisions involve trade-offs between protecting privacy and advancing research, and thus attempt to guide researchers and RECs when the use and transfer of data is contemplated.[50] There is a conflict between respecting individual autonomy by keeping data confidential and advancing the possibility of public beneficence by sharing data for socially and scientifically valuable research. A key consideration for researchers is how to find a balance between these competing interests.

With regard to re-identifiability, the Guidelines acknowledge the possibility of re-identification, with specific reference to groups rather than individuals, through genetic markers. It is the responsibility of researchers to pay attention to eliminating or at least minimizing privacy and autonomy risks resulting from re-identification and RECs are equally responsible to check that this is adequately addressed by the researcher.[51] Therefore, the new Guidelines attempt to address some of the challenges that have developed through the enactment of new legislation regarding the protection of personal information, and include added guidance for RECs on how to manage these challenges.

It is evident that privacy governance in South Africa has developed at a rapid pace over the past 30 years. From being developed under the common law, included as a fundamental right within the Bill of Rights and solidifying patient confidentiality within legislation and policy guidelines, to safeguarding the protection of personal information and developing a Code of Conduct for research, it is submitted that South Africa has made significant strides in line with international best practice. However, the development of new privacy laws, particularly data protection laws, has come at a time when open science and the wide sharing of data for research purposes is gaining momentum. South Africa has aligned itself with the open science trend. To this end, the Draft National Open Science policy which encourages open science, open data, and open access was approved for stakeholder consultation in the first quarter of 2022.[52] In addition, in 2021 the Draft National Data and Cloud policy[53] was published with a vision to transform South Africa into a data-driven digital economy. Both these policies encourage open data sharing. On the face of it, POPIA may appear to create underlying challenges between achieving an open science framework for research against its strict privacy protections geared towards the processing of personal information. However, POPIA is not a research framework per se; therefore, these challenges need to be balanced with the progress of research in the era of open science. The first challenge which needs to be addressed is the cross-border transfers of personal information.

Underlying challenges

Managing cross-border information flows

In accordance with section 72 of POPIA, international personal information transfers may take place under five circumstances, three of which appear relevant for research purposes, including for health research:

1. When the participant consents to the transfer (S72(1)(b)). Meeting the requirements for the withdrawal of consent (as required per s 11(2)(b) of POPIA) may not be practical because withdrawal may not be possible after the transfer has taken place. Furthermore, the details of the third party with whom the personal information will be shared, including the risks associated with the sharing, may not be known at the time initial consent is provided.[54]

2. When the transfer is for the benefit of the participant and where consent is not reasonably practicable to obtain, recognizing that if consent were possible, the research participant would likely provide it (S72(1)(e)). This ground seems impractical and even impossible when large data sets are transferred across borders because a decision regarding the transfer being for the benefit of each individual participant would in effect need to be made, per participant.[55]
3. When the recipient in the foreign country is subject to a law, binding corporate rules, or binding agreement that provides for an adequate level of protection that upholds principles that are substantially similar for the processing of personal information (S72(1)(a)). This appears to be the most practical basis for international transfers of personal information. Thus, a binding contractual agreement, such as a DTA that uphold the principles for the processing of personal information as set out in POPIA, seems to provide a realistic solution for the transfers of personal information outside South Africa.[56]

Currently, the South African Material Transfer Agreement template, gazetted into law in July 2018, provides some guidance for researchers regarding the transfers of materials and data outside South Africa. However, as the template was published prior to POPIA coming into effect, it is limited with regard to the transfers of personal information. Therefore, the fact that a binding DTA appears to be the most practical solution for the international transfers of personal information, together with the fact that the current MTA template is limited in its application to personal information, has prompted a call for the development of a national DTA template to facilitate and safeguard the transfers of personal information outside South African borders.[57] This then prompts a second challenge: how much is too much when personal information is processed?

Data minimization in the era of open science

Section 10 of POPIA states that personal information "may only be processed if, given the purpose for which it is processed, it is adequate, relevant and not excessive". To this end, POPIA appears to be focused on a minimalistic approach—the less personal information processed, the better. This seems to be contrary to the Draft National policy on Open Science, which encourages scientists to embrace open science and ensure "optimal use and reuse of research data",[58] and the Draft Data and Cloud policy, which aims to transform South Africa into a data-intensive and data-driven digital economy with data sharing being encouraged between multiple users. The Draft policy on open science follows the principle of "as open as possible, as closed as necessary" to ensure that "maximum benefit is derived from all publicly funded research".[59] It applies to research generated from public funds, yet section 4.1 indicates that it will be applied on a best-effort basis when research is funded by the private sector or by philanthropic funders and is made subject to contractual conditions requiring open science. In addition, under its rewards and incentives section, the Draft policy encourages private sector funding for open science projects through appropriate tax incentives.

The Draft Data and Cloud policy applies to everyone, including public and private institutions, and (controversially) states that any data generated in the country will be the property of South Africa, regardless of where the technology company is domiciled.[60] In addition, the Draft Data and Cloud policy concedes under its background and context that "the digital economy is a sharing economy" with the integrity of any digital economy depending on the extent to which sharing advantages are delivered among its ecosystem partners. It also proposes the development of a national open data strategy, which incorporates principles that data should be open by default, accessible, usable and reusable, comparable, and interoperable and trusted.[61] Wide accessibility and re-usability of data is thus a core objective of both draft policies. Thus, while both draft policies respect privacy protections, the language used appears to be much broader than the minimalist approach taken by POPIA where personal information is subject to limitations depending on the purpose for which it is processed.

While POPIA provides for exceptions from its strict processing requirements in the context of research, the practical implication of its minimalistic approach to processing personal information remains to be seen.[62] The reference to "the purpose for which it [personal information] is processed"[63] should be read together with section 15 of POPIA, which allows for further processing for research purposes where the data subject consents to the further processing. This may occur if it is necessary to mitigate a serious threat to public health or the life or health of a data subject or another individual or where the responsible party (researcher or research institution) ensures that the further processing is carried out solely for research purposes and where the information will not be published in an identifiable form. Therefore, the amount and types of data collected, used, and stored would depend on the context of the research project underway. In order to provide guidance to researchers, the ASSAf's Code of Conduct for Research developed a minimality assessment to assess whether the processing of identifiable personal information is necessary and proportional.[64]

Although POPIA takes a more cautious approach to the processing of personal information, it does include exceptions from its strict provisions when processing is for research purposes. However, with the Draft National Policy on Open Science and the Draft Data and Cloud policy recognizing the significance of South Africa being part of a globally inclusive digital economy, with the latter appreciating data as the "new oil",[65] questions around practically managing the sharing of personal information in an open access space arise. Furthermore, POPIA is specific to protecting personal information, while the Draft Policy on Open Science does not distinguish between personal and non-personal information/data. Yet, the Draft Data and Cloud policy appears to extend the application of POPIA to data and international data transfers that are currently not under its remit.[66] The rationale behind distinguishing personal information from non-personal information is now considered.

Distinguishing personal information from non-personal information

To determine the scope of POPIA's application, the difference between personal information and non-personal information needs to be established. In accordance with POPIA, personal information broadly covers all information related to an identifiable, living person and an identifiable, existing juristic person where applicable.[67] Thus, POPIA is only applicable to data that fits within this definition of personal information. De-personalized data, for example, data that was once personal information but manipulated into anonymous data where the data subject is no longer identifiable,[68] is theoretically not considered personal information under the Act.

However, questions remain around how to treat data that can potentially be re-identified and no specific guidance is provided by POPIA on how de-identification can be achieved.[69] The Code of Conduct attempts to provide clarity to this issue and defines de-identification to mean: the deletion of personal information that identifies research participants; personal information that can be manipulated to identify research participants; or personal information that can be linked by a reasonably foreseeable method to other information that identifies research participants.[70] The Code of Conduct further acknowledges that complete de-identification is difficult, if not impossible to achieve, considering technological advancements and the fact that increasing volumes of personal information are in the public domain. Categorizing information as personal or non-personal depends on the context and has practical ramifications beyond theoretical debate. Depending on the circumstances, the same data point can be personal or non-personal, thus subject to the strict processing requirements of POPIA or not.[71]

Other than acknowledging that personal information should be safeguarded and treated in accordance with the provisions of POPIA, the Draft Policy on Open Science does not distinguish between personal and non-personal information. According to the Draft Data and Cloud policy, any cross-border transfer of citizen data (not only personal information) must comply with POPIA and international best practice and provides that ownership and control of personal information and data shall be in line with POPIA—thus extending the application of POPIA to data and international data transfers currently not under its scope.

It is clear that there are challenges that have been brought forth by POPIA, which have implications for the practical management of data in the era of open science. A careful balance needs to occur when drawing the line between overstepping privacy of patients or participants on the one hand, and promoting optimal healthcare and health research for the common good of humankind, on the other. It is difficult to provide exact boundaries as the nature of technologies are always developing and changing rapidly. These boundaries have blurred even further with the advent of artificial intelligence (AI) in healthcare. As such, a discussion regarding the underlying challenges to the right to privacy would not be complete without touching on the role and risks associated with AI in healthcare.

Role and risks of AI in healthcare

Currently, the use of AI in health and medicine is continually expanding. Usable data has flourished specifically in the healthcare sector, being collected from numerous sources, including wearable technologies, genetic information generated by genome sequencing, electronic healthcare records (EHRs), radiological images, and hospital rooms.[72] Although the application of AI in low- or middle-income countries (LMICs) may be limited due to varying factors, including a lack of infrastructure, digital health technologies are already widely used in LMICs for data collection, dissemination of health information by mobile phones, and extended use of electronic medical records on open-software platforms and cloud computing (among others).[73]

An important area of health research utilizing AI is centred around the use of data generated from EHRs. However, using such data can prove challenging if the underlying information technology system and database do not discourage the production of heterogeneous or low-quality data. Nevertheless, AI can be effectively applied to EHRs for biomedical research, quality improvement, and optimization of clinical care. Additionally, AI can assist in analysing clinical practice patterns derived from EHRs to develop new clinical practice models. The collection, analysis, and use of health data, including from clinical trials, laboratory results, and medical records, are the foundation of medical research and the practice of medicine. However, over the past two decades, what qualifies as health data has expanded dramatically, now including massive quantities of personal information from various sources, such as genomic data, radiological images, medical records, and non-health data converted into health data.[74] Collectively known as "biomedical big data", these various types of data form a health data ecosystem that includes data from standard sources (e.g. health services, public health, clinical research) and further sources (environmental, lifestyle, socioeconomic, behavioural, and social). Consequently, there are now many more sources of health data, entities that wish to make use of such data, and commercial and non-commercial applications for the data.[75]

It is clear that with the encouragement of wider data sharing, including through the use of EHRs, comes an increased risk of data breaches. As a result, protections and safeguards must be available to prevent (in as far as possible) any threats to data security which could have devastating effects for patients, participants, researchers, institutions, and the scientific research space in general.

Data breaches in healthcare

The healthcare sector accounts for the highest number of security breaches compared to other industries.[76] Healthcare data is more valuable than any other type of data on the black market because it usually takes longer for healthcare fraud to be discovered. Thus, the data may be used for longer periods compared to data extracted from a stolen credit card for example, which can be stopped immediately when the breach is discovered.[77] Healthcare databases are usually large, making them perfect targets for hackers. The risks associated with data breaches and subsequent informational harms increased during the COVID-19 pandemic, providing cybercriminals with the opportunity to exploit cybersecurity vulnerabilities and launch cyber-attacks within the healthcare sector.[78]

According to IBM Security's annual *Cost of Data Breach Report*, the average data breach cost for South African organizations reached a record breaking R49.5 million in 2023.[79] In addition, it was found that South African companies had the highest percentage of organizations that had not used security automation that allowed security technologies to enhance or replace human intervention. Furthermore, there are several issues that hospitals face with regard to storing, sharing, and distributing health records and the most common issues in hospital information systems include human errors, hackers, missing or stolen paper, and software errors.[80] A few examples of data breaches in South Africa include those reported by the Life Healthcare Group in 2020, the second largest private hospital operator in South Africa which was hit by a malicious cyber-attack in the midst of the pandemic; and Experian, a consumer, business, and credit information services agency which exposed the personal information of as many as 24 million South Africans and almost 800,000 business entities.[81]

Prior to the Cybercrimes Act 19 of 2020, the Electronic Communications and Transactions Act 25 of 2000 (ECTA) was the main piece of legislation that enabled and facilitated electronic communications and transactions in the public interest.[82] Section 86 of the ECTA outlined that unauthorized access to, interception of, or interference with data is an offence. The Cybercrimes Act, which offers comprehensive legislation dealing exclusively with cybercrimes and related issues, was signed into law in June 2021, with certain sections of the act coming into operation with effect from

December 2021. While data protection and cybercrimes are two distinct areas of information communications technology, there is a correlation between these two areas in that the law now has an opportunity to remedy situations of vulnerability.[83] Given that data has been described as the "new oil"[84] and that the commission of crimes across physical borders has become easier, it would seem that the relationship between the laws relating to cybercrimes and data protection will only strengthen over time.[85]

It is also submitted that the Cybercrimes Act provides more clarity in relation to the unlawful use of and crimes committed in respect of data and/or computers. A contravention of the Act may result in a fine and/or imprisonment up to 15 years, depending on the nature of the contravention. Direct imprisonment is mandatory for, inter alia, unlawful access or unlawful interference with data or a computer programme if the offence was committed by a person or with the collusion or assistance of another person who as part of their duties, functions, or lawful authority were in charge of, in control of, or had access to data, a computer programme, a computer data storage medium, or a computer system belonging to another person in respect of which the offence in question was committed.[86]

Similarly, POPIA sets out offences,[87] penalties,[88] and fines[89] where its provisions are infringed and places a duty on responsible parties to disclose breaches of personal information. Section 22 of POPIA deals with the notification of security compromises and indicates that where the personal information of a data subject has been accessed or acquired by any unauthorized person, the Regulator and data subject (unless the data subject's identity cannot be established or if notification impedes a criminal investigation) must be informed as soon as reasonably possible. Notably, POPIA makes it an offence to pass on personal information to a third party without the authority of the data subject.

However, while POPIA and the Cybercrimes Act provide more stringent measures where breaches of personal information/data takes place, effectively enforcing these measures remains a challenge. It is imperative that responsible parties have the requisite technical and organizational protections in place to safeguard personal information. In addition, the duty to safeguard personal information or data entails cybersecurity measures aimed at identifying internal and external security threats and vulnerabilities.[90] The Code of Conduct for Research provides comprehensive guidance regarding responsible parties' obligations when it comes to technical and organizational safeguards. Furthermore, if the safeguards cannot be implemented, responsible parties need to document why this is the case.[91]

The regulation of data breaches and penalties associated thereto are contained within POPIA, and further safeguarded under the Cybersecurity Act and in the ECTA. A practical explanation of how to safeguard personal information and what to do in the event of a security compromise is set out in the

Code of Conduct for Research. However, the risks associated with breaches in privacy of data are very real, and although safeguards and reporting procedures may assist with preventing and managing these risks, the impact of informational harms as a result of data breaches can be very severe. With regard to research that involves the extensive networking of samples and data, privacy infringements of personal information may only take place years after the initial research is carried out. Therefore, a robust mechanism which translates the theoretical legal privacy framework into practice, and which aims to safeguard the integrity of participants' data, is paramount.

Conclusion

South Africa has made significant strides towards the development of a comprehensive ethico-regulatory framework that aims to protect the privacy and confidentiality of patients and research participants in the healthcare setting. Both the Draft National Open Science Policy and the Draft National Policy on Data and Cloud are data-driven, with core objectives of fostering access to data, its re-use and reproducibility, while the protection of personal information under POPIA appears to be suffused with promoting the individual autonomy of data subjects. However, the Code of Conduct for Research attempts to address certain tensions that POPIA creates, which have an impact on existing research practices. Nevertheless, AI and its advances pose significant challenges that South Africa will need to consider as its privacy protections further evolve. In addition, an increase in local data breach incidents, particularly in the healthcare setting, point to the urgent need to appropriately translate and enforce the legal framework for data sharing and transfer in South Africa into practice. This includes providing ethically sound practices, flexible infrastructure, and appropriate governance policies. While there are already calls for a national DTA template to manage the transfer of data across South Africa's borders, any practical data management tool that is developed to regulate data flows should be adapted in line with appropriate safeguards that respect the dignity of people, particularly considering the pre-democratic South African context.

Notes

1 Aspects of this chapter are based, in part, on the author's PhD thesis entitled *An ethico-legal framework for the regulation of biobanks in South Africa* (University of the Witwatersrand, South Africa 2018).
2 World Medical Association (WMA) Declaration of Helsinki—Ethical Principles for Medical Research Involving Human Subjects adopted by the 18th WMA General Assembly, Helsinki, Finland, June 1964 and amended by the 64th WMA General Assembly, Fortaleza, Brazil, October 2013; The International Ethical Guidelines for Health-related Research Involving Humans prepared by the

Council for International Organizations of Medical Sciences in collaboration with the World Health Organization prepared by the Council for International Organizations of Medical Sciences (CIOMS) in collaboration with the World Health Organization (WHO) Geneva 2016; WMA Declaration of Taipei on Ethical considerations regarding Health Databases and Biobanks adopted *by the 53rd WMA General Assembly*, Washington, DC, USA, October 2002 and revised by the 67th WMA General Assembly, Taipei, Taiwan, October 2016; OECD Guidelines on Human Biobanks and Genetic Research Databases (OECD Guidelines) (2009).

3 Ames Dhai and David McQuoid-Mason, *Bioethics, Human Rights and Health Law Principles and Practice* (2nd edn, Juta 2020), 97–98.

4 Safia Mahomed and others, "Managing Human Tissue Transfer Across National Boundaries: An Approach from a South African Institution" (2016) 6 *Developing World Bioethics* 29; Safia Mahomed and Ian Sanne, "Benefit Sharing in Health Research" (2015) 8 *South African Journal of Bioethics and Law* 60.

5 Jerome Amir Singh, "Project Coast: Eugenics in Apartheid South Africa" (2008) 32 *Endeavour* 5.

6 Trefor Jenkins and Graeme McLean, "The Steve Biko Affair" (2004) 364 Suppl 1 *The Lancet* s36.

7 Ibid., 36–37.

8 Konanani Happy Raligilia, "Beyond Foot-Dragging: A Reflection on the Reluctance of South Africa's National Prosecution Authority to Prosecute Apartheid Crimes in Post-Transitional Justice" (2020) 41 *Obiter* 63.

9 Dhai and David McQuoid-Mason, n 3, 118.

10 See e.g. section 7 of the Choice of Termination of Pregnancy Act 92 of 1996; sections 12, 13, 133, and 134 of the Children's Act 28 of 2005; and section 14 of the National Health Act 61 of 2003.

11 The Constitution of the Republic of South Africa (South African Government 1996).

12 Melodie Nothling Slabbert, "Genetic Privacy in South Africa and Europe: A Comparative Perspective. Part 2" (2008) 71 *Tydskrif vir Hedendaagse Romeins-Hollandse Reg (Journal of Contemporary Roman-Dutch Law)* 81: "In subsequent cases such as *Universiteit van Pretoria* v *Tommie Meyer Films (Edms) Bpk*, [1977 4 SA 376 (T) 384] *National Media Ltd* v *Jooste*, [1996 3 SA 262 (A) 271] *Bernstein v Bester NO* [1996 2 SA 751 (CC) 789] and *Swanepoel v Minister van Veiligheid en Sekuriteit*, [1999 4 SA 549 (T) 553] privacy has been referred to as an "individual condition of life characterised by seclusion from the public and publicity", which "embraces all those personal facts which the person concerned has himself determined to be excluded from the knowledge of outsiders and in respect of which he has the will that they be kept private. It follows from this that a person's privacy can only be infringed when others learn of true private facts about this person against his or her will and determination.".

13 Chapter 2 of the Constitution of the Republic of South Africa, 1996.

14 As a common law right, the right to privacy is limited by the legitimate interests of others and the public interest. As a fundamental right enshrined within the Bill of Rights, the right to privacy is subject to limitation by section 36 of the Constitution, 1996.

15 Section 36 of the Constitution of the Republic of South Africa, 1996.

16 Section 14(2) NHA.

17 Section 15(1) NHA.

18 Sections 16 and 17 NHA.

19 Regulation (EU) 2016/679 of the European Parliament and of the Council of 27 April 2016 on the protection of natural persons with regard to the processing of personal data and on the free movement of such data, and repealing Directive 95/46/EC (General Data Protection Regulation) [2016] OJ L 119/1.

20 Third edition of the National Health Research Ethics Committee (NHREC) Guidelines, Principles, Structures & Processes 2023.

21 ASSAf Update on the *Code of Conduct for Research* to Stakeholders, dated 14 December 2023.

22 The eight conditions set out in POPIA are: (i) accountability; (ii) processing limitation; (iii) purpose specification; (iv) further processing limitation; (v) information quality; (vi) openness; (vii) security safeguards; and (viii) data subject participation.

23 Section 3.1.9 of the third edition of the NHREC Guidelines, 2023.

24 *O'Keeffe v Argus Printing and Publishing Co Ltd* [1954] 3 SA 244 (C).

25 Helen Scott, "Liability for the Mass Publication of Private Information in South African Law: *NM v Smith* (Freedom of Expression Institute as Amicus Curiae)" (2007) 18 *Stellenbosch Law Review* 387.

26 Slabbert, n 12.

27 *Seetal v Pravitha* [1983] (3) SA 827 (D).

28 *Jansen van Vuuren NNO v Kruger* [1993] (4) SA 842(A).

29 Adila Hassim, Mark Heywood, and Jonathan Berger, 'The Rights and Duties of Users of the Health Care System", in Adila Hassim, Mark Heywood, and Jonathan Berger (eds), *Health & Democracy: A Guide to Human Rights, Health Law and Policy in Post-Apartheid South Africa* (SiberInk 2007), 254.

30 Ibid., 254.

31 *NM and Others v Smith and Others* (CCT69/05) [2007] ZACC 6; 2007 (5) SA 250 (CC); 2007 (7) BCLR 751 (CC) (4 April 2007).

32 Anne Hughes, *Human Dignity and Fundamental Rights in South Africa and Ireland* (Pretoria University Law Press 2014).

33 Ibid., 265.

34 Ibid., 265.

35 *National Coalition for Gay and Lesbian Equality and Another v Minister of Justice and Others* CCT11/98) [1998] ZACC 15; 1999 (1) SA 6; 1998 (12) BCLR 1517 (9 October 1998).

36 Bertalan Meskó and Brennan Spiegel, "A Revised Hippocratic Oath for the Era of Digital Health" (2022) 24 *Journal of Medical Internet Research* e39177.

37 Health Professions Act 56 of 1974.

38 HPCSA Guideline 5.

39 HPCSA Guideline 4.2.

40 HPCSA Guideline 7.4.

41 Hassim, Heywood, and Berger, n 29, 255.

42 HPCSA Guideline 7.5.

43 HPCSA Guideline 8.2.

44 HPCSA Guidelines 8.2.2, 8.2.3 & 8.2.4.

45 HPCSA Guideline 11.

46 Third edition of the National Health Research Ethics Committee Guidelines, Principles, Structures & Processes 2024.

47 Section 72(6)(a) of the NHA.

48 Third edition of the National Health Research Ethics Committee Guidelines, Principles, Structures & Processes 2024, section 3.1.9.

49 Ibid., section 4.2.2.1.

50 Ibid., section 3.4.3.

51 Ibid., section 4.1.4.

52 Department of Science and Innovation, Draft National Open Science Policy, v19. 24/01/2022. (Obtained from the Open Science Stakeholder workshop co-hosted by the DSI, ASSAf & USAf on 22 February 2022).
53 Draft National Policy on Data and Cloud, Government Notice 306, Government Gazette 44389 of 1 April 2021.
54 Safia Mahomed, Glaudina Loots, and Ciara Staunton, "The Role of Data Transfer Agreements in Ethically Managing Data Sharing for Research in South Africa" (2022) 15 *South African Journal of Bioethics and Law* 26.
55 Ibid., 27.
56 Ibid., 27.
57 Ibid. See also Lee Swales and others, "Towards a Data Transfer Agreement for the South African Research Community: The Empowerment Approach" (2023) 16 *South African Journal of Bioethics and Law* 13.
58 Department of Science and Innovation, Draft National Open Science Policy, v19. 24/01/2022, section 8.2.5.
59 Ibid., section 11.
60 Ibid., section 10.4.4.
61 Draft National Policy on Data and Cloud, section, 10.2.2.
62 Ciara Staunton and Elizabeth de Stadler, "Protection of Personal Information Act No.4 of 2013: Implications for Biobanks" (2019) 104 *South African Medical Journal* 232.
63 Section 10 of POPIA.
64 Annexure D of the POPIA Code of Conduct for Research, Government Notice 3409, Government Gazette 48589 of 21 April 2023.
65 Draft National Open Science Policy, section 10.1.
66 Draft National Policy on Data and Cloud, sections 10.4.2 and 10.4.4.
67 Section 1 of POPIA.
68 Michèle Finck and Frank Pallas, "They Who Must Not Be Identified— Distinguishing Personal from Non-Personal Data Under the GDPR" (2020) 10 *International Data Privacy Law* 11.
69 Lee Swales, "The Protection of Personal Information Act and Data De-Identification" (2021) 117 *South African Journal of Science* 1.
70 Annexure A of the POPIA Code of Conduct for Research, Government Notice 3409, Government Gazette 48589 of 21 April 2023.
71 Finck and Pallas, n 68.
72 Laurie Flynn, "When AI Is Watching Patient Care: Ethics to Consider" Bill of Health, 18 February 2020, available at: https://blog.petrieflom.law.harvard.edu/2020/02/18/when-ai-is-watching-patient-care-ethics-to-consider.
73 World Health Organization, *Ethics and Governance for Artificial Intelligence for Health* (WHO Guidance) (WHO 2021) available at: https://www.who.int/publications/i/item/9789240029200.
74 Effy Vayena and Alessandro Blassime, "Biomedical Big Data: New Models of Control Over Access, Use, and Governance" (2017) 14 *Bioethical Inquiry* 501.
75 WHO, n 75, 35.
76 The HIPAA Journal, Healthcare Data Breach Statistics, available at: https://www.hipaajournal.com/healthcare-data-breach-statistics/.
77 Ibid.
78 Anthony Minnaar and Friedo Herbig, "Cyberattacks and the Cybercrime Threat of Ransomware to Hospitals and Healthcare Services During the COVID-19 Pandemic" (2022) 35 *ACTA Criminologica* 155.
79 South African Data Breach Cost almost R50 million, July 2023, available at: https://www.businesstechafrica.co.za/security/2023/07/27/south-africa-data-breach-cost-almost-r50-million/.

80 Tumiso Thulare, Marlien Herselman, and Adele Botha, "Data Integrity: Challenges in Health Information Systems in South Africa" (2020) 14 *International Journal of Computer and Information Engineering* 423.

81 Safia Mahomed and Melodie Labuschaigne, "The Evolving Role of Health Research Ethics Committees in the Era of Open Data" (2022) 15 *South African Journal of Bioethics and Law* 80.

82 Section 2(1) of the Electronic Communications and Transactions Act 25 of 2000.

83 Sizwe Snail ka Mtuze, "The Convergence of Legislation on Cybercrime and Data Protection in South Africa: A Practical Approach to the Cybercrimes Act 19 of 2020 and the Protection of Personal Information Act 4 of 2013" (2022) 43 *Obiter* 536, 539: "Vulnerability in the cybercrimes area takes various forms, such as fraud, forgery and uttering, whereas in the area of data protection, it may take the form of data breaches".

84 Draft National Policy on Data and Cloud, section 10.1.

85 Mtuze, n 83, 560.

86 Section 19(6) of the Cybercrimes Act 19 of 2020.

87 Sections 100–106 of POPIA.

88 Sections 107 and 108 of POPIA.

89 Section 109 of POPIA.

90 Mtuze, n 83, 568.

91 POPIA Code of Conduct for Research, Government Notice 3409, Government Gazette 48589 of 21 April 2023, section 4.3.7.1.3.

7

IS HEALTH PRIVACY WORTH THE COST?

Mark A. Rothstein

Introduction

The privacy of health information—or lack of it—affects many aspects of daily life both within and beyond healthcare settings, and advances in health information technology are raising new questions about the goals, methods, and feasibility of protecting health privacy. Of special concern, the costs of protecting health privacy, in both financial and non-financial terms, are substantial, as are the costs of failing to protect health privacy.

Financial expenditures incurred by healthcare institutions, professionals, and their business associates include payments to technology suppliers, security consultants, staff hiring and training, compliance with legal regulations, and reduced healthcare productivity associated with the use of frequently changing and multiple passwords, role-based access controls, encryption, audit trails, and de-identification.

Non-financial burdens are more difficult to quantify and include both healthcare and other environments, such as difficulty in accessing individual health information in clinical settings and limitations on health information disclosures for public health, health research, and various public purposes, such as law enforcement.

Conversely, the reality or perception of inadequate privacy safeguards undermines the relationships between health professionals and their patients, causing some patients to decline sharing sensitive information, forego diagnostic procedures or preventive care, or refuse to participate in health research. Inadequate health privacy also may result in personal harm ranging from identity theft and economic loss to embarrassment and emotional distress.

Beyond healthcare, when individual health information, especially if obtained without consent, is widely accessible for commercial purposes or government uses, individuals could suffer from stigma or discrimination; experience a lack of access to employment, insurance, and financial opportunities; and have their trust in government and other institutions seriously undermined.

DOI: 10.4324/9781003394518-10

This chapter explores the costs and benefits of health privacy considering health information technology, healthcare systems, legal provisions, and societal attitudes. To answer the question of whether health privacy is "worth the cost", the chapter will trace the history of health privacy and the related concepts of confidentiality and security and assess the consequences of various methods of protecting privacy. Although health privacy has several forms, including physical privacy, this chapter focuses on informational health privacy.

The chapter highlights several less known or discussed aspects of health privacy. Even though it is not possible to explore these myriad issues in depth in a single chapter, the composite picture that emerges is of substantial, diverse, and new challenges that, at least in the United States, are evolving faster than efforts to protect health privacy.

Notwithstanding the word "cost" in the title of the chapter, it is not an economic analysis. Instead, it considers the ethical, legal, and policy implications of health privacy issues and challenges. Furthermore, the legal analysis in the chapter is primarily based on the laws and practices in the United States, although some of the discussion has wider applicability.

Health privacy, confidentiality, and security

Definitions of privacy and related terms vary, and in this chapter the terms have the following meanings. *Privacy* is a condition of limited access to an individual or information about an individual. *Confidentiality* means a condition in which a possessor of information disclosed in confidence does not redisclose the information without authorization. *Security* involves physical, electronic, and other means used to grant access to information to those authorized and deny access to those not authorized.

Confidentiality of personal health information, a bedrock principle of medical ethics, traces its origins to the Oath of Hippocrates in the fourth century, BCE. The Oath reads in pertinent part:

> What I may see or hear in the course of treatment or even outside of the treatment in regard to the life of men, which on no account must be spread abroad, I will keep to myself, holding such things shameful to be spoken about.[1]

At the time of Hippocrates there were no hospitals or medical offices and patients were treated in public places or homes. Patients had little or no physical privacy because treatment was often conducted in the open and controlled by male heads of households, but Hippocratic physicians pledged not to redisclose health or other information obtained in the course of treatment, such as observations in a home where a patient was treated.[2] In effect, physicians and patients implicitly entered into a "Hippocratic bargain" in which patients allowed physicians access to their person and health information, and physicians pledged to conduct examinations in a professional manner and to maintain the confidentiality of patient health status or other information unless disclosure was authorized by the patient or others with authority to do so.[3] Maintaining the confidentiality of health information respects the dignity of patients, and without confidentiality patients would be reluctant to disclose medically significant but personally embarrassing or sensitive information.

Formal organization of the medical profession in the 19th century led to the codification of physicians' obligations to protect their patients' privacy and maintain the confidentiality of their health information. Thomas Percival's code of medical ethics in 1803[4] and the American Medical Association's first code of medical ethics in 1847[5] expanded the commitment to professionalism and confidentiality first described in the Hippocratic Oath.[6] Eventually, these professional requirements were incorporated into state medical practice laws[7] and health privacy laws in the United States.[8]

Although the fundamental "bargain" continues today,[9] Hippocratic-era medical practice involved a single patient and physician. By contrast, and as discussed below, modern healthcare in many countries involves huge integrated delivery systems; multiple types of healthcare providers; longitudinal, comprehensive, electronic health records (EHRs); and numerous individuals with access to health information for payment and other nonclinical purposes. Privacy, confidentiality, and security, as both abstract concepts and basic legal and ethical precepts, are broadly supported by health professionals and patients, but the methods and effectiveness of current approaches, several of which are discussed below, have been called into question. Indeed, some modern assessments of healthcare practices and legal protections have called confidentiality a "decrepit concept"[10] and health privacy a "broken promise"[11] and an "illusion".[12]

Electronic health records

By the end of the 20th century digital information technology had revolutionized many aspects of daily life, with the notable exception of healthcare.[13] To improve healthcare efficiencies and outcomes federal legislation was enacted in the United States in 2009,[14] and in other countries around the same time,[15] to provide direct subsidies or other incentives to adopt EHRs. In the United States, by 2017, 86% of office-based physicians[16] and 94% of hospitals[17] had adopted an EHR system. There were at least five compelling reasons for replacing paper health records with newly developed EHRs.[18]

1 Paper health records were often handwritten and illegible, leading to errors in diagnoses, patient instructions, filling prescriptions, and other aspects of care.
2 Paper health records were incomplete and decentralized, with information scattered in the files of numerous providers over time and by medical specialty.
3 Paper health records were inefficient, requiring vast storehouses, and difficulty in accessing them resulted in the duplication of health histories, diagnostic tests, and imaging.
4 Paper health records were unavailable when a patient travelled from home and needed medical care in an emergency.
5 Paper health records were labour-intensive to analyse, thereby impeding quality improvement and research.

The adoption of EHRs in the United States has had a mixed record of success in eliminating the problems associated with paper records for both patients and clinicians. For example, many patients still need to provide detailed medical histories when seeking care from different physicians in the same health system,[19] interoperability of EHRs has been thwarted by the commercial interests of EHR vendors and healthcare institutions,[20] and remote access to EHRs in medical emergencies remains a largely unrealized goal.[21] Furthermore, the economic efficiencies in billing and payment have come at a high cost to physicians, whose increased time needed to document care in EHRs has contributed to alarming rates of burnout.[22] Some EHR vendors are attempting to use generative artificial intelligence to relieve some of these burdens, but it is not clear whether doing so will resolve the problem of physician overload or possibly create other problems.

Despite some unfulfilled promises, the digitization of health information also has had several extraordinary successes in facilitating better informed clinical management of patients, unprecedented levels of public health monitoring, and tremendous progress in health research. The challenge is to maximize the benefits of increased health data while simultaneously protecting wide-ranging privacy interests.

In what follows, I outline two key privacy concerns associated with EHRs: first, those that arise in relation to the longitudinal nature of EHRs (and then consider whether the "right to delete" health information adequately addresses these concerns); and second, those that arise in relation to the comprehensive nature of EHRs (and then consider whether segmentation and de-identification adequately address these concerns). I conclude the section by looking at privacy risks associated with dependents' health information in explanations of benefits and patient portals.

Privacy risks in longitudinal records

Many significant health privacy issues result from two important technical features of EHRs—they are longitudinal and comprehensive. Unlike paper records, EHRs, at least in theory, are "cradle to grave", including data collected and recorded by multiple healthcare providers over a patient's lifetime, and they are generally retained indefinitely. There are clinical advantages in longitudinal records, including detailing progression of disease, recording the effects of various treatment modalities, documenting adverse drug reactions, and supporting continuity of care. Nevertheless, there are downsides to all-inclusive records.

A leading privacy concern about longitudinal EHRs is that sensitive, old health information without any continuing clinical utility never goes away. Two examples follow.

1 A male PhD candidate in his mid-20s, to celebrate the oral defence of his dissertation, embarked on an evening of heavy drinking that ended with an encounter with a commercial sex worker. Realizing the health risks associated with this one-time, indiscreet behaviour, the student went to his doctor and was tested for a battery of sexually transmitted infections, and all the tests were negative.
2 A female PhD candidate in her mid-20s saw her physician after she suffered mild physical abuse at the hands of her brief, romantic companion. The minor injuries resolved shortly with no long-term medical significance, and she immediately terminated this abusive relationship.[23]

Medical records from these clinical encounters are likely to contain both objective findings, such as laboratory results, and narratives explaining the reasons for the office visits. According to current legal requirements and professional practices, this embarrassing, easily accessible information will remain in the EHRs of these two individuals for the rest of their lives.

Some clinicians and others, no doubt, would argue that this health information should remain in both EHRs because one can never be sure when some bit of medical history will have future clinical utility. Such a position has three flaws. First, it assumes that current longitudinal health records are overwhelmingly complete and error free, and that is certainly not the case.[24] Errors and omissions are common, and clinicians are trained to probe patients about other possibly relevant information and not to rely exclusively on medical records. Second, the likely psychological benefit of excluding this information dwarfs any remote chance that the information will have medical benefits and would be otherwise unavailable. Of course, if the medical facts in the prior two examples were varied, then there might be a different calculus of risks and benefits. Third, the physician–patient relationship is based on confidentiality and trust, and inflexibly recording and retaining highly sensitive information over the objection of patients will likely have adverse consequences on individual and even public health.

Assuming the benefits of exclusion outweigh the benefits of retention, what, if anything, can be done to reform the present situation?

Right to delete health information

In the United States, in the mid-20th century several states enacted laws prohibiting the deletion of any information from medical records to prevent some healthcare providers from removing evidence of malpractice.[25] Today, it is physicians, their institutions, and malpractice insurers who would strenuously object to giving patients a right to delete any health information. They want to ensure that complete clinical information, including imaging results and referrals to specialists, remains in patient records to protect against possible claims of malpractice or inappropriate care.

In contrast to the largely theoretical malpractice implications of incomplete records, serious health privacy issues persist from too much unnecessary information. To bolster health privacy, older laws could be repealed and replaced with new legislation giving patients a limited right to delete certain items from their EHRs based on the age of the information or other criteria. Such laws would be analogous to "right to be forgotten" (or "right to erasure") legislation enacted in the United Kingdom[26] and the European Union,[27] which applies in certain situations for one's personal data. (Segmentation, discussed below, also would protect against certain disclosures of sensitive information without need for deletions.)

It is possible that, if permitted, some patients would imprudently delete health information of possible clinical utility. However, this risk is likely to be less than the current risk of individuals deferring medical care for sensitive conditions or self-censoring relevant medical information they disclose to physicians due to concerns about privacy.

Furthermore, it is well established that competent adults have a legal right to refuse even life-sustaining medical care.[28] Consistent with a societal commitment to autonomy in healthcare, patients ought to have some right to control the records on which their healthcare is based. The specifics of such a right would need to be determined, but recognizing the importance and feasibility of the right are the first steps.

Privacy risks in comprehensive records

The second feature of EHRs raising important privacy concerns is that the records are comprehensive and include information about healthcare provided by diverse clinicians for a wide range of conditions. Unquestionably, medical benefits derive from clinicians being able to access records generated by all of a patient's past and current providers, but comprehensive EHRs also increase the risk of unnecessary disclosure. Consolidation of healthcare practices into increasingly large, multi-specialty or integrated delivery systems with a single EHR used by all providers heightens this risk by expanding the number of people with access to a patient's complete EHR.

Healthcare personnel without a need to access the EHR of an individual who is not their patient can be blocked or deterred by password protection, role-based access controls, encryption, audit trails, and other security measures. These procedures have been adopted and enforced with varying levels of rigour by healthcare institutions. However, the main privacy concern caused by comprehensive EHRs is that, in general, a patient's authorized, treating health professionals have access to a patient's complete EHR, even if all-inclusive records are unnecessary for a particular health problem.[29]

For example, physicians and nurses treating a patient in a hospital emergency department for a sprained ankle injured in a sporting event ordinarily do not need access to information about that patient's genetic test results, reproductive health, substance use, mental health, history of abuse or neglect, or other sensitive information. Virtually all healthcare providers do not have the time or inclination to scroll through a patient's EHR to view sensitive health information unrelated to their present condition. Nevertheless, occasional stories of inadvertent or intentional access to sensitive information unrelated to a patient's current healthcare as well as accessing the health records of celebrities, ex-spouses, and other patients of interest increase the level of patients' emotional distress.[30] Merely knowing that one's sensitive health information remains accessible by numerous healthcare staff members during every clinical encounter can be the source of continuing anxiety.

Segmentation

One way of protecting sensitive health information is actually enabled by EHRs. With modified EHR architecture patients could elect to separate or segment one or more types of sensitive information from a predetermined list of categories, such as reproductive health or mental health.[31] Clinicians providing care for non-sensitive conditions like a sprained ankle would have access only to the non-segmented portions of the EHR. However, if necessary for treatment, patients could supply additional passwords or otherwise consent for clinicians to access the segmented portions of their record. A "break-the-glass" feature could also allow broader access in emergencies. In addition, electronic clinical decision support aided by artificial intelligence could scan the entire EHR to determine if there is medically valuable information in a segmented file, such as the risk of a drug interaction involving medication prescribed for a condition in a segmented category.

Segmentation represents a trade-off between a patient's right to delete certain information and the status quo of all-inclusive health record availability. Segmentation is technically feasible, and even though it would involve some additional costs and inconvenience it is likely to provide significant privacy benefits. It has been used without reported problems to protect the confidentiality of psychotherapy notes.[32] Nevertheless, to date there has been little recognition of the need for or benefits of segmentation from patients, EHR vendors, healthcare institutions, payers, or regulators in adopting this enhanced health privacy measure.

De-identification

A more easily adoptable strategy to increase privacy in EHRs involves excluding identifying information from health records when they are used for purposes other than treatment. For example, financial personnel typically submit charges for healthcare services in electronic form using the patient's name and other overtly identifying information. Even if claims only use a diagnostic or billing code to describe the services provided, sensitive health information can be disclosed. There is no need for the many dozens of clerical and administrative staff overseeing payment information for hospitals and other providers or health insurance companies and other payers to know the identity of the patient. Every patient already has a unique medical or insurance identification number, and if necessary, the identity of the patient can be easily obtained.

De-identification also could be used by covered entities when they review health records for quality control, professional licensing, and other purposes to generate aggregate data or information about the appropriateness of care provided by specific healthcare providers. (These uses and disclosures are considered "healthcare operations" under the HIPAA Privacy Rule, discussed below.) The identities of individual patients are unnecessary in such instances. The HIPAA Privacy Rule uses the "minimum necessary" standard for disclosures of health information,[33] but it does not incorporate a "least identifiable form" requirement. Despite the ease and low cost of de-identification, this measure to protect health privacy also has received little or no support from healthcare organizations, professionals, or regulators, primarily because the issue has received scant attention.

Dependents' health information in explanations of benefits and patient portals

Standard health insurance billing practices in the United States pose privacy risks to anyone insured as a dependent, such as a minor, young adult child, or spouse, on another person's health insurance policy. Insurance-related disclosures often occur through explanation of benefits forms (EOBs), which are notices sent to the policyholder whenever a claim for medical services is processed. EOBs typically include the name of the individual receiving services, the name and profession of the provider, the date of service, and the general category of services received. With this billing practice, developed to protect against fraud and abuse, policyholders are notified each time a dependent receives medical care and is provided with general information about the care received. In addition to breaching confidentiality, the disclosure of health information to a policyholder may increase the risk of spousal abuse.[34] For example, because pregnancy can trigger or escalate intimate partner violence, disclosure of an individual's visit to an obstetrician could lead to physical or emotional abuse.[35]

Legal protection from disclosures through EOBs is sparse. With the patient's consent, usually obtained through an authorization form signed annually, providers are permitted by the HIPAA Privacy Rule to release health information to obtain payment. The HIPAA Privacy Rule allows dependents to request that EOBs are withheld, but insurance companies are not required to comply with the request unless the patient or a third party pays for the services in full.[36] Fourteen US states have enacted laws to protect the confidentiality of insurance policy dependents, but only four states have EOB-specific confidentiality laws.[37]

For minors, multi-user patient portals can also lead to the inadvertent disclosure of medical information. Although the details vary by state, minors and young adults are legally able to consent to a variety of sensitive services, such as those related to sexually transmitted infections, pregnancy, contraception, and mental health, without parental consent.[38] Many healthcare institutions in the United States, however, offer patient portals accessible by both the patient and their parent or guardian.[39] Such multi-access portals could disclose a minor's sensitive health information to the parent or guardian when a provider enters a new medication or orders a laboratory test or when the minor schedules a referral to a certain type of specialist. There is no standardized approach to protecting the health information of minors with EHRs; some providers utilize features of EHRs, such as entering a confidential note, but it is not clear how widespread, or effective, such efforts are.[40]

Expanding the scope of health data

Besides being longitudinal and comprehensive, EHRs are more expansive than paper records because the variety of health information now included in EHRs is unprecedented in scope and continues to grow. It is beyond dispute that "all our data will be health data one day",[41] and it is important to consider the reasons for and nature of this growth, as well as the implications for health privacy.

Big data, artificial intelligence, and precision medicine

New health information technology has enabled advances in big data, artificial intelligence, and precision medicine.[42] All of these new developments rely on tremendous amounts of diverse data, and all serve to operationalize the view that more data is always a good thing, even if its relevance or significance is currently unknown. To clarify the nomenclature, big data is "a large collection of disparate data sets that, taken together, can be analysed, to find unusual trends".[43] Artificial intelligence includes an extensive range of computing technologies that emulate human intelligence and utilize massive amounts of data storage and computing power.[44] Precision medicine is the application of clinically relevant, finer, and more accurate stratification of patients aided by genomics and other technologies.[45]

These new information-intensive technologies and medical approaches require extensive data beyond traditional clinical information, and they may include the following:

1 Health histories and vital statistics of family members, including birth and death certificates, and marriage, divorce, and adoption records.
2 Military service records, which may include health records and data on hazardous exposures.
3 Employment records, including exposure to toxic substances and biological monitoring data.
4 Financial information, including consumer data generated by credit cards and consumer loyalty programmes.
5 Educational records, including behavioural health information and student health service records.
6. Travel information and geo-location data obtained from mobile phones, as well as geographically related exposures.
7 Social media posts, including behavioural and mental health self-reports.
8 Personal health data from biological monitoring devices and wearable devices, including smart watches and smart clothing.
9 Government records, such as Social Security/national insurance data, records of military veterans and other government-provided health services, criminal justice information, professional licensure data, driving licence information, and passport information.[46]

There is virtually no limit to the data that might be considered relevant to some potential aspect of healthcare, public health, or research.[47]

Once health-related information is collected, it may be difficult to protect it from disclosure. Beyond collection, health privacy issues are raised by the aggregation, storage, use, and redisclosure of wide-ranging, nonclinical data. Some of these data come from publicly available sources, such as social media posts and birth and death records. Other information is derived from government files that are not publicly accessible, such as income tax and passport records. Still other data are proprietary, including consumer information and geo-location data maintained by mobile phone companies and information generated by health apps. As these non-traditional sources of data have increased value in big data analytics, there will be more interest by diverse entities in obtaining access to them, thereby raising concerns about whether individual consent is needed for access and the implications of monetizing personal data. It is not clear whether or when the marginal benefits of obtaining and using such immense data sets, including potentially sensitive information, outweigh the privacy risks. Nevertheless, entities in a strong economic position are likely to demand access to personal information in the absence of legal prohibitions.

Nonclinical uses of health data

Health data have many valuable uses beyond the treatment of individuals. Although public policy supports such beneficial uses, it does not do so unconditionally. Informational health privacy remains important in these contexts in the acquisition, use, and disclosure of the information.

Public health

Health information has tremendous value beyond individual clinical uses. Laws enacted in every US state require healthcare providers to report to state or local public health departments or law enforcement agencies all cases of certain types of infectious diseases, sexually transmitted infections, child abuse, gunshot wounds, and other conditions. This information is essential for statistical analysis, epidemiology, contact tracing, and other government interventions to protect public health and safety. The reports are in individually identifiable form to enable follow-up. As noted in the section on "legal protections" (discussed below), the law does not require covered entities disclosing public health information to notify or obtain consent from the individuals identified in the reports. Despite periodic concerns about the confidentiality of sensitive health information, public health departments have an excellent record of safeguarding the confidentiality and security of these reports.[48]

Research

Biological specimens and health information from biobanks, clinical records, and other sources are extremely important for health research. The amount, granularity, and scientific utility of these data sources and compilations all have increased substantially in recent years. In the United States, biobanks range from the All of Us research programme of the Department of Health and Human Services, eventually containing data and biospecimens from one million Americans,[49] to small hospital pathology repositories with several thousand specimens, although even small biobanks increasingly are part of large networks.[50]

Laws around the world have attempted to balance individual interests in privacy with societal interests in promoting health research.[51] Two issues, identifiability and consent, have been especially important to research policies.

First, regarding identifiability, if the source of the biospecimens and medical records cannot be identified at all (e.g. data were collected anonymously) or cannot be readily identified (e.g. data are coded), then legal restrictions on uses and disclosures usually do not apply and, theoretically, there is little or no privacy risk to the individuals whose specimens or data are used. Unfortunately, the value of the data declines significantly if individuals cannot be identified for verifying or updating health information, follow-up examination, or notification of critical research findings.

Furthermore, de-identification is not a panacea, and various ethical concerns remain, especially where no consent has been obtained. These include the possibility of re-identification by sophisticated computer techniques using publicly available sources; group harms when studies are published with data categorized by race, ethnicity, sex, religion, or other criteria; objectionable uses if samples obtained from a known source are used for research that some patients consider morally unacceptable; commercial exploitation if individuals object to their data or specimens being monetized without their consent; and undermining of trust in healthcare institutions if researchers are seen as taking steps to avoid notice and consent in their research.[52]

Second, problems associated with obtaining or avoiding traditional, specific consent for each research use of specimens or data have encouraged researchers to explore alternative models of consent in biobanks. The options include: (1) blanket consent (participants agree to all subsequent research uses of their specimens and data); (2) broad consent (participants provide wide consent and ethics review determines whether a specific protocol is within the bounds of the consent); (3) tiered consent (participants indicate what types of research, such as genetic research or mental health research, are permitted); (4) dynamic consent (participants are recontacted electronically for each new research proposal); and (5) registered access (researchers with prior approval are granted access without detailed assessments of each protocol). All these methods attempt to accommodate the autonomy and privacy interests of the participants without placing excessive burdens on the research enterprise.[53] The use of increasingly technical and multifaceted forms of consent further increases demands on the informed consent process, whose ability to satisfy current requirements has been questioned.[54]

Compelled authorizations

Many patients erroneously believe that health information maintained by a healthcare provider or entity is protected from disclosure. Even if stringent security measures protect against unauthorized access, a significant—but underappreciated—threat to privacy comes from patient-authorized, compelled disclosures. As a condition of applying for employment, various types of insurance, and certain government benefits, each year Americans sign an estimated 25 million authorizations for the disclosure of their health information to third parties.[55] Although individuals are not required to authorize such disclosures, if they fail to do so they will be declined financial benefits or other valuable opportunities when they apply for employment, life insurance, disability insurance, and long-term care insurance; submit claims for Social Security disability, veterans disability, and workers' compensation; or seek compensation for injuries caused by automobile accidents or other mishaps.

The entities requiring access to the health records usually have a legitimate reason, such as determining the cause or severity of an individual's medical condition. Yet, mostly for reasons of convenience, complete health records are often disclosed regardless of the purpose for disclosure. Unfortunately, there are few laws or guidelines regarding security measures to safeguard this information or regulating whether the records may be redisclosed to other individuals or entities.

Genetic discrimination in life insurance

The compelled disclosure of genetic test results for life insurance underwriting illustrates how nonmedical use of health information can result in serious, unintended health consequences. In the United States, life insurance companies do not perform their own genetic testing, but for policies over a minimum level many require access to applicants' complete health records that may contain the results of genetic tests performed in clinical settings. Although precise estimates are unavailable, informal surveys of genetic counsellors indicate that about 5% of individuals with a familial risk of genetic-related disorders, including certain types of cancer, decline genetic testing because of concern about the economic consequences of a positive test result. For example, one study of individuals who declined to participate in genomic sequencing research cited fear of insurance discrimination as their primary reason.[56]

Individuals with a genetically confirmed increased risk are more likely to engage in vigilant prevention and surveillance measures that lower their risk and detect cancer at an earlier stage.[57] As a group, their prognosis is much better than individuals who do not have genetic testing and are diagnosed at a later stage.[58] Accordingly, to encourage genetic testing by at-risk individuals it is extremely important to remove the economic disincentives to genetic testing by prohibiting the use of genetic test results in life insurance underwriting.[59]

The federal Genetic Information Nondiscrimination Act of 2008 prohibits discrimination based on genetic information only in employment and health insurance.[60] Several states also have enacted laws dealing with genetics and life insurance, but these laws have negligible value. For example, laws requiring informed consent for genetic testing are currently irrelevant because there is no insurer-mandated genetic testing. Similarly, laws requiring that any use of genetic information must be actuarially justified are superfluous because actuarial justification already is required by consumer protection laws. Only Florida prohibits life insurers from using genetic test results in underwriting.[61] In all other states, the lack of genetic privacy and non-discrimination legislation can result in higher rates of morbidity and mortality.[62]

The United States is an outlier among high-income countries by not prohibiting the use of genetic information in life insurance underwriting.[63] Australia, Canada, France, Germany, South Korea, the United Kingdom, and other countries have enacted legislation or have ratified insurance industry-developed moratoria on using genetic information. There is no evidence that any of these measures has resulted in increased costs or decreased availability for individuals, or financial distress for life insurance companies.[64]

Comprehensive legal protections

A variety of comprehensive, extensive, and innovative laws, such as the European Union's General Data Protection Regulation (GDPR),[65] have been enacted by nations around the world to protect personal data, including health information. By contrast, in the United States, there is no comprehensive, national law protecting personal health information. By default, the main applicable law is the Health Insurance Portability and Accountability Act (HIPAA) of 1996,[66] with its well-known Privacy Rule.[67] Other HIPAA regulations address security,[68] breach notification,[69] interoperability,[70] and administrative requirements.[71] In general terms, the EU's GDPR prohibits the use or disclosure of personal data unless there is a specific provision authorizing it; the HIPAA Privacy Rule permits such disclosures unless there is a specific provision prohibiting it.

HIPAA privacy rule

The HIPAA statute was designed to promote mobility in employment by requiring that employment-based health coverage is portable when an employee moves from one employer to another. Because its statutory focus is health insurance, the HIPAA Privacy Rule only applies to entities in the healthcare payment chain: health providers (e.g. hospitals), health plans (e.g. health insurers), health clearinghouses (technology companies that put health claims in standard electronic formats), and the business associates of covered entities (businesses that assist covered entities perform functions related to the payment chain, such as claims processing). It does not cover life, disability, or long-term care insurance companies; employers outside of healthcare; banks, mortgage companies, and other financial institutions; educational institutions; medical websites; or mobile health app developers. However, some of these entities (e.g. educational institutions[72]) are covered under other federal or state laws.

Besides limited coverage, the Privacy Rule also has limited protections. It only applies to individually identifiable health information. After a covered entity provides individuals with a notice of its privacy practices, no additional consent or authorization is necessary for uses and disclosures of health information for treatment, payment, or a broad category of healthcare operations including quality assessment, accreditation and licensing, and general administrative activities. The Privacy Rule does not afford special protection for sensitive information other than psychotherapy notes. Furthermore, individuals have no right to bring a private lawsuit to obtain compensation for harm caused by a violation of the Privacy Rule; they are merely permitted to file a complaint with the US Department of Health and Human Services.[73]

The HIPAA Privacy Rule's 12 public purpose exceptions exemplify the balancing of costs and benefits in health privacy regulations. In attempting to ensure the flow of health information to benefit the public, the Privacy Rule permits a healthcare provider or other covered entity to disclose individual health information in the following categories without specific notice to or consent, or authorization from the individual whose records are disclosed.

1   If required by law.
2   For public health activities, such as vital statistics and public health surveillance.
3   About victims of abuse, neglect, or domestic violence.
4   For health oversight activities.
5   For disclosures for judicial or administrative proceedings.
6   For law enforcement.
7   For uses and disclosures about decedents.
8   For uses and disclosures for cadaveric organ, eye, or tissue donation.

9   For some research purposes.
10 For uses and disclosures to avert a serious threat to health or safety, such as when a mental health patient discloses an intent to murder another person.
11 For uses and disclosures for specialized government functions, including national security.
12 For disclosures for workers' compensation.[74]

The Privacy Rule does not mandate any of these disclosures. A legal obligation to disclose information must come from another source, such as a public health law or a domestic violence reporting law. In addition, a covered entity may voluntarily disclose information under one of the exceptions. By broadly defining the scope of these permissive disclosures by covered entities, the Privacy Rule has accorded greater importance to the disclosure of health information than health privacy in these categories.[75]

For example, few people would question the national security exception permitting a hospital to disclose to government officials the health records of suspected terrorists who received treatment for their wounds after an explosion and then staged a violent escape from the hospital. But many people might question using the broad law enforcement exception (which does not require a warrant, court order, or other legal process) to give police access to numerous hospital records to aid in a preliminary search for information about a suspected shoplifter who might have received treatment after a scuffle with a shopkeeper.[76]

Consumer privacy and reproductive health privacy laws

In the last decade, at least 16 US states have enacted consumer privacy protection acts,[77] inspired by the GDPR and the perceived need to protect privacy and prevent the non-consensual monetization of online and other consumer information. The first and most stringent of these laws, enacted in California,[78] establishes rules for the collection, use, disclosure, sale, and retention of the personal information of consumers. Regrettably, it exempts healthcare providers (presumably because they are covered by the HIPAA Privacy Rule or a state health privacy statute) and thus it provides greater protection for the records of common consumer transactions than sensitive health information.[79]

New state laws also attempt to protect reproductive health privacy. A highly controversial decision of the US Supreme Court in 2022[80] overruled nearly 50 years of precedent[81] and held that there is no longer a federal constitutional right to abortion (see also Chapter 1 in this volume by Graeme Laurie), which resulted in about half the states severely limiting or prohibiting abortions. Some states in which abortion remains legal have enacted reproductive health privacy laws to prevent anti-abortion groups from identifying women, including those from out of state, who obtain lawful abortions.[82] Among the provisions of these laws are protections against the non-consensual disclosure of reproductive health information, information about medication used for abortions, and disclosure of mobile phone geolocation information indicating an individual's proximity to an abortion clinic ("geofencing"). Thus, the continuing political debate about abortion also has important health privacy implications.

Age-related differences in health privacy concerns

A common argument by individuals who oppose expanding or even maintaining current levels of health privacy protection is that doing so is a waste of time and money because younger generations do not have the same concerns about privacy—including health privacy—as older generations. They point to the extensive online sharing of highly personal information, photos, and videos by young people, and they also note the increased technical, practical, and financial burdens of protecting privacy.

An online survey of 1,319 individuals published in 2017 attempted to determine whether there are substantial intergenerational differences in views about the importance of health privacy.[83] The answers to one question were especially revealing. The following percentage of respondents, divided by age cohort, indicated they were "somewhat concerned" or "very concerned" about health privacy (Table 7.1).

These responses support two important inferences. First, although respondents in an online survey might be assumed to have fewer concerns about privacy (including health privacy) than the general population, all age groups, including the youngest group, indicated a significant level of concern, with the oldest three groups having about the same level of concern. Second, a more granular analysis of the views of the youngest respondents indicated a significant increase in concern as they approached age 30. This is the age

TABLE 7.1 Concerns about Health Privacy by Age Group. $n = 1319$.

Age	Percent
18–28	58
29–35	73
36–51	71
52–70	74

Source: Stacey Pereira and others, "Do Privacy and Security Regulations Need a Status Update? Perspectives from an Intergenerational Survey" (2017) 12 *PLoS One* e0184525, http://doi.org/10.1371/journal.pone.0184525

when many people become concerned about their ability to obtain various types of insurance, a home mortgage, or consumer credit.

The realization by young adults of the possible economic consequences of health information could help to explain an increased concern about health privacy by people as they neared age 30. Thus, rather than confirming the hypothesis of intergenerational differences, another interpretation of the data is that relatively less concern about health privacy by 18- to 28-year-olds reflects the life stage of the youngest group and that, over time, the level of concern for health privacy by this cohort is likely to be comparable to that of older generations.

Conclusion: Costs and benefits in context

This chapter explored a wide sample of topics on the costs and benefits of health privacy, including the role of technology, healthcare systems, legislation, and individual values. Two main conclusions flow from this far-flung discussion.

First, there are significant costs associated with health privacy as well as a lack of it. Therefore, policies addressing health privacy should consider myriad financial and non-financial costs along with tangible and intangible benefits.

Second, the question of whether health privacy is "worth the cost" is complicated by the numerous circumstances in which it arises. On a societal level, the answer depends on the overall risks and benefits of disclosing certain types of health information, including to whom, in what form, and for what purpose. On a personal level, the answer may depend on the individual's age, health status, socio-economic position, cultural background, psychological disposition, and risk tolerance.

Challenges to one's health of a sensitive nature are inescapable elements of the human condition. EHRs, big data analytics, consolidation in healthcare, and other factors have increased the risks and magnitude of harm from nonclinicians accessing, using, storing, and disclosing highly personal health information. Unfortunately, at least in the United States, minimal legal protections and vague principles of professional ethics are inadequate to address the crucial, complex, and constantly evolving issues of health privacy.

Comprehensive health privacy laws are unlikely to be enacted in the United States unless there is a public consensus that the cost of safeguarding health privacy is a reasonable price to pay for living in a society that respects the dignity, autonomy, emotional well-being, and personal space of every individual. In the absence of such legislation, even more modest, limited measures as outlined in this chapter can still make a vital and significant improvement to informational health privacy. Yes, health privacy is worth the cost.

Acknowledgements

Kelly Carty Zimmerer, J.D. 2024, Louis D. Brandeis School of Law, University of Louisville, provided outstanding research assistance.

Notes

1 "Oath of Hippocrates," reprinted in Warren Thomas Reich (ed), *Encyclopedia of Bioethics* (rev. edn, vol. 5, Simon & Schuster MacMillan 1995), Appendix, at 2632.
2 Steven Miles, *The Hippocratic Oath and the Ethics of Medicine* (Oxford University Press 2004), at 149.
3 Mark A Rothstein, "The Hippocratic Bargain and Health Information Technology" (2010) 38 *Journal of Law, Medicine & Ethics* 7.
4 Thomas Beauchamp and James Childress, *Principles of Biomedical Ethics* (8th edn, Oxford University Press 2019), at 13.
5 American Medical Association, *Code of Medical Ethics of the American Medical Association* (American Medical Association 2017), at xiii.
6 Robert Gelman, "Prescribing Privacy: The Uncertain Role of the Physician in the Protection of Patient Privacy" (1984) 62 *North Carolina Law Review* 255.
7 Health Information & the Law, George Washington University Hirsh Health Law and Policy Program. States, available at: http://www.healthinfolaw.org/state.
8 James Coleman and others, "Seyfarth. 50-State Survey of Health Care Information Privacy Laws" (2021), available at: https://www.seyfarth.com/a/web/77459/50-State-Survey-of-Health-Care-Information-Privacy-Laws.pdf.
9 Anne Slowther and Irwin Kleinman, "Confidentiality", in Peter Singer and Adrien Viens (eds), *The Cambridge Textbook of Bioethics* (Cambridge University Press 2008), at 4–5; William Winslade, "Confidentiality," in Warren Thomas Reich (ed), *Encyclopedia of Bioethics* (rev. edn, vol. 1, Simon & Schuster MacMillan 1995), at 453.
10 Mark Siegler, "Confidentiality in Medicine—A Decrepit Concept" (1982) 307 *New England Journal of Medicine* 1518.
11 Paul Ohm, "Broken Promises of Privacy: Responding to the Surprising Failure of Anonymization" (2010) 57 *UCLA Law Review* 1701.
12 Mark A Rothstein, "The Illusion of Health Privacy in Obstetrics-Gynecology" (2023) 66 *Clinical Obstetrics and Gynecology* 267.
13 Chen Hsi Tsai and others, "Effects of Electronic Health Record Implementation and Barriers to Adoption and Use: A Scoping Review and Qualitative Analysis of the Content" (2020) 10 *Life (Basel)* 327; Samara Rosenfeld, "U.S. Is Lagging Behind in Digital Health Technology Adoption", Chief Healthcare Executive, 2019, available at: https://www.chiefhealthcareexecutive.com/view/us-is-lagging-behind-in-digital-health-technology-adoption.
14 Health Information Technology for Economic and Clinical Health Act (HI-TECH Act) of 2009, part of the American Recovery and Reinvestment Act of 2009, 42 U.S.C. § 1320d.
15 R Scott Evans, "Electronic Health Records: Then, Now, and in the Future" (2016) (Suppl 1) *Yearbook of Medical Informatics* S48.
16 Office of the National Coordinator for Health Information Technology. Office-based Physician Electronic Record Adoption. Health IT website, 2019, available at: http://www.healthit.gov/data/quickstats/office-based-phsician-electronic-health-record-adoption.

17 Office of the National Coordinator for Health Information Technology. Hospitals' Use of Electronic Health Records Data, 2015–2017 (2019), available at: https://www.healthit.gov/sites/default/files/page/2019-04/AHAEHRUseDataBrief.pdf.

18 Ofir Ben-Assuli, "Electronic Health Records, Adoptions, Quality of Care, Legal and Privacy Issues and their Implementation in Emergency Departments" (2015) 119 *Health Policy* 287; Jonathan Carter, "Electronic Medical Records and Quality Improvement" (2015) 26 *Neurosurgery Clinics of North America* 245; Brian Rothman, Joan Leonard, and Michael Vigoda, "Future of Electronic Health Records: Implications for Decision Support" (2012) 79 *Mount Sinai Journal of Medicine* 757.

19 Annie Burky, "Majority of Patients Repeatedly Provide Duplicate Health Information, Carta Healthcare Survey Finds", Fierce Healthcare (30 January 2023), available at: https://www.fiercehealthcare.com/health-tech/carta-healthcare-survey-finds-83-patients-repeatedly-providing-duplicate-health.

20 David Blumenthal, "A Step Toward Interoperability of Health IT" (2022) 387 *New England Journal of Medicine* 2201; Eric Setterlund and Melissa Soliz, "If You Build It, They Will Come: Implementing the CMS Patient Access APR and Payer-to-Payer Exchange Requirements" (2021) 15 *Journal of Health and Life Sciences Law* 30.

21 Katie Walker, Tim Dwyer, and Heather Heaton, "Emergency Medicine Electronic Health Record Usability: Where to from Here?" (2021) 38 *Emergency Medicine Journal* 408; Alexandra Mullins and others, "Health Outcomes and Healthcare Efficiencies Associated with the Use of Electronic Health Records and Hospital Emergency Departments: A Systematic Review" (2020) 44 *Journal of Medical Systems* 200.

22 Clemens Scott Kruse, "Physician Burnout and the Electronic Health Record Leading Up to and During the First Year of COVID-19: Systematic Review" (2022) 24 *Journal of Medical Internet Research* e36200, doi: 10.2196/36200.

23 Mark A Rothstein, "Health Privacy in the Electronic Age" (2007) 28 *Journal of Legal Medicine* 487.

24 Sigall Bell and others, "Frequency and Types of Patient-Reported Errors in Electronic Health Record Ambulatory Care Notes" (2020) 3 *JAMA Network Open* e205867; Amy Linsky and Steven Simon, "Medical Discrepancies in Integrated Electronic Health Records" (2013) 22 *BMJ Quality & Safety* 103.

25 Milton Corn, "Archiving the Phenome: Clinical Records Deserve Long-term Preservation" (2009) 16 *Journal of the American Medical Informatics Association* 1; State Medical Record Laws: Minimum Medical Record Retention Periods for Records Held by Medical Doctors and Hospitals. Health IT, available at: https://www.healthit.gov/sites/default/files/appa7-1.pdf.

26 United Kingdom Information Commissioner's Office, "Right to Erasure" (2023), available at: https://ico.org.uk/for-organisations/uk-gdpr-guidance-and-resources/individual-rights/individual-rights/right-to-erasure/.

27 Eugenia Politou and others, "The 'Right to Be Forgotten' in the GDPR: Implementation Challenges and Potential Solutions", in Eugenia Politou and others (eds), *Privacy and Data Protection Challenges in the Distributed Era* (Springer 2021), at 41–68.

28 *Cruzan* v *Director, Missouri Department of Health*, 497 U.S. 261 (1990).

29 Julie Agris, "Extending the Minimum Necessary Standard to Uses and Disclosures for Treatment" (2014) 42 *Journal of Law, Medicine & Ethics* 263.

30 Denis Campbell, "Warnings Over NHS Data Privacy after 'Stalker' Doctor Shares Woman's Records" *The Guardian* (14 May 2023), available at: https://www.theguardian.com/society/2023/may/14/nhs-england-data-privacy-confidentiality-records-addenbrookes-hospital.

31 Mark A Rothstein and Stacey Tovino, "Privacy Risks of Interoperable Electronic Health Records: Segmentation of Sensitive Information Will Help" (2019) 47 *Journal of Law, Medicine & Ethics* 771.

32 45 C.F.R. § 164.508(a)(2).

33 45 C.F.R. § 164.506(b).

34 Rachel Benson Gold, "Unintended Consequences: How Insurance Processes Inadvertently Abrogate Patient Confidentiality" (2009) 12 *Guttmacher Policy Review* 12, available at: https://www.guttmacher.org/gpr/2009/11/unintended-consequences-how-insurance-processes-inadvertently-abrogate-patient.

35 Monica Lutgendorf, "Intimate Partner Violence and Women's Health" (2019) 134 *Obstetrics & Gynecology* 470.

36 Society for Adolescent Health and Medicine and the American Academy of Pediatrics, "Confidentiality Protecting for Adolescents and Young Adults in the Health Care Billing and Insurance Claims Process" (2016) 58 *Journal of Adolescent Health* 374.

37 Protecting Confidentiality for Individuals Insured as Dependents, Guttmacher Institute (1 July 2023), available at: https://www.guttmacher.org/state-policy/explore/protecting-confidentiality-individuals-insured-dependents.

38 B Jessie Hill, "Minors' Right to Access Sexual and Reproductive Health Care" (2023) 113 *American Journal of Public Health* 350.

39 Rachel Goldstein and others, "Providers' Perspectives on Adolescent Confidentiality and the Electronic Health Record: A State of Transition" (2020) 66 *Journal of Adolescent Health* 296.

40 Howard Dubowitz and Susan J Kressly, "Documenting Psychosocial Problems in Children's Electronic Health Records" (2023) 177 *JAMA Pediatrics* 881.

41 Christophe Schneble, Bernice Elger, and David Shaw, "All Our Data Will Be Health Data One Day: The Need for Universal Data Protection and Comprehensive Consent" (2019) 22 *Journal of Medical Internet Research* e16879.

42 Bhavneet Bhinder and others, "Artificial Intelligence in Cancer Research and Precision Medicine" (2023) 11 *Cancer Discovery* 900; Mark A Rothstein, "Big Data, Surveillance Capitalism, and Precision Medicine: Challenges for Privacy" (2021) 49 *Journal of Law, Medicine & Ethics* 666; Giovanni Rubeis, "Liquid Health. Medicine in the Age of Surveillance Capitalism" (2023) 322 *Social Science & Medicine* 115810, doi: 10.1016/j.socscimed.2023.

43 John Halamka, "Early Experiences with Big Data at an Academic Medical Center" (2014) 33 *Health Affairs* 1132.

44 Silvana Secinaro and others, "The Role of Artificial Intelligence in Healthcare: A Structured Literature Review" (2021) 21 *BMC Medical Informatics and Decision Making* 125.

45 Inke König and others, "What Is Precision Medicine?" (2017) 50 *European Respiratory Journal* 1700391.

46 Mark A Rothstein, "Structural Challenges of Precision Medicine" (2017) 45 *Journal of Law, Medicine & Ethics* 274, 276.

47 Sharona Hoffman, *Electronic Health Records and Medical Big Data* (Cambridge University Press 2016).

48 Jeremy Wacksman, "Digitization of Contract Tracing: Balancing Data Privacy with Public Health Benefit" (2021) 23 *Ethics and Information Technology* 855.

49 United States Department of Health and Human Services, National Institutes of Health, All of Us Research Program. Available at: https://allofus.nih.gov/about/program-overview.

50 Heather Harrell and Mark A Rothstein, "Biobanking Research and Privacy Laws in the United States" (2016) 44 *Journal of Law, Medicine & Ethics* 106.

51 Edward S Dove, "Biobanks, Data Sharing, and the Drive for a Global Privacy Governance Framework" (2015) 43 *Journal of Law, Medicine & Ethics* 675; Mark A Rothstein, Bartha Knoppers, and Heather Harrell, "Comparative Approaches to Biobanks and Privacy" (2016) 44 *Journal of Law, Medicine & Ethics* 161.

52 Mark A Rothstein, "Is Deidentification Sufficient to Protect Health Privacy in Research?" (2010) 10 *American Journal of Bioethics* 3.

53 Yann Joly, "Are Data Sharing and Privacy Protection Mutually Exclusive?" (2016) 167 Cell 1150; Rasmus Bjerregaard Mikkelsen and others, "Broad Consent for Biobanks Is Best—Provided It Is Also Deep" (2019) 20 *BMC Medical Ethics* 71.

54 PJ Fortun and others, "Recall of Informed Consent by Healthy Volunteers in Clinical Trials" (2008) 101 *QJM: An International Journal of Medicine* 625.

55 Mark A Rothstein and Meghan Talbott, "Compelled Disclosure of Health Records: Updated Estimates" (2017) 45 *Journal of Law, Medicine & Ethics* 149.

56 Robert Green, Denise Lautenbach, and Amy McGuire, "GINA, Genetic Discrimination, and Genomic Medicine" (2015) 372 *New England Journal of Medicine* 397.

57 Allison Kurian and others, "Genetic Testing and Counseling among Patients with Newly Diagnosed Breast Cancer" (2017) 317 *Journal of the American Medical Association* 531.

58 Tal Hadar and others, "Presymptomatic Awareness of Germline Pathogenic BRCA Variants and Associated Outcomes in Women with Breast Cancer" (2020) 6 *JAMA Oncology* 1460.

59 Mark A Rothstein, "Can Genetic Nondiscrimination Laws Save Lives?" (2021) 51 *Hastings Center Report* 6.

60 42 U.S.C. § 2000ff.

61 Fla. Stat. § 627.4301.

62 Mark A Rothstein and Kyle Brothers, "Banning Genetic Discrimination in Life Insurance: Time to Follow Florida's Lead" (2020) 383 *New England Journal of Medicine* 2099; Mark A Rothstein, "Time to End the Use of Genetic Test Results in Life Insurance Underwriting" (2018) 46 *Journal of Law, Medicine & Ethics* 794.

63 Jean-Christophe Belisle-Pipon and others, "Genetic Testing, Insurance Discrimination and Medical Research: What the United States Can Learn from Peer Countries" (2019) 25 *Nature Medicine* 1198.

64 Yann Joly and others, "Looking Beyond GINA: Policy Approaches to Address Genetic Discrimination" (2020) 21 *Annual Reviews of Genomics and Human Genetics* 491.

65 Regulation (EU) 2016/679 of the European Parliament and of the Council of 27 April 2016 on the protection of natural persons with regard to the processing of personal data and on the free movement of such data, and repealing Directive 95/46/EC (General Data Protection Regulation); Edward S Dove, "The EU General Data Protection Regulation: Implications for International Scientific Research in the Digital Era" (2018) 46 *Journal of Law, Medicine & Ethics* 1013.

66 42 U.S.C. §§ 300gg-300gg-2.

67 HIPAA Administrative Simplification, 45 C.F.R. Pts. 160, 164E.

68 Security and Privacy, General Provisions, 45 C.F.R. Pt. 164A.

69 Notification in the Case of Breach of Unsecured Protected Health Information, 45 C.F.R. Pt. 164D.

70 Centers for Medicare and Medicaid Services, "Interoperability and Patient Access Final Rule" (2020) 85 *Federal Register* 25510–25640.

71 Administrative Requirements, 45 C.F.R. Pt. 162.

72 Family Educational Records and Privacy Act of 1974, 20 U.S.C. § 1232g.

73 U.S. Department of Health and Human Services, Summary of the HIPAA Privacy Rule, available at: http://hhs.gov/hipaa/for-professionals/privacy/laws-regulations/index.html.
74 45 C.F.R. § 164.512.
75 Richard Sobel, "The HIPAA Paradox: The Privacy Rule That's Not" (2007) 37 *Hastings Center Report* 40.
76 Eileen Baker and others, "Law Enforcement and Emergency Medicine: An Ethical Analysis" (2016) 68 *Annals of Emergency Medicine* 599.
77 California, Colorado, Connecticut, Delaware, Florida, Iowa, Indiana, Maryland, Montana, New Jersey, Oregon, Tennessee, Texas, Utah, Vermont, and Virginia.
78 California Consumer Privacy Act of 2018, Cal. Civ. Code § 1798.100-.192.
79 Mark A Rothstein and Stacey Tovino, "California Takes the Lead on Data Privacy Law" (2019) 49 *Hastings Center Report* 4.
80 *Dobbs* v *Jackson Women's Health Organization*, 597 US 215 (2022).
81 *Roe* v *Wade*, 410 US 113 (1973).
82 The states include California, Connecticut, Maryland, Nevada, New York, and Washington.
83 Stacey Pereira and others, "Do Privacy and Security Regulations Need a Status Update? Perspectives from an Intergenerational Survey" (2017) 12 *PLoS One* e0184525, doi: 10.1371/journal.pone.0184525.

8

MISUSE OF PRIVATE INFORMATION AND THE COMMON LAW RIGHT OF PRIVACY

A new frontier in biomedicine?

Edward S. Dove

Introduction

In the United Kingdom (UK), health information relating to identifiable individuals is protected under several legal regimes. This includes confidentiality law, as reflected in the common law duty of confidentiality (protected under equitable obligation and sometimes also a contractual obligation) and data protection law, as reflected primarily in legislation such as the Data Protection Act 2018 and UK General Data Protection Regulation. Health information is also protected under human rights law, as reflected in the Human Rights Act 1998 (HRA 1998), which domesticates the European Convention on Human Rights (ECHR)[1] and provides protection against a public authority for violating a Convention right.[2] Specifically, Article 8(1) ECHR provides that everyone has a "right to respect for his private and family life, his home and his correspondence". Case law has long established that this right to private life extends to one's health information.[3]

While there are several regimes of legal protection today, it was not always this way. Gaps existed for decades. The UK was something of an outlier in common law jurisdictions for failing to protect citizens' privacy in a broader sense, including one's sphere of non-intrusion into their private life and protection against misuse of their personal information. In recent years, however, and in particular since the 2004 House of Lords *Campbell* case that I discuss below, a new legal frontier has emerged in the UK that is seen as beginning to seal these gaps: "a civil wrong for intrusions of privacy".[4] Specifically, English common law now affords protection against the misuse of one's private information through domestic tort law, and in Scotland, there is also now recognition of a

DOI: 10.4324/9781003394518-11

stand-alone "right of privacy" in the common law that appears to be justiciable.

This raises several points of query. What caused this new form of legal protection to emerge, and what is this new regime's relationship with the longer-standing regimes of legal protection? As we will see, legal development was largely spurred by the coming into force of the HRA 1998, but as Rowbottom notes, "While Article 8 [ECHR] and the HRA 1998 allowed for the interpretation taken in *Campbell*, it did not mandate the development of a new tort".[5] This, then, also raises questions about the relationship between human rights law and tort law. We know that in UK jurisdictions, the ECHR is not directly effective in "horizontal" cases (i.e. cases between private parties not involving the state or its institutions), but that it is indirectly effective, operating through existing domestic legal mechanisms such as common law doctrines. But what does this mean in practice? Can an aggrieved individual whose health information has been wrongfully accessed and misused sue, in principle, on the multiple-headed claims of data protection breach, breach of confidentiality, violation of Article 8 ECHR (as a sui generis cause of action arising directly out of the HRA 1998 against a public authority[6]), *and* misuse of private information? If so, what is the nature of this multi-headed hydra, and what are the implications for the reach of privacy-related rights?

For years, legal scholars and judges recognized that confidentiality and privacy ought to be seen as distinct concepts deserving different kinds of legal protection, with the former focused more (but not exclusively) on the relationship between the parties and the latter more on the nature of the underlying object deserving privacy protection. In its 1981 report, for example, the Law Commission of England and Wales observed legal differences between the "duty of confidence" and a "right of privacy":

> [...]once information has been entrusted in circumstances giving rise to an obligation of confidence, that information is in effect impressed with a duty of confidence owed to the person who has entrusted it. By contrast, a right of privacy in respect of information would arise from the nature of the information itself: it would be based on the principle that certain kinds of information are categorised as private and for that reason alone ought not to be disclosed.[7]

Yet while English law has long protected confiders of information by impressing a common law (and equitable) duty on the confidant, if not already stipulated in a contract, it has struggled to afford protection to a person whose information is wrongly used, regardless of whether a relationship exists between the individual and others. Only recently have courts given credence to the view that UK domestic law gives effect to different aspects of information pertaining to an individual: (1) a duty of confidence (often but not always established from a pre-existing relationship); (2) a human right to respect the sphere of one's private (and family) life; and (3) a gradual move towards a stand-alone right to privacy, through the tort of misuse of private information, which, at least to date, attaches only to information. This latter development puts the UK on a jurisprudential path that may deviate from the ECHR and jurisprudence from the Strasbourg judges.[8] This has significant implications in the health context.

In this chapter, I make two substantive contributions that add insight and value to this area of health privacy law. First and foremost is an effort to rationalize the law to show a way through, which hitherto has remained elusive. I explore the jurisprudential development of the emerging tort of misuse of private information (MOPI), the influence of human rights law on privacy in the biomedical domain (in particular Articles 8 and 10 ECHR[9]), and how some nations within the UK (specifically Scotland[10]) may be taking divergent approaches to a common law right of privacy, namely by significantly expanding the scope of such a right. In so doing I explain how MOPI differs from the long-standing breach of confidence claim. I argue that breach of confidence should continue to be grounded in equity, meaning a duty of trust and honour, and a duty to be of good faith that fastens on the conscience of a party which often (but not absolutely) arises out of their relationship with the confider.

Second is an effort to unpack MOPI to analyse where legal gaps might remain. I argue that both the MOPI tort and a common law right of privacy as additional forms of legal protection may be partially welcomed as "gap-filling" measures to address long-standing concerns about lack of full coverage from the other legal regimes, and this is especially valuable in a health context given the general sensitivity of much information generated, collected, and used in this area. However, these developments also raise implications for legal divergence and uncertainty within the UK. As such, these developments might thwart effective use of such information in socially and scientifically valuable cross-border national data sharing and international research endeavours.

In what follows, I begin with an overview of the development of the MOPI tort and the common law right of privacy.

The evolution of the right of privacy and MOPI under *Campbell*

As Bennett says, "the doctrine of [MOPI] has developed in a rather haphazard and undeniably murky fashion".[11] Tracing the evolution of the MOPI tort should begin prior to its "birth", which we might date to 2004, and commence with a discussion of the historic position regarding a common law right of privacy.

Through the early 21st century, UK courts refused to recognize a stand-alone right to privacy, reflecting a conservative, cautious approach to common law judicial creation of a right.[12] For example, in the "notorious"[13] 1990 case of *Kaye* v *Robertson*[14]—"a low point in the protection of privacy"[15]—and the 2003 case of *Wainwright* v *Home Office* that involved intrusive strip searches of prison visitors,[16] two higher courts, the Court of Appeal and House of Lords, respectively, took the view that "in English law there is no right to privacy, and accordingly there is no right of action for breach of a person's privacy",[17] and privacy was not "in itself a legal principle which is capable of sufficient definition to enable one to deduce specific rules to be applied in concrete cases. That is not the way the common law works".[18] In *Wainwright*, Lord Hoffmann opined that past court judgments were "flat against a judicial power to declare the existence of a high-level right to privacy" and, as such, did not "think that they suggest that the courts should do so".[19] In his view, there was "[...] a great difference between identifying privacy as a value which underlies the existence of a rule of law (and may point the direction in which the law should develop) and privacy as a principle of law in itself".[20]

And yet, both in the year before and year after *Wainwright*, the jurisprudential door began to open in recognizing privacy not just as a value but a possible legal right, particularly in the ongoing absence of legislative reform and the growing recognition that the UK *somehow* needed to give domestic legal effect to the rights delineated in the ECHR following the coming into effect of the HRA 1998 in October 2000. Further, as Rowbottom explains, "...as the issue of privacy and press ethics moved off the political agenda, the courts became more willing to take the initiative in developing the law".[21] The "unsatisfactory" outcome in cases like *Kaye* "may have helped to spur changes in the common law".[22]

First, predating *Campbell*, in the 2002 case of *A* v *B plc*,[23] Lord Woolf CJ, giving the judgment of the Court of Appeal, stated that Articles 8 and 10 ECHR provided "new parameters"[24] within which the court would decide actions for breach of confidence, and that the court could act in a way that was compatible with ECHR rights, as they were required to do under section 6 of the HRA 1998, by "[...] absorbing the rights which articles 8 and 10 protect into the long-established action for breach of confidence. This involves giving new strength and breadth to the action so that it accommodates the requirements of those Articles".[25] But why breach of confidence? Lord Woolf CJ did not say, but again, we can assume it is because English law lacked another existing (and more appropriate) cause of action to remedy a wrongful invasion of privacy. In other words, then, breach of confidence claims would have to take stock of the jurisprudence of Articles 8 and 10 ECHR and those articles would form, as a subsequent case put it, "the very content of the domestic tort that the English court has to enforce", which was the "new" misuse of private information read into the "old" existing breach of confidence.[26] Elsewhere, Lord Woolf CJ explained:

> It is most unlikely that any purpose will be served by a judge seeking to decide whether there exists a new cause of action in tort which protects privacy. In the great majority of situations, if not all situations, where the protection of privacy is justified, relating to events after the Human Rights Act came into force, *an action for breach of confidence now will, where this is appropriate, provide the necessary protection.* This means that at first instance it can be readily accepted that it is not necessary to tackle the vexed question of whether there is a separate cause of action based upon a new tort involving the infringement of privacy.
>
> [...]
>
> A duty of confidence will arise whenever the party subject to the duty is in a situation where he either knows or ought to know that the other person can reasonably expect his privacy to be protected. [...] If there is an intrusion in a situation where a person can reasonably expect his privacy to be respected then that intrusion will be capable of giving rise to liability in an action for breach of confidence unless the intrusion can be justified.[27]

This statement, of course, raises several points of contention. As breach of confidence is historically grounded in equity,[28] it is unclear what happened to this basis and whether the cause of action wholly moved from equity to common law (tort) and if not, what the relationship between equity and tort might be (recognizing that generally in law, equity is seen as a corrective to the "harshness" of common law rules). Indeed, one can query whether in cases such as this, just after the coming into effect of the HRA 1998, there was some degree of unknowing judicial sleight of hand, injecting conceptual confusion between confidentiality and privacy and their protection under the law. This is evidenced in Lord Woolf's CJ mixing of "reasonable expectation of privacy" and "liability in an action for breach of confidence" in the same breath, and it becomes further apparent in later cases such as *McKennitt* v *Ash*, in which Buxton LJ observed that:

> [...] in developing a right to protect private information, including the implementation in the English courts of articles 8 and 10 of the European Convention on Human Rights, the English courts have to proceed through *the tort of breach of confidence*, into which the jurisprudence of articles 8 and 10 has to be "shoehorned" *Douglas v Hello! (No3)* [2006] QB 125 [53].[29]

But the real watershed in the strange development of MOPI, and of the right of privacy more generally in England, can be traced to the case of *Campbell v MGN Ltd*.[30] In this case, the House of Lords considered whether the media publishing company MGN Ltd had breached supermodel Naomi Campbell's right of confidentiality when it published details about her drug addiction and therapy at Narcotics Anonymous in the tabloid newspaper *The Mirror*, and whether a duty of confidence arose at all and if so, on whom did it fall.[31] Their Lordships were unanimous on the principles to be applied and all concluded that the newspaper in question had been justified (in light of Ms Campbell's public profile and previous public claims) in publishing the fact that she was a drug addict and was receiving treatment. A majority also held that the newspaper in question had *not* been justified in publishing further information relating to the name of the clinic at which she was receiving treatment, the details of that treatment, and a photograph of her leaving a specific meeting with other addicts.

The question arose, however, whether—and if so, how—the common law action for breach of confidence was to be interpreted in line with Article 8 ECHR. The judges struggled to differentiate confidentiality and privacy, both conceptually and in law. In the decision, the judges split in interesting ways, ultimately ruling 3–2 in favour of Ms Campbell that her privacy interests had been violated (note, however, that the actual cause of action pleaded was breach of confidence and a violation of data protection law). In leading speeches for the majority, Lord Hope and Baroness Hale held that Ms Campbell's privacy interests in the detailed information about her treatment, as well as the photographs, were protected by an action for breach of confidence.[32]

For the purposes of this chapter, I want to highlight the judgments of Lord Nicholls and Lord Hoffmann. Under the heading "Breach of Confidence: Misuse of Private Information", Lord Nicholls charted an entirely new path for the long-standing breach of confidence claim. While re-asserting that there was no overarching, all-embracing cause of action for "invasion of privacy" in the UK (being fully aware of the House of Lords' *Wainwright* decision just a few months earlier), he observed that "protection of *various aspects* of privacy is a fast developing area of the law, here and in some other common law jurisdictions".[33] Immediately in his judgment Lord Nicholls framed the facts of the case as involving "one aspect of invasion of privacy: wrongful disclosure of private information".[34]

Lord Nicholls was clearly concerned with the breach of confidence action historically being grounded in an established relationship between confider and confidant, as well as publication of information, and the limitations this could impose on claimants whose privacy was violated in some way without there necessarily being a relationship between them and the defendant, and without there necessarily being publication.[35] For Naomi Campbell, there was no confidential relationship between her and *The Mirror* (although the information about Campbell's attendance at Narcotics Anonymous had been communicated to *The Mirror* in breach of confidence from an unknown source and it was held that *The Mirror* must have known that the information was confidential). There was, however, publication of her intimate details and accompanying photographs.

In Lord Nicholls' view, the common law long afforded protection to the wrongful use of private information by means of the cause of action in breach of confidence, but that this nomenclature was now "misleading" in the 21st century. And more than just nomenclature, the fundamental nature of the cause of action had changed: Lord Nicholls opined that the confidence referred to in the phrase "breach of confidence" was historically the confidence arising out of a *confidential relationship*, but this was now a "limiting constraint" no longer needed in the 21st century and since the HRA 1998 came into force. Now, the law ought to recognize a duty (and corresponding right) "whenever a person receives information he knows or ought to know is fairly and reasonably to be regarded as [private]".[36] "The essence of the tort", Lord Nicholls continued, without explaining how the underlying basis would shift from equity to tort,[37] "is better encapsulated now as misuse of private information".[38] Harking back to *Wainwright*, Lord Nicholls explained that this tort "[…] affords respect for one aspect of an individual's privacy. That is the value underlying this cause of action. An individual's privacy can be invaded in ways not involving publication of information. Strip-searches are an example".[39] Lord Nicholls did not clarify whether this new misuse of private information tort, grounded in the value (and human right) of respect for one's privacy, could cover other kinds of invasions to one's privacy, including intrusions upon their person such as strip searches. As he put it:

> The extent to which the common law as developed thus far in this country protects other forms of invasion of privacy is not a matter arising in the present case. It does not arise because, although pleaded more widely, Miss Campbell's common law claim was throughout presented in court exclusively on the basis of breach of confidence, that is, the wrongful publication by the 'Mirror' of private information.[40]

Lord Nicholls was suggesting a common law expansion of recognizing privacy as a value *and* right to be protected, albeit under certain "forms" and not as a stand-alone, overarching right. He was also suggesting folding this into an *expanded* breach of confidence claim that would *encompass* misuse of private information, itself one form of invasion of privacy, assessed in light of Article 8 ECHR (as well as freedom of the press under Article 10 ECHR),[41] and with a key consideration being that, "Essentially the touchstone of private life is whether in respect of the disclosed facts the person in question had a reasonable expectation of privacy".[42]

For his part, Lord Hoffmann also considered there to be a step-change in the legal recognition of protecting private information its own right and that this ought to *differ* from older forms of breach of confidence claims:

> In recent years, however, there have been two developments of the law of confidence, typical of the capacity of the common law to adapt itself to the needs of contemporary life. One has been an acknowledgement of the artificiality of distinguishing between confidential information obtained through the violation of a confidential relationship and similar information obtained in some other way. The second has been the acceptance, under the influence of human rights instruments such as article 8 of the European Convention, of the privacy of personal information as something worthy of protection in its own right.[43]

Lord Hoffmann appeared to agree in some ways with Lord Nicholls regarding the shift in breach of confidence as a cause of action, suggesting a move away from confidentiality law's focus on the conscience of the defendant and to a rights-based focus, thanks to the HRA 1998, which identified "private information as something worth protecting as an aspect of human autonomy and dignity".[44] He did not, however, go so far as to explicitly reframe breach of confidence as a tort encapsulated as the misuse of private information, although he did openly question why Article 8 ECHR's protection of private information "should be worth protecting against the state but not against a private person"[45] and as such could "see no logical ground for saying that a person should have less protection against a private individual than he would have against the state for the publication of personal information for which there is no justification".[46] Lord Hoffmann thus wanted breach of confidence to *extend* beyond its traditional confines and apply to situations like Naomi Campbell's, but without the need for creating a new common law tort as Lord Nicholls appeared to do. For him, breach of confidence should no longer be based "upon the duty of good faith applicable to confidential personal information and trade secrets alike"; instead, it ought to focus "upon the protection of human autonomy and dignity — the right to control the dissemination of information about one's private life and the right to the esteem and respect of other people".[47] Either way, Lord Hoffmann evidently also favoured pulling breach of confidence away from its equitable moorings.

At least three pertinent questions emerge from Lord Nicholls' and Lord Hoffmann's judgments. First, even if an expansion of breach of confidence was accepted as necessary in light of the HRA 1998, what was the precise legal basis for this? Was the basis grounded in confidentiality itself (and thus an expansion of equity), was it something happening in tort law linked to breach of confidence, and/or was it something emerging from human rights law that acted as a kind of trump card? Second, what were the precise drivers of this evolution and change? Again, it seems apparent that the impetus was the HRA 1998 rather than the particular facts of *Campbell* and growing judicial recognition that domestic effect in some manner of Article 8 ECHR was needed, but this is more implied than explicitly declared. Third, what would be the (new) relationship between the different areas of law implicated in this development?

What we see is that the HRA 1998 and its underlying ECHR rights slowly but surely began to take foot to address this domestic legal gap in privacy protection, albeit it in uncertain ways. In the early years subsequent to the HRA 1998 coming into force, courts struggled with how to domesticate the right to respect for private life, and seemed to suggest the long-existing equitable action for breach of confidence could be *extended* (or "absorbed" or "shoehorned", as different courts termed it) to cover the underlying value of privacy.[48] In other words, the courts seemed steadfast in their view that misuse of private information would *not* be treated as a separate cause of action; instead, the more flexible breach of confidence claim would now be modified and operate as a kind of hybrid equitable-tortious action. This cause of action would now no longer require a pre-existing relationship between claimant and defendant (even though this had already been long recognized in law, dating back to at least since *Stephens* v *Avery*[49] and the *Spycatcher* case[50])— although it would remain an important consideration—and an obligation of confidentiality could be inferred from the private nature of the information per se (so long as the claimant could show a "reasonable expectation of privacy" thereto). Questions of scope were to be determined on a case-by-case basis. As Baroness Hale put it in *Campbell*:

> Clearly outside [the] scope [of breach of confidence] is the sort of intrusion into what ought to be private which took place in *Wainwright*. Inside its scope is what has been termed 'the protection of the individual's informational autonomy' by prohibiting the publication of confidential information.[51]

In the first few years following *Campbell*, this expanded scope of the breach of confidence cause of action appeared to be the new legal position.

Yet, it has since become apparent that this expansive reading of a "new" kind of breach of confidence reflected a confused attempt by courts to give appropriate effect to the HRA 1998 and fasten Article 8 ECHR onto an existing but not perfectly fitting common law hook—rather than explicitly create a new (sui generis) tort addressing a private information misuse—and breach of confidence appeared the most appropriate. This was, as I go on to argue, only a temporary but rather unfortunate blip in the jurisprudence, roughly covering a decade following *Campbell*. We can see this play out in three key cases in this era, which I call the "decade of jurisprudential confusion". This era mixed the concepts of confidentiality and privacy and, more incoherently and damaging to the coherence of law, mixed principles of equity and tort.

The decade of jurisprudential confusion (2005–2015)

Not long after *Campbell*, there was early putative discomfort expressed by some judges in shifting away from the "old-fashioned breach of confidence",[52] which focused on conduct inconsistent with a *pre-existing relationship*, rather than "simply [...] the purloining of private information" and with no pre-existing relationship established between the parties.[53] Moreover, the elision of privacy and confidentiality through grounding a duty of *confidentiality* in tort and by reference to a reasonable expectation of *privacy* seemed to cause a fair bit of violence to the underlying principles of the duty historically grounded in equity.

The earliest of these confusing cases dates to the 2001 case of *Douglas* v *Hello! Ltd* (which became a multi-year saga of cases). This involved the actors Michael Douglas and Catherine Zeta-Jones, as well as *OK! Magazine*, who each sued the publisher that printed unauthorized photos of their wedding in *Hello!* magazine, which specializes in celebrity news and human-interest stories. The photographs had been taken surreptitiously (by an intruder), without the claimants' permission, and then sold to *Hello!*. The Douglases had earlier entered into an agreement with *OK! Magazine* (a rival of *Hello!*) granting it temporary exclusive rights to publish photographs approved by them of their wedding. The claims concerned, inter alia, breach of confidence. In the earlier cases in this judicial saga,[54] just as the HRA 1998 went into effect, we see, for instance, the Court of Appeal struggling to recognize invasion of privacy. There was no mention of "misuse of private information"; as Sedley LJ stated, the photographer who crashed their wedding likely was an intruder with whom no relationship of trust or confidence had been established, which meant the court would have to explore the law relating to privacy when it is not bolstered by considerations of confidence. But how? The court had no ready answer, and the case suggests the judges were fumbling in the dark trying to work through invasion of privacy and the relationship, if any, to breach of confidence. Sedley LJ sought to distinguish breach of confidence as long understood from the nascent right to privacy, and in ways that Lord Hoffmann would similarly take up three years later in *Campbell*:

> What a concept of privacy does, however, is accord recognition to the fact that the law has to protect not only those people whose trust has been abused but those who simply find themselves subject to an unwanted

intrusion into their personal lives. The law no longer needs to construct an artificial relationship of confidentiality between intruder and victim: it can recognise privacy itself as a legal principle drawn from the fundamental value of personal autonomy.[55]

At most, the Court could acknowledge that it and other courts, as per the HRA 1998, were obliged to develop the breach of confidence action consistently with Article 8 ECHR and that there was a growing sense that an individual *could* have a right to privacy outside the bounds of a breach of confidence action. Ultimately, the couple's attempt to gain an injunction to prevent the publication of unauthorized photographs failed because they could not expect privacy at a wedding with 250 guests: they were seeking not so much to protect their privacy as instead to control the form of publicity which ensued.

Yet by 2007, just a few years following *Campbell*, and in a later version of the *Douglas v Hello! Ltd* case (*OBG Ltd v Allan*), the House of Lords ruled 3–2, in a judgment led by Lord Hoffmann, that there was indeed a breach of confidence to *OK! Magazine* (*OK!* had sued *Hello!* for breach of confidence and for the tort of causing loss by unlawful means. The Douglases brought separate proceedings against *Hello!* and recovered modest damages, but these are not in issue in the 2007 appeal, and to which the Douglases were not parties). This was because the Douglases, by the way they arranged their wedding, were in a position to impose an obligation of confidence, the obligation was imposed for the benefit of *OK!* as well as the Douglases, and the intruding photographer was subject to that obligation in respect of the pictures which he took and sold to *Hello!*, and in turn the obligation of confidence was binding upon *Hello!* (which knew that *OK!* had an exclusive contract).

What is interesting here is Lord Nicholls' minority opinion, in which he clearly states that breach of confidence and MOPI were in fact after all *two distinct causes of action*, and that this jurisprudential development had all occurred in the span of just a couple of years:

As the law has developed breach of confidence, or misuse of confidential information, now covers *two distinct causes of action, protecting two different interests: privacy, and secret ("confidential") information*. It is important to keep these two distinct. In some instances information may qualify for protection both on grounds of privacy and confidentiality. In other instances information may be in the public domain, and not qualify for protection as confidential, and yet qualify for protection on the grounds of privacy. Privacy can be invaded by further publication of information or photographs already disclosed to the public. Conversely, and obviously, a trade secret may be protected as confidential information even though no question of personal privacy is involved.[56]

Lord Nicholls' statement above understandably would cause the judicial uncertainty reflected in subsequent cases such as *Tchenguiz* and *W, X, Y and Z*, which I discuss below. After all, in the same breath as stating there were two distinct causes of action, he also stated that these two distinct causes of action were in fact covered under the same (broad) heading of breach of confidence—"or misuse of confidential information". How could parties and legal counsel, not to mention judges, "keep these two distinct" if they fell under the same heading, a heading which historically had an equitable rather than tortious jurisdiction? Notwithstanding, the decision in *OBG Ltd* v *Allan* was significant because it, like *Tchenguiz* three years later, indicated growing judicial recognition that privacy and confidentiality had different features that ought to be treated differently under the law—this despite the fact that the ruling itself continued to muddy legal waters about the nature of ongoing developments.

And indeed, another key case demonstrating the odd judicial conflation of confidentiality and privacy comes from the Court of Appeal case of *Tchenguiz* v *Imerman*,[57] which also tentatively suggested a questioning of the rhetoric of "old" and "new" breach of confidence claims, with the latter "absorbing" misuse of private information claims. In this case, the claimant husband sued the brother of his former wife, with whom he shared an office, for breach of confidence after the ex-brother-in-law accessed the claimant's computer without his permission, obtained and copied information which was stored there, and then passed the information and documents to the wife and her solicitors. The husband claimed, among other things, an order for the delivery up of the documents, and an injunction restraining the use of the information in those documents. The access aspect is important, and I return to this below; the case establishes as authority that acquiring information (leaving aside whether it is better qualified as "private" or "confidential") about a person can, subject to important qualifiers, be actionable. Although opining that "with the 1998 [Human Rights] Act now in force, privacy is still classified as part of the confidentiality *genus*",[58] Lord Neuberger MR went on to state that:

> [...]the law should be developed and applied consistently and coherently in both privacy and "old fashioned confidence" cases, even if they sometimes may have different features. Consistency and coherence are all the more important given the substantially increased focus on the right to privacy and confidentiality, and the corresponding legal developments in this area, over the past twenty years.[59]

A final example from the decade of conceptual confusion comes from the Court of Appeal case of *W, X, Y and Z* v *The Secretary of State for Health*.[60] This case concerned a judicial review of guidance issued by the Secretary of

State for Health on implementing the National Health Service (Charges to Overseas Visitors) Regulations 2011. The claimants were four non-UK residents, who, at the stage of the issue of the claim, had been or were liable to be charged in excess of £1,000 each for NHS services they used, and were, therefore, liable to immigration sanctions if they failed to pay the charges due. The claimants challenged the lawfulness of part of the guidance, including the way in which certain non-clinical information relating to non-resident patients was transmitted by NHS Trusts and NHS Foundation Trusts to the Secretary of State, who then passed it on to the Home Office. The information included the name, date of birth, and gender of the patient, and (if known), their current address, the nationality and travel document number with expiry dates, as well as the amount and date of the debt and the NHS body to which it was owed. Among other arguments, the claimants claimed this information was "private and confidential"[61].

Under the heading "Is the Disclosure of the Information in Breach of the Claimants' Common Law Rights to Privacy/Confidentiality?", and writing for the Court, Lord Dyson MR held that:

> It is common ground that the test as to whether the disclosure of the Information to the Secretary of State and then to the Home Office breaches the claimants' common law rights to privacy and confidentiality involves two questions. The first is whether the claimants have a reasonable expectation of privacy in relation to the Information. This question is judged objectively by reference to the reasonable person of ordinary sensibilities. If they do have a reasonable expectation of privacy, the second question is whether there has been a breach of their rights to privacy and confidentiality. This requires a balancing exercise of weighing the public benefit that would be attained by the transmission of the Information against the harm that would result from the interference with the rights.[62]

As will be discussed below, this is, respectfully, an incorrect formulation of the test, even for MOPI tort claims, and unhelpfully merges "common law rights" to privacy and confidentiality (the former of which, as already discussed, has not ever been recognized in England as a stand-alone common law right) and the bases for assessing their claimed breach by a wrongdoer.

The Court held that the information in this context was neither private nor confidential by applying the MOPI test only. It considered that while the relevant information was "inherently private information", particularly because it revealed information of substance about the health "of the data subjects",[63] namely that the claimants were unwell to the extent that they had to seek medical care at a particular point in time from one or more NHS bodies, (1) there was no breach of confidence because doctors, nurses, and ancillary staff were entitled, without being in breach of that duty, to pass the relevant information to hospital administrators for the purpose of record keeping and of recovery of the charges,[64] and (2) a patient *liable to charges* would reasonably expect that, in the event of default, steps would be taken to enforce payment, which may include informing others of the fact, duration, and cost of their stay at the hospital concerned; and that to this extent their stay at the hospital "would not necessarily be kept confidential".[65] The Court went on to state that:

> We do not see how overseas visitors who, before they are treated in an NHS hospital, *are made aware of the fact that*, if they incur charges in excess of £1,000 and do not pay them within 3 months, the Information may be passed to the Secretary of State for onward transmission to the Home Office for the stated immigration purpose can have any, still less any *reasonable*, expectation that the Information will not be transmitted in precisely that way. They will, however, have a reasonable expectation of privacy in relation to the Information vis-à- vis anyone else.[66]

Concerningly, this was despite the fact that the guidance stated that

> [...] [w]hilst it is not necessary to seek the patient's consent before sharing their personal information with the Home Office, it is best practice—if possible or appropriate—to inform [the patient] that you have done so or are going to do so and why,

and that, as the Court noted three paragraphs later,

> We do not know whether all or any of the claimants were [in fact] notified in accordance with the Guidance that the Information would be disclosed to the Secretary of State and the Home Office, or whether there were any special circumstances which made such notification impracticable in their case.[67]

In other words, the basis for their judgment—the claimants were made aware in advance that their information may be shared with various bodies, including the Home Office, and thus could not assert a reasonable expectation of privacy—was not evidenced as a finding of fact.

For the purposes of this chapter, the point of emphasis to stress is that the judicial pronouncements in these cases contributed to an unfortunate conflation of confidentiality and privacy—largely the courts own doing—and that breach of confidence could transform from an equitable to tortious cause of action. Respectfully, it is my view that the *W, X, Y and Z* case especially demonstrates jurisprudential (and doctrinal) incoherence by treating privacy and confidentiality as synonymous concepts and failing to consider the relevant legal test for each. Indeed, it could hardly be said that it was "common ground" that the "the test" to determine whether a claimant's "common laws rights to privacy and confidentiality" comprised the same two-part test asking the same questions. The case has only further injected incoherence into the law and how healthcare professionals ought to uphold their duty of confidentiality *and* not misuse private information. As I will discuss in the following sections, still to date, the courts have not provided definitive guidance on working through these two concepts and how the two causes of action ought to operate in relationship to each other.

Yet, more promisingly, some judgments like *Tchenguiz* also suggested recognition that privacy and confidentiality do have distinct features that the law ought to recognize, even if they were unclear on what those distinct features were and how exactly the law was to proceed. Through 2015, then, the legal position appeared to be that breach of confidence was refashioned after the coming into force of the HRA 1998 and could encompass claims covering *both* confidentiality and privacy violations, and the jurisdictional basis for this was both equity *and* tort, or simply tort.

Yet this was not, thankfully, a long-lasting position, as Lord Nicholls himself would come to clarify just a few years after his earlier pronouncement in *Campbell*. Indeed, in years subsequent to *Campbell*, after some time of uncertainty well through the second decade of the 2000s, we now have confirmation that there are at least three firmly established, distinct heads now protecting various privacy-related interests of individuals: (1) a claim in breach of confidence; (2) a claim in MOPI; (3) a claim of a violation of data protection law. A potential fourth claim of a sui generis cause of action against a public authority for a violation of Article 8 ECHR may be possible, but is outside the scope of this chapter. What I proceed to discuss below, and what courts in the UK recognize, belatedly but more clearly, is that the concepts of confidentiality and privacy are not the same and protect different interests. Might we be entering a new era of conceptual clarity?

An emerging era of conceptual clarity (2015–): Equity returns?

In this section, I discuss several key cases, the last of which emanates from Scotland, as a means to argue that courts in the UK are belatedly coming round to the recognition that MOPI is a cause of action distinct from breach of confidence, protecting similar but different interests, and that there is growing judicial recognition of a full-standing "right to privacy". This signals that equity has not disappeared from breach of confidence. Rather, jurisprudential coherence is emerging that delineates the relationship between confidentiality and privacy and the causes of action particular to each. At the same time, I suggest that Scotland may be taking a divergent approach to a common law right of privacy, namely by significantly expanding the scope of such a right.

Some clarity would come in the 2015 case of *Vidall-Hall* v *Google*,[68] in which the Court of Appeal upheld Tugendhat J's determination[69] that MOPI was a tort rather than equitable cause of action and held that it was "[...] clear that, contrary to the submissions of the defendant, there are now two separate and distinct causes of action: an action for breach of confidence; and one for misuse of private information".[70] In the judgment of McFarlane LJ and Sharp LJ, not only did they correctly observe that

> [...] there are problems with an analysis which fails to distinguish between a breach of confidentiality and an infringement of privacy rights protected by article 8, not least because the concepts of confidence and privacy are not the same and protect different interests,[71]

they also went on to state that:

> [...] we cannot find any satisfactory or principled answer to the question why misuse of private information should not be categorised as a tort for the purposes of service out of the jurisdiction. *Misuse of private information is a civil wrong without any equitable characteristics.* We do not need to attempt to define a tort here. But if one puts aside the circumstances of its "birth", there is nothing in the nature of the claim itself to suggest that the more natural classification of it as a tort is wrong.[72]

This ruling, of course, was only somewhat helpful in clarifying the situation. It confirmed that MOPI is a separate cause of action and the basis is tort, but did not clarify whether breach of confidence still rested firmly in equity, much less what the relevant tests were to establish each cause of action. *Vidall-Hall* was a case concerned with the rules providing for service of proceedings out of the jurisdiction; it did not involve, nor need to involve, the relationship between breach of confidence and the MOPI tort. As such, the case cannot be said to adequately address the questions that emerged from the earlier long decade of jurisprudential confusion discussed above.

A bit more clarity would come, however, in the 2016 Supreme Court case of *PJS* v *News Group Newspapers Ltd.*[73] This case concerned PJS and his husband YMA, both of whom were well-known individuals in the entertainment business and together had two young children. Between 2009 and 2011, PJS had a sexual relationship with AB and, on one occasion, with AB and CD. In January 2016 the editor of the *Sun on Sunday* newspaper notified PJS that he proposed to publish AB's account of the relationship. PJS issued proceedings against the publisher, alleging that the proposed publication would be a misuse of private information and a breach of confidence.

PJS applied for an interim injunction to restrain publication pending the trial of his claim (although it should be noted that various details had already been published in magazines in the US, Canada, and Scotland and on various websites). This application required the court to balance PJS's Article 8 rights with the publisher's right to freedom of expression under Article 10 ECHR. It was also subject to section 12 of the HRA 1998, which provides that an interim injunction can only be granted if a claimant is likely to establish at trial that publication should not be allowed. Section 12 further provides that the court must have particular regard to the importance of freedom of expression and, in relation to journalistic material, to the extent to which the material has or is about to become available to the public, to the public interest in the material being published, as well as to any relevant privacy code.

By a majority of 4–1, the Court allowed PJS's appeal, and held that, inter alia, it was essential to distinguish between the claims for breach of respect for private life and for breach of confidence. As stated by Lord Neuberger:

> If PJS's case was simply based on confidentiality (or secrecy), then, while I would not characterise his claim for a permanent injunction as hopeless, it would have substantial difficulties. The [already existing] publication of the story in newspapers in the United States, Canada, and even in Scotland would not, I think, be sufficient of itself to undermine the claim for a permanent injunction on the ground of privacy.
>
> [...]
>
> However, claims based on respect for privacy and family life do not depend on confidentiality (or secrecy) alone. As Tugendhat J said in *Goodwin v News Group Newspapers Ltd* [2011] EMLR 27, para 85, "[t] he right to respect for private life embraces more than one concept". He went on to cite with approval a passage written by Dr Moreham in *Law of Privacy and the Media* (2nd ed (2011), edited by Warby, Moreham and Christie), in which she summarised "the two core components of the rights to privacy" as "unwanted access to private information and unwanted access to [or intrusion into] one's ... personal space"—what Tugendhat J characterised as "confidentiality" and "intrusion".[74]

At first glance, Lord Neuberger's statement would suggest that a majority of the Supreme Court was not only accepting of MOPI as separate from breach of confidence, but also that such a privacy breach, read under Article 8 ECHR, might in fact encompass at least two core features: misuse of private information and unwanted intrusion into one's personal space. Subsequent case law, however, has thrown cold water on this reading. As Senior Master Fontaine noted in the High Court case of *Pryor* v *Liverpool Women's NHS Foundation Trust*:

[*PJS* concerned] a claim under Art 8 of the ECHR, and for misuse of private information. The breach of confidence and invasion of privacy claims were made under Art 8. The claimant sought to protect information about his private life from publication. It is clear from the judgments that the injunction was continued to prevent misuse of private information (and breach of the right to respect for private and family life) and the *references in the judgments to "intrusion" relate to the consequences of that tort*, rather than that "intrusion" was recognised as a freestanding tort. There is also no suggestion in *PJS* that *McKennitt*, *Campbell* or *Wainwright* were no longer good law.[75]

Finally, it is worth noting an intriguing recent judgment from the Outer House of the Court of Session in Scotland. In *C v Chief Constable of the Police Service of Scotland*,[76] the ten petitioners were individual police officers against whom misconduct proceedings had been brought under the Police Service of Scotland (Conduct) Regulations 2014. The officers sought orders from the court, including: finding and declaring that the use by constables in the Police Service of Scotland of WhatsApp messages sent to, from, and among the officers for the purpose of bringing misconduct proceedings against them was incompatible with their right to respect for their private and family life in terms of Article 8 ECHR.

In his opinion, Lord Bannatyne drew heavily on Lord Nicholls' judgment in *Campbell*, and to a more limited extent the Scottish case of *Henderson v Chief Constable of Fife*.[77] He appeared to place significant weight on privacy as a "core value"[78] and a "fundamental right"[79] in Scottish society, holding that:

In the context of whether there is a right to privacy in Scots common law the above analysis of the English position [especially *Campbell*] is of assistance.

The English courts' approach to the development of the common law of privacy in *Campbell* has been to use the values which form the basis of Article 8 rights and to accept that these should be reflected in the common law.

This approach of developing the common law in light of Convention rights and in particular the development of the common law by seeking to reflect in it the values which underlie the Convention rights would in my view find favour in the Scottish courts.[80]

This holding is somewhat questionable as we know the English courts' approach to the development of the common law of privacy since *Campbell* has been haphazard, but nonetheless firmly limited to privacy in respect of personal information. Yet, based on his analysis, Lord Bannatyne held that a broad right to privacy exists in the common law of Scotland:

> I would adopt Lord Nicholls' characterisation of the importance of a right of privacy [in *Campbell*]. It is a right which can I think be described as a core value and one which is inherent in a democratic and civilised state.[81]

Moreover, Lord Bannatyne held that Article 8 ECHR would not supersede a right of privacy in common law, but that Article 8 and the European Court of Human Rights jurisprudence flowing therefrom could be used to inform and develop the common law in the area of the right to privacy.

It is important to emphasize here that Lord Bannatyne *did not* qualify this right in any way. Unlike the courts in England, there was no discussion of a separate tort (or delict, to use Scots law terminology) for "misuse of private information", in this case being the officers' WhatsApp messages. Instead, Lord Bannatyne indicated that in Scotland, all individuals are entitled to a right to privacy in all its dimensions, including intrusions upon one's personal space,[82] meaning that the outcomes in *Kaye* v *Robertson* and *Wainwright* v *Home Office* would be very different if tried in Scotland: "The nature and scope of that right would I believe be the same as that protected in terms of Article 8 [ECHR] except that it would apply to bodies other than public authorities",[83] presumably meaning private bodies and individuals as well.

So far, then, what we see is a mixed picture emerging with respect to judicial recognition of a common law "right to privacy" and the MOPI tort, and their relationship to breach of confidence. English courts, as well as the UK Supreme Court, have provided some clarity in confirming that MOPI and breach of confidence are two distinct causes of action, but have not explicated the conceptual, much less legal, differences between each in terms of the underlying values and interests they protect. Meanwhile, Scottish courts might be veering off in a different direction completely, giving unbridled judicial recognition of a common law right of privacy that fills in any gaps where breach of confidence might not suffice. Given the above discussion, and applying this analysis to the biomedical domain, we ought now to consider where we are today in the UK with protecting health information and privacy interests, and what these legal developments mean for the collection of use of such information for clinical and scientific research purposes.

Where are we today with breach of confidence and MOPI?

Before zeroing in on the significance of the MOPI tort and common law right to privacy in the biomedical domain, it is worth clarifying what the legal position is today. The contours still have yet to become solidified and in consequence, it is more important than ever to chart what pertains to a breach of confidence claim and what pertains to a MOPI claim. While these two causes of action are certainly often related, and at times might overlap, it is possible to discern differences in the individual cores and it is important to identify these in order to understand the overall legal picture. As we will see, privacy in English law remains focused on the informational domain and hitherto courts remain reluctant to protect broader, (meta)physical privacy interests.

Let us begin with the cause of action with the greatest longevity and ask what it looks like in the wake of all of the above developments. As a starting point, we must be careful to distinguish breach of confidence from MOPI and the broader label of "breach of privacy" claims. In breach of confidence claims, and particularly in the biomedical context, we are concerned with circumstances where the information would, in ordinary usage, be called "confidential information" and there would be nothing strained about recognizing a "duty of confidence" from one party to another. It is strongly arguable that, despite all of the above judicial developments, the cause of action remains grounded in equity, with the duty, once established, fastening on the conscience of one party that can be enforced as an equitable right exercisable by the other party.

In the Supreme Court case of *Bloomberg LP* v *ZXC*,[84] writing for the Court in its unanimous opinion, Lord Hamblen and Lord Stephens affirmed that MOPI "is a distinct cause of action from breach of confidence. It rests on different legal foundations and protects different interests".[85] They went on to explain that:

> The recognition that the causes of action for misuse of private information and for breach of confidence are distinct means that *there is no necessary overlap between them*. Information may be private but not confidential, or confidential but not private. To prove that information is private it is not necessary to show that it is confidential. Often, however, confidentiality and privacy will overlap and confidentiality may well be relevant to whether there is a reasonable expectation of privacy. In particular, if information is confidential that is likely to support the reasonableness of an expectation of privacy.[86]

It is also strongly arguable, then, that the basis for breach of confidence continues to rest on the three requirements set out in the foundational case of *Coco* v *AN Clark (Engineers) Ltd*,[87] which have been clarified and somewhat modified in subsequent case law.[88] This means: first, the obligation is one that is focused upon *confidential* information. Only where the relevant information is "confidential" will the law restrain a person from disclosing it; and not all information that is generated in a given context, e.g. even a clinical or clinical research encounter, always will have the necessary quality of confidence about it. Second, the information must be imparted in particular circumstances importing an obligation of confidentiality. Ordinarily, pre-existing relationships would establish such a circumstance, but there need not always be a pre-existing relationship, as jurisprudence has established.[89] In the biomedical context, one would assume the doctor-patient relationship and researcher-participant relationship to constitute circumstances in which confidential information is disclosed. Third, the confidential information must have been misused or is threatened to be misused. It is not enough that information has the necessary quality of confidence about it and is imparted in particular circumstances; something wrongful must be done with that information for the law to intervene.

By contrast, with respect to the MOPI tort, a different legal test arises, untethered to equity and ostensibly much more firmly grounded in tort law and influenced by human rights law. In assessing a MOPI claim, courts generally adopt a two-stage test addressing two broad issues:[90]

(1) whether a privacy interest (or right) is engaged at all depends on whether the claimant objectively had a "reasonable expectation of privacy" in respect of the relevant information;

(2) if this is shown, then the issue to consider is whether that reasonable expectation of privacy is outweighed by other relevant considerations and countervailing interests of the defendant, such as the defendant's own rights (e.g. Article 10 ECHR), the rights of others, and/or a public interest in receiving (via e.g. publication) the information.

In *Bloomberg*,[91] Lord Hamblen and Lord Stephens endorsed this two-stage framework, which will be further explained below. The language in the framework also confirms that whereas in the earliest stages of the emerging doctrine, MOPI was considered an "interright conflict" between Article 8 and Article 10 ECHR, it has since evolved, pulling away from ECHR language, to encompass actions well outside contexts "involving high-profile claimants seeking to restrain publication of personal information by tabloid defendants",[92] including individuals who wish to protect their health information against misuse.

This is not to say, however, that *Bloomberg* has clarified all the issues. Indeed, the case in my view unfortunately generates as many questions as it answers. In particular, it is somewhat unclear why counsel for ZXC pleaded the case as a MOPI tort rather than a breach of confidence. After all, the facts evidenced that Bloomberg published information surreptitiously obtained from a UK law enforcement body's confidential Letter of Request sent to a foreign state. The Supreme Court noted that the likely source for the information published in the Bloomberg article was someone employed by the UK law enforcement body, and the Letter of Request itself was headed "CONFIDENTIAL LETTER OF REQUEST" and contained therein a statement under the heading "Confidentiality" that the information in the letter was to be treated confidentiality. In other words, there was every reason to think the cause of action most relevant in this case was breach of confidence rather than MOPI. In the High Court judgment, Mr Justice Nicklin observed only that "The Claimant originally included also claims for breach of confidence and breaches of the Data Protection Act 1998, but these claims have fallen away".[93]

One can surmise that given the ongoing jurisprudential uncertainty regarding the relationship between the two causes of action, and perhaps uncertainty about the relevant test to establish breach of confidence, ZXC's counsel felt more confident pleading the cause of action in tort rather than equity. Moreover, perhaps because the author of the letter, the UK law enforcement body itself, did not pursue a breach of confidence claim against Bloomberg, ZXC's counsel felt more secure relying on MOPI (even though it could be argued ZXC was as much the subject of the letter as the law enforcement agency's employee). As Mr Justice Nicklin opined in the High Court judgment:

> Even if UKLEB [the UK law enforcement body] had the appetite for litigation against the Defendant (and a willingness to spend its limited resources on legal proceedings), the reality was that the Article had already been published. In practical terms, the damage to the confidentiality of the [Letter of Request] had been done; in legal terms, given the publication, UKLEB may well have been pessimistic at the prospects of a Court granting an injunction based on breach of confidence.[94]

Be that as it may, equitable compensation for breach of confidence may well still have been awarded. Finally, it may be that because the confidential information contained in the Letter of Request was not "owned" by ZXC, there was concern about ZXC's standing to sue for breach of confidence.

The Supreme Court did not directly address this point in its discussion of the two causes of action, leaving it only to state in the facts that the trial court judge "found that [the Letter of Request] had been given to the [Bloomberg] journalist 'in what must have been (and should have been recognised as) a serious breach of confidence by the person who originally supplied it' (para 125)";[95] and later on in the judgment to opine that:

> It is correct that the judge treated the confidentiality of the information as being a relevant and important factor at both stage one and stage two but he did not treat it as being determinative. The Court of Appeal rightly held that such an approach was justified and involved no error of law.[96]

This suggests that confidentiality may well indeed be relevant to determining whether there is a reasonable expectation of privacy to establish the first element of the MOPI test, but the scope of that relevance remains uncertain. Clearly, questions remain in the law about the relationship between confidentiality and privacy, and the respective causes of action.

The above jurisprudential concerns aside, evidence that MOPI is now used by claimants to protect against misuse of their health information can be seen, for example, in recent case of *Prismall* v *Google UK*.[97] This involved a class action MOPI lawsuit against Google for enabling its subsidiary artificial intelligence firm DeepMind Technologies to obtain patient data from the Royal Free London NHS Trust to develop a mobile app designed to analyse medical records and detect acute kidney injuries.[98] This case did not involve a media publisher or any Article 10 ECHR claim. Though the lawsuit was struck out at the High Court because each member of the claimant class did not have a realistic prospect of establishing a reasonable expectation of privacy in respect of their relevant medical records, it demonstrates the potential for MOPI to serve as a powerful cause of action in the context of health information.[99] Indeed, Williams J was careful to comment that "I am not concerned with whether some of those [individual patients] whose medical records were transferred to DeepMind in 2015 would have a viable claim in MOPI if their individual circumstances were taken into account".[100]

As Williams J noted in *Prismall*, the purposes for which private information came into the hands of the alleged wrongdoer is a relevant factor to take into account when considering whether there was a reasonable expectation of privacy,[101] and it is relevant to take account of the alleged wrongdoer's purpose(s) at the point when the MOPI is said to have occurred.[102] "Misuse" of private information may include unintentional use, although a "use" does require a positive action; and intentionally obtaining information can amount to "misuse" for these purposes, as can storing information.[103] Thus, liability for MOPI is imposed if the defendant knew or ought to have known that the claimant had a reasonable expectation of privacy in the information.

For the first stage of the MOPI test, whether there is a reasonable expectation of privacy is an objective question, although there is some indication that it is a modified objective test comprising an amalgam of objective and subjective factors.[104] The expectation is that of a reasonable person of ordinary sensibilities placed in the same position as the claimant and faced with the same publicity. The question of whether there is a reasonable expectation of privacy is a broad one that takes account of all the circumstances of the case. As stated in *Murray*, such circumstances are likely to include, but are not limited to, what are now known as "*Murray* factors", comprising:

(1) the attributes of the claimant;
(2) the nature of the activity in which the claimant was engaged;
(3) the place at which it was happening;
(4) the nature and purpose of the intrusion;
(5) the absence of consent and whether it was known or could be inferred;
(6) the effect on the claimant; and

(7) the circumstances in which and the purposes for which the information came into the hands of the publisher (noting that this last factor may not be applicable in a biomedical context).

Moreover, as Senior Master Fontaine noted in *Pryor*:

> If the information, or similar information about the claimant, is in the public domain, or is about to become available to the public, the court must have regard to that. In such a case it is a matter of fact and degree as to whether the legitimate expectation of privacy has been lost. Privacy rights can survive a degree of publicity for the information or related information.[105]

In *Bloomberg*, Lord Hamblen and Lord Stephens observed that while all the circumstances of each case must be considered, there are certain types (or categories) of information which will normally, but not invariably, be regarded as giving rise to a reasonable expectation of privacy so as to be characterized as being private in character. These include the state of a person's physical or mental health or condition, meaning that most kinds of medical or health information will ordinarily be presumed to be private:

> There can of course be exceptions even in relation to information concerning the state of an individual's health, but generally, details as to an individual's health are so obviously intimate and personal that a consideration of all the circumstances will result in that information being appropriately characterised as private under the stage one test unless there are strong countervailing circumstances.[106]

In their Lordships view, this consequentially means that:

> In respect of those categories of information [that generally result in a determination that there is a reasonable expectation of privacy] it is appropriate to state that there is a *legitimate starting point* that there is an expectation of privacy in relation to that information. We prefer the terminology of "a legitimate starting point" to emphasise the fact specific nature of the enquiry and to avoid any suggestion of a legal presumption [...]. [...] This means that once the claimant has set out and established the circumstances, the court should commence its analysis by applying the starting point.[107]

This also means, though, that blanket categorization of all health information as per se private (or confidential) ought to be avoided. Similar to the first element in establishing a breach of confidence, there will be no reasonable expectation of privacy in trivial or anodyne information.[108] This might include, for example and depending on the circumstances, information that an individual is suffering from a common cold or a migraine. Thus, while breach of confidence is still very much about "confidential" information, the role of the publicness of information appears particularly relevant in MOPI claims. Also, while claims in breach of confidence focus on the nature of confidence and is linked mostly to an actual relationship, this "objectivization" of privacy expectations in MOPI necessarily throws the net much wider.

But not infinitely wider. In *Prismall* v *Google UK*, Williams J observed that "[…] not every disclosure of medical information will give rise to a reasonable expectation of privacy and/or involve an unlawful interference".[109] To be actionable, the information in a MOPI claim "must reach a level of seriousness".[110] In her words:

> I do not accept that *all* patient-related information that is derived from the doctor-patient context *inevitably* gives rise to a reasonable expectation of privacy (outside of direct care situations). Where information of this nature is involved, I agree that it will be a highly relevant factor to take into account in applying the [stage one] approach [outlined in *Bloomberg* and *Murray*]. But it does not follow that a reasonable expectation of privacy will always exist, irrespective of the circumstances and the content.[111]

Among the other reasons Williams J provided for this finding[112] was that the MOPI tort is "derived" from Article 8 ECHR, in which it is well established that there is a threshold of seriousness that applies and is considered on a fact-sensitive case-by-case basis, rather than it being understood that a particular category of information, even health or medical information, is exempt from the application of this threshold or treated as *always* surmounting it.

Moreover, a reasonable expectation of privacy would not arise in relation to health or medical information that is used for the direct care of patients and where it is established that there was explicit or implied consent for use in this context.[113] Williams J observed in *Prismall* that

> Whether a particular activity is capable of being regarded as direct care is relevant both to whether a reasonable expectation of privacy can be established and to whether a wrongful interference with the information can be shown.[114]

Generally then, it may be difficult for a claimant to establish a reasonable expectation of privacy in health information that is used for the direct care of that claimant, assuming explicit or implied consent to such use has been provided. Conversely, use of that health information for, say, various research or planning purposes, may lead to more open questions about whether a reasonable expectation of privacy exists in the information.

With respect to the second stage of the MOPI test, there is no fixed judicial formula to determine which interest should prevail in a given case, be it Article 8 interests, such as those interests (i.e. exceptions) listed under Article 8(2), or other interests, including Article 10 interests (namely publication of information considered to be in the public interest), or rights and freedoms of others. In other words, and noted above, the balance is not *necessarily* always against Article 10 ECHR, but nonetheless, a *balancing exercise is* carried out in each instance to determine which interest should prevail.

Lord Steyn noted in *In re S* that the balancing exercise involves "an intense focus on the comparative importance of the specific rights being claimed in the individual case", the "justifications for interfering with or restricting each right", and the proportionality of the respective interference or restriction.[115]

So, as with confidential information, it does not follow that partial publication or disclosure of private information is to be treated as being in the public domain for *all* purposes. This said, information that has been accepted to have entered the public domain cannot be confidential, but may yet remain private (e.g. intimate photographs, social media posts about a person's mental or physical health condition, newspaper stories with lurid or prurient details).[116]

MOPI as a new frontier in biomedicine?

What does all of the foregoing analysis, broadly sketched and mostly without specific application to the biomedical context, really mean for the information of patients and research participants? In short, it means that patients and research participants now have added legal protection regarding their health information (and beyond), covering gaps in confidentiality law (often but not exclusively focused on pre-existing relationships between parties; losing protection once information is in the public domain) and where data protection law (focused on "categories" of "personal data" that are "processed") might not apply. There is no indication in law that a claimant cannot seek both civil remedies in some cases where both breach of confidence and MOPI apply. As breach of confidence and MOPI may apply to the same facts, the remedies likely would apply to the same loss. Given multiple causes of action in respect of the same loss do not result in multiple recoveries, and only provide concurrent grounds on which to base the same award, it would not be the case that a claimant would be "double-recovering" by seeking remedies on these two grounds.

Publication, or threatened publication, of private information is not only covered under MOPI, but so too are a swathe of various acts by healthcare professionals, data stewards (i.e. those responsible for managing datasets), researchers, and others that may be construed as wrongful, including unwarranted access to information and unwanted intrusion into one's personal space, such as watching, listening to, or physically encroaching on a person against their wishes.[117] Just as Scots law seemingly now recognizes a broad, all-encompassing right to privacy more firmly aligned with Article 8 ECHR, so too English common law is *moving* in the direction where the privacy tort covers MOPI and (meta)physical interests that enable one to exert informational autonomy and exist in a sphere of non-interference.

But English law is not there yet; as noted above, courts are reluctant to recognize a tort of invasion of physical privacy (unlike in most of the US and Canada, and New Zealand, for instance). The ghosts of *Wainwright* continue to haunt claimants. English courts continue to ground the action in information rather than sensory and physical aspects of the privacy interest.[118] Senior Master Fontaine re-affirmed in *Pryor* v *Liverpool Women's NHS Foundation Trust*, for instance, that "a tort of 'invasion of privacy' or 'breach of privacy rights' or 'breach of physical privacy' is not a tort recognised in English law".[119] The Court of Appeal decisions in *Gulati* v *MGN Ltd*[120] and *NTI* v *Google LLC*[121] constitute authority that there is not

> a basis for establishing a new tort of invasion of privacy, as both cases were claims for misuse of confidential information/breach of Art 8 [ECHR]. [...] In other words, breach or invasion of privacy is an overarching term for a number of torts, including misuse of private information.[122]

Thus, while there might in the future be a tort of breach of physical privacy, which might involve, say, a hospital porter wrongfully watching a patient undress,[123] such a tort does not exist in English law and claimants must continue to ground the wrong in information-publication or information-acquisition principles, or try for another claim such as harassment[124] or rely on an argument that the porter is employed by an entity that is a "public authority" for the purposes of the HRA 1998. On the other hand, in Scots law, the open nature of Lord Bannatyne's finding of a common law right of privacy in *C* v *Chief Constable* suggests there is more willingness to recognize a general claim for breach of privacy, including for sensory and physical aspects.

That does not mean, however, that English law is not inching towards greater recognition of a swathe of privacy interests. In the biomedical context, the continuing focus in English law on informational aspects only is not cause for too much concern, as the jurisprudential widening since *Gulati* v *Mirror Group Newspapers Ltd* in 2015[125] to apply MOPI to informational acquisition and not just disclosure or publication provides much-needed added protection to claimants.[126] As Moreham observes, "Although it is called 'misuse of private information', at least before *Gulati*, the English privacy action had only ever been applied to one type of misuse, the *disclosure* of private information".[127] This approach through 2015 was unduly narrow given that, as we saw from the 1981 Law Commission report, privacy torts like MOPI aim to protect the *content* of information, providing protection against unwarranted incursions into private spaces and activities, regardless of whether the underlying information is "moved" in some sense.

Indeed, in biomedical contexts, wrongful "disclosure" often may not occur through publication or other form of active dissemination of disclosed facts (e.g. taking information and publishing it to others), but rather through various means of wrongful access (i.e. viewing) to the information that are more akin to punishing the *entry* to the private sphere and access to information therein rather than acts of publishing or publication, which are *ex post* actions. This is particularly the case in modern healthcare and data-intensive science and medicine, where a number of (third) parties may access a patient's or research participant's health information for a variety of purposes. In principle, then, MOPI would go further than breach of confidence in protecting downstream access of private information as the focus is on reasonable expectations of privacy rather than the existence of a relationship importing an obligation of confidentiality. The broadening in *Gulati* at least opens the door to recognizing that information acquisition can be as actionable as information dissemination, although as Moreham persuasively argues, "[...] even if some information is obtained in physical privacy cases, the significance of the information is unlikely to reflect the seriousness of the intrusion".[128] Given that both breach of confidence and MOPI claims will not protect trivial or anodyne information, there remains a significant limitation in the law to afford protection to people who feel their sphere of privacy, their "sanctity of a realm in which [they] can reveal themselves (both physically and emotionally without instruction from [an] outsider",[129] will be overlooked. This is unfortunate as the nature of what is being protected—a sense of a larger private sphere and not just private information (or confidential information for that matter) is more akin to Article 8's protection of one's private and family life and as such deserves stronger legal recognition (and remedy) for the loss that is felt, a loss akin to injury to feelings.

The begs the question, then: what might "wrongfulness" in both confidence and MOPI look like in the biomedical context? By way of analogy, were the 2010 *Tchenguiz* case[130] discussed above to be heard today, I suspect that rather than resting the action in breach of confidence, both counsel and the court would likely instead establish as authority that acquiring private information about a person can be actionable under the MOPI tort, even if that information is not disclosed to (or published by) a third party. To borrow an example from Moreham, we could find the MOPI tort's expansion to cover obtaining of information (and not only publication) being of value to a patient who finds her information wrongfully obtained by an anti-abortion campaigner operating a surveillance campaign at an abortion clinic.[131] But it may provide cold comfort to a clinical trial participant whose (anodyne) demographic details are surreptitiously glanced over by a nurse on the ward, or who "merely" observes the patient-participant undressing and receiving the investigational medical device. As the class action against Google and its DeepMind AI division suggest, the MOPI action will continue to rest on claims of wrongful use of individuals' private information (in this case, their medical records in the NHS). We are far from arriving at a point, then, where we can authoritatively state that the courts of England and Wales will favourably look upon a MOPI claim to address alleged violations equivalent to an intrusion upon seclusion or solitude.

There are three other gaps worth highlighting.

First, it is unclear what the scope is of existing statutory frameworks in England that seek to carve out the duty of confidence from attaching in certain circumstances where confidential patient information is used. For example, Section 251 of the NHS Act 2006 provides a power to ensure that patient identifiable information needed to support essential NHS activity can be used without patient consent. The Health Service (Control of Patient Information) Regulations 2002 (known colloquially as the COPI Regs) were passed in June 2002 under the provision re-enacted as Section 251 and they remain in force. Subject to the restrictions contained within Regulation 7, Regulation 5 grants the Secretary of State the power to authorize the processing of "confidential patient information" for

> medical purposes' in circumstances set out in the Schedule of the COPI Regs. Regulation 4 states in full that "Anything done by a person that is necessary for the purpose of processing confidential patient information in accordance with these Regulations shall be taken to be lawfully done despite any obligation of confidence owed by that person in respect of it.

What of privacy, though? It remains an open question, given Regulation 4 does not address MOPI, whether a patient can seek legal regress against a person or organization who misuses their private patient information, even if they could not under a claim for breach of confidence. There has not been consideration of the relationship between legal support for processing under Section 251 and MOPI, as well as other frameworks and guidelines promulgated by the Department of Health and Social Care, NHS England, and professional regulators such as the General Medical Council that consider breach of confidence but not MOPI. However, as I have written with a colleague elsewhere, an argument can be made that given, at least insofar as the COPI Regs are concerned, it "was passed when Convention obligations were already established, it seems highly likely that support under the scheme would be positively considered by a court reviewing a MOPI claim".[132] Thus, even though Section 251 is restricted to providing an exemption from the common law duty of confidentiality and does not provide any kind of exemption from the requirements of the Data Protection Act 2018 or UK GDPR, it and the underlying 2002 COPI Regs, as well as potentially other guidelines and frameworks, may be argued to have extended coverage to MOPI. This does remain an open question, however.

Second, the evolving scope of a common law right to privacy, ostensibly more broadly recognized in Scotland than (so far) in the other three nations of the UK, suggests that there is risk of uncertainty and jurisprudential divergence. This is problematic for cross-UK data sharing initiatives, not to mention those also involving international partners. We have seen a number of concerns raised by data protection legal divergence within the EU and internationally and how this hampers (if not prohibits) data flows from one site to another.[133] While divergence in privacy law is less likely to cause immediate concern (if only because the UK operates a common law regime contingent on litigation and judicial action), it is nonetheless problematic from the perspective of ensuring smooth data flows that both patients and participants, and health-related information concerning them, may receive different levels of legal protection within the UK. This may promote arbitrage, whereby researchers and clinicians limit cross-border data flows to ensure they adhere to the legal regimes within one jurisdiction alone (e.g. one that protects against MOPI but not one that protects a broader right of privacy); it may also temporarily inhibit data-driven initiatives in health until the legal regime is further clarified in case law, given the ongoing development in this area and its relatively unclear attributes, as compared to data protection law, for example.

A third gap is that the existing doctrine of MOPI, as with, it must be said, the other existing privacy legal regimes, fails to adequately protect the interests of third parties (e.g. communities) whose privacy interests may also be adversely affected by some form of misuse.[134] I am not speaking in this context of individuals (e.g. family members) whose privacy has been invaded by the same actions; here they can likely co-join in a tort action and be the subject of the private information in their own right. Rather, I am speaking of contexts in which a larger cohort of people are affected by private information misuse, raising, inter alia, questions of proximity. This gap is, of course, partly due to the traditional bilateral structure of tort claims. We know not just how important these interests are in the biomedical (especially genetic) context, where health-related information about an individual very likely implicates connected others, such as children, siblings, and parents, but also their relevance to potential legal proceedings. And yet, just as data protection law continues to treat "data subjects" as atomized individuals in relation to their "personal data", with legal rights and duties belonging to them alone, so too does MOPI (and confidentiality law for that matter) largely disregard rights and duties of extended groups and communities. While some cases indicate that courts are willing to consider third-party interests as relevant,[135] it remains that this is done on an unprincipled basis; no "third party interests doctrine", as Bennett calls it,[136] has yet emerged in the jurisprudence relating to MOPI. This means that groups or community members whose private information has been misused in some collective manner are unlikely to have recourse to a MOPI claim, and courts are reluctant to consider whether a group or community unit as a whole has a reasonable expectation of privacy in respect of the information.[137] For the foreseeable future, third-party interested community group members would have to make their own individual claims, and a viable case seems unlikely.

Conclusion

In this chapter, I have aimed to inject conceptual coherence into the law regarding breach of confidence and MOPI (and, to an extent, a wider common law right of privacy), with some focus on the biomedical context. I have done this by charting the jurisprudential development of the MOPI tort that emerged from the HRA 1998 and contrasting it with the long-established breach of confidence claim, which I argue remains grounded in equity. Further, I explained that some nations within the UK, namely Scotland, appear to now recognize a free-standing, general common law right to privacy. Applied to the biomedical context, I argued this is, generally speaking, a welcome development and opens a new frontier in biomedicine. It means patients and research participants, not to mention all users of the healthcare system (such as the National Health Service), will have added protection against any misuse of their health information through a cause of action that attaches to reasonable expectations of privacy in relation to their information rather than (only) protection against misuse of information imparted in a circumstance importing an obligation of confidentiality (most often in the context of pre-existing confidential *relationships*).

However, I have also argued that the contours of the MOPI cause of action (including as a tort) as well as the contours of the common right to privacy in Scotland remain in development. We are still, some years later, in a muddle where courts go to great rhetorical lengths to stress they must preserve established principles of law while at the same time, with some judicial chicanery, craft new, arguably sui generis causes of action. In the absence of legislative will and in the social recognition of significant gaps in legal protection, gap-filling to remedy an injustice is no bad thing—provided there is transparency of process and well-reasoned substantive justification. To date, in the realm of privacy, that has not happened. As Hartshorne has aptly opined:

... one is left wondering whether the root of the difficulties present in this area lies in the fact that the MOPI action is essentially a sui generis claim forged out of a desire to offer protection to a right contained in an international human rights instrument, but which has nevertheless been forced into a straightjacket of a "tort" for reasons of domestic necessity.[138]

The solution to this ongoing muddle, I suggest, lies in careful, coherent judgments from courts of law across the UK that explicate what confidentiality and privacy are and are not, and what each, as legal concepts, protect as core values, rights, and duties. It is my hope, too, that courts will eventually expand the existing contours of privacy law to afford protection to violations equivalent to an intrusion upon seclusion or solitude,[139] and grant scope for a "third party interests doctrine" to afford better legal protection to groups and communities whose privacy interests may be adversely affected by information misuse and intrusions upon seclusion. We can only hope that new frontiers in biomedicine continue to unfold.

Acknowledgements

I thank Graeme Laurie and Mark Taylor, as well as the participants in the seminars held at the University of Edinburgh, University of Melbourne, and University of Birmingham, for their insightful comments on previous drafts of this chapter. The usual disclaimer for any errors applies.

Notes

1 Opened for signature 4 November 1950, 213 UNTS 221 (entered into force 3 June 1952).
2 See also International Covenant on Civil and Political Rights, opened for signature 19 December 1966, 999 UNTS 171, 6 ILM 368 (entered into force 23 March 1976), Article 17. The UK has signed and ratified the Covenant. Article 17 provides, *inter alia*, that "No one shall be subjected to arbitrary or unlawful interference with his privacy [...]".
3 See e.g. *LL* v *France* (Application No. 7508/02 2006) ECtHR; *LH* v *Latvia* (Application No. 52019/07 2014) ECtHR; *PT* v *Republic of Moldova* (Application No. 1122/12 2020) ECtHR.
4 *Gulati* v *Mirror Group Newspapers Ltd* [2015] EWCA Civ 1291 [88] (Arden LJ).
5 Jacob Rowbottom, "A Landmark at a Turning Point: *Campbell* and the Use of Privacy law to Constrain Media Power", in Thomas DC Bennett and Daithí Mac Síthigh (eds), *The Campbell Legacy: Reflections on the Tort of Misuse of Private Information* (Routledge 2018), 21–45, at 28.
6 While the action must be against a "public authority" as per ss. 6 and 7 of the HRA 1998, this may concern alleged breaches of one's private life committed by another individual, given Article 8 ECHR encompasses positive obligations by the state to respect and promote the interests of private life. See generally *X and Y* v *The Netherlands* (1985) 8 EHRR 235.

7 Law Commission, *Breach of Confidence* (Law Com No 110, 1981), para 2.2–2.3.
8 See e.g. *HRH Duchess of Sussex* v *Associated Newspapers Ltd* [2020] EWHC 1058 (Ch). The European Court of Human Rights is an international court of the Council of Europe which interprets the European Convention on Human Rights. It sits in Strasbourg, France.
9 Article 10(1) ECHR states: "Everyone has the right to freedom of expression. This right shall include freedom to hold opinions and to receive and impart information and ideas without interference by public authority and regardless of frontiers. [...]" Both Articles 8 and 10 are qualified human rights: Articles 8(2) and 10(2) stipulate the circumstances in which these two human rights may be lawfully circumscribed.
10 In this chapter, I use English law terminology rather than Scots law terminology, e.g. "tort" rather than "delict"; "claimant" rather than "pursuer"; "defendant" rather than "defender"; "injunction" rather than "interdict".
11 Thomas DC Bennett, "*PJS v News Group Newspapers Ltd* (2016)", in Paul Wragg and Peter Coe (eds), *Landmark Cases in Privacy Law* (Hart 2023), 301–326, at 301.
12 We can compare the long-standing judicial conservatism in the UK with other jurisdictions, where privacy has long received greater judicial support. We see this, for example, in the US, where in the 1902 case of *Roberson* v *Rochester Folding Bos Co.* 171 N.Y. 538; 64 N.E. 442 (1902), the dissenting judge declared that the claimant had a right to be protected against the use of their image for the defendant's commercial advantage and "Any other principle of decision [...] is as repugnant to equity as it is shocking to reason". Following general discontent in society with the judgment, the State of New York enacted a statute to make it unlawful to make unauthorized use of an individual's name or image for advertising or trade purposes. Moreover, three years later, the Supreme Court of Georgia adopted the dissenting judge's reasoning in *Roberson* in the case of *Pavesich* v *New England Life Insurance* Co., 122 Ga. 190; 50 S.E. 68 (1905). In short, across the US, a "right to privacy" has long existed, either in general form (e.g. in state constitutions) or as a grouping of separate but related torts.
13 *Mills* v *News Group Newspapers* [2001] EMLR 41 [22] (Lawrence Collins J).
14 (1991) FSR 62.
15 Jacob Rowbottom, "*Kaye v Roberston* (1990)", in Wragg and Coe, n 11, 85–105, at 85.
16 [2003] UKHL 53; [2004] 2 AC 406. The facts in *Wainwright* arose before the HRA 1998 came into force, meaning reliance could not be placed Article 8 ECHR to obtain a domestic remedy.
17 *Kaye* v *Roberston* (1991) FSR 62, at 66 (Glidewell LJ).
18 *Wainwright* v *Home Office* [2003] UKHL 53 [31] (Lord Hoffmann).
19 Ibid., [26].
20 Ibid., [31].
21 Rowbottom, n 15 (*Kaye*), at 99.
22 Ibid., 105.
23 [2002] EWCA Civ 337; [2003] QB 195.
24 Ibid., [4].
25 Ibid. Moreham describes *A v B plc* as falling in a "transition point" of English law and one of a handful of cases that "kickstarted the transformation of the breach of confidence action from its traditional incarnation into the misuse of privacy tort that we know today". See N A Moreham, "*A v B & C* (2002)", in Wragg and Coe, n 11, 137–157, at 137. The open question, though, and what

I hope to address in this chapter, is whether this "transition point" has ended and whether breach of confidence has been indefinitely transformed (or transmogrified) solely into a MOPI tort. I argue against this view.

26 *McKennitt* v *Ash* [2006] EWCA Civ 1714 [11] (Buxton LJ). However, as I go on to argue, courts have moved away from this position and carved out MOPI as a distinct English domestic tort, increasingly untethered to Article 8 ECHR. See e.g. *Gulati* v *Mirror Group Newspapers Ltd* [2015] EWCA Civ 1291 [89] ("First, the conditions of the [MOPI] tort are governed by English law and not the Convention") (Arden LJ).

27 *A* v *B plc*, n 23, [11vi, ix–x] (emphasis added).

28 See generally Megan Richardson, *Breach of Confidence: Social Origins and Modern Developments* (Edward Elgar 2012).

29 *McKennitt*, n 26, [8ii].

30 [2004] UKHL 22; [2004] 2 AC 457.

31 As noted by Lord Hoffmann at [42], Campbell issued proceedings for damages for "breach of confidence and/or invasion of privacy". The conjunction "and/or" and the claim for "invasion of privacy" demonstrate the legal uncertainty of the relevant cause of action at that time. At the House of Lords, however, the claim was exclusively presented on the basis of breach of confidence.

32 Ibid., [82] (Lord Hope) and [132–133] (Baroness Hale).

33 Ibid., [11] (emphasis added).

34 Ibid., [12].

35 Lord Hoffmann also expressed concerns at [44]:
But although the action for breach of confidence could be used to protect privacy in the sense of preserving the confidentiality of personal information, it was not founded on the notion that such information was in itself entitled to protection. Breach of confidence was an equitable remedy and equity traditionally fastens on the conscience of one party to enforce equitable duties which arise out of his relationship with the other.

36 Ibid., [14]. The actual word used in the quote is "confidential", but Lord Nicholls in the same paragraph went on to comment that
Even this formulation is awkward. The continuing use of the phrase 'duty of confidence' and the description of the information as 'confidential' is not altogether comfortable. Information about an individual's private life would not, in ordinary usage, be called 'confidential'. The more natural description today is that such information is private.

37 Ibid. And as Bennett notes, as outlined in *Campbell*, MOPI adopted a bilateral structure in alignment with other torts (i.e. interpersonal wrongdoing between private persons whereby the claimant sues those they identify as their injurers) and with the equitable doctrine of confidentiality, and "laid the groundwork for the doctrine to be treated as a tort, even when it was unclear that it was properly regarded as being of the tort *genus*". See Bennett, n 11, at 304.

38 *Campbell*, n 30, [14].

39 Ibid., [15].

40 Ibid., [15].

41 As per Lord Nicholls at [17]: "The time has come to recognise that the values enshrined in articles 8 and 10 are now part of the cause of action for breach of confidence.".

42 Ibid., [21].

43 Ibid., [46].

44 Ibid., [50].

45 Ibid.

46 Ibid.

47 Ibid., [51].
48 See e.g. *Douglas* v *Hello! Ltd* [2001] QB 967; *Douglas* v *Hello! Ltd* [2005] EWCA Civ 595, [2006] QB 125; and *Douglas* v *Hello! (No3)* [2006] QB 125.
49 [1988] Ch. 449.
50 *Attorney-General* v *Guardian Newspapers (No 2)* [1990] AC 109.
51 *Campbell*, n 30, [134].
52 *Mosley* v *News Group Newspapers Ltd* [2008] EMLR 20 at [7] (Eady J).
53 Ibid., [8].
54 *Douglas* v *Hello! Ltd* [2001] QB 967.
55 Ibid., [126].
56 *Douglas* v *Hello! Ltd* (also known as *OBG Ltd* v *Allan*) [2007] UKHL 21 [255] (Lord Nicholls) (emphasis added).
57 [2010] EWCA Civ 908.
58 Ibid., [67].
59 Ibid. This said, Lord Neuberger MR went on to suggest that "a reasonable expectation" (whether of privacy or confidentiality) was a good test to apply when considering either cause of action.
60 [2015] EWCA Civ 1034.
61 Ibid., [7].
62 Ibid., [26].
63 Ibid., [35]. "Data subjects" itself is a confusing term in the judgment that comes from the separate legal regime of data protection law. The Court flipped terminology at [37] and in subsequent paragraphs [38]-[40], affirming that while the information contained details on the debt owed, "it *also* contain[ed] confidential information" (emphasis in original), and proceeded to discuss various professional guidance on sharing confidential patient information.
64 Ibid., [42].
65 Ibid., [43].
66 Ibid., [44] (emphasis added).
67 Ibid., [47].
68 [2015] EWCA Civ 311. The question of whether MOPI was a tort was specifically for the purposes of the rules providing for service of proceedings out of the jurisdiction. This was an important legal question in the case because if a MOPI claim was not a tort for the purposes of service out of the jurisdiction, but is classified as a claim for breach of confidence, then on the basis of binding precedent (*Kitechnology BV* v *Unicor*), the claimants Vidall-Hall and others would not have been able to serve their MOPI claim on the defendant Google Inc.
69 [2014] EWHC 13 (QB).
70 [2015] EWCA Civ 311 [21].
71 Ibid.
72 Ibid., [43] (emphasis added).
73 [2016] UKSC 26.
74 *PJS*, n 73, [57–58].
75 *Pryor* v *Liverpool Women's NHS Foundation Trust* [2021] EWHC 2911 (QB) [34] (emphasis added).
76 [2019] CSOH 48.
77 1988 SLT 361 (Court of Session, Outer House).
78 *C* v *Chief Constable*, n 76, [106].
79 Ibid., [116].
80 Ibid., [111–113].
81 Ibid., [106].
82 Ibid., [121–122].
83 Ibid., [123].

84 [2022] UKSC 5. See also *Various Claimants* v *MGN Limited* [2022] EWHC 1222 (Ch).

85 Ibid., at [45].

86 Ibid., [150] (emphasis added).

87 [1969] RPC 41.

88 See e.g. *Attorney-General* v *Guardian Newspapers (No 2)* [1990] AC 109.

89 Ibid. In the alternative formulation of Lord Goff at 281: "I start with the broad general principle (which I do not intend in any way to be definitive) that a duty of confidence arises when confidential information comes to the knowledge of a person (the confidant) in circumstances where he has notice, or is held to have agreed, that the information is confidential, with the effect that it would be just in all the circumstances that he should be precluded from disclosing the information to others." See also *Hellewell* v *Chief Constable of Derbyshire* [1995] 1 W.L.R. 804 at 808 (Laws J): "[...] a duty of confidence may be created simply out of the relationship between the parties with no requirement of any express notice from confider to confidant.".

90 See *Murray* v *Express Newspapers Plc* [2008] EWCA Civ 446. See also *Prismall* v *Google UK* [2023] EWHC 1169 (KB) at [66]; *ZXC* v *Bloomberg LP* [2022] UKSC 5 [26].

91 N 84. See also *Various Claimants* v *MGN Limited* [2022] EWHC 1222 (Ch).

92 Rebecca Moosavian, "A Just Balance or Just Imbalance? The Role of Metaphor in Misuse of Private Information", in Bennett and Mac Síthigh, n 5, 46–74, at 47.

93 *ZXC* v *Bloomberg LP* [2019] EWHC 970 (QB) [2].

94 Ibid., [68].

95 *Bloomberg*, n 84, [18].

96 Ibid., [148].

97 *Prismall*, n 90.

98 See Reuters, "Google Asks London Court to Throw Out Lawsuit Over Medical Records" (21 March 2023), available at: https://www.reuters.com/technology/google-asks-london-court-throw-out-lawsuit-over-medical-records-2023-03-21/.

99 *Prismall*, n 90.

100 Ibid., [186].

101 Ibid., [139].

102 Ibid., [140].

103 Ibid., [79–80]. See also *Tchenguiz*, n 57, [68]; *Amann* v *Switzerland* (2000) 30 EHRR 843 [69].

104 See NA Moreham, "Unpacking the Reasonable Expectation of Privacy Test" (2018) 134 *Law Quarterly Review* 651–674, in which she argues that the first part of the test in English law is underpinned by two previously unarticulated principles, both of which should be considered: (1) a claimant will have a reasonable expectation of privacy if such an expectation is consistent with *societal attitudes* to the information or activity in question (a society-focused route); and (2) a claimant will have a reasonable expectation of privacy if they made it clear to the defendant through their *privacy signals* (if any) that disclosure or observation of the information or activity in question was unwelcome and that society would usually expect such a signal to be respected (a claimant-focused route).

105 See also *Pryor*, n 75, [30]; *Prismall*, n 90, [136]: "The fact that information is already in the public domain may impact on whether there is a reasonable expectation of privacy; it is well established that this is a relevant circumstance to take into account [...].".

106 *Bloomberg*, n 84, [72].

107 Ibid., [144] (emphasis added).

108 *Ambrosiadou v Coward* [2011] EWCA Civ 409 [30] (Lord Newburger): "Just because information relates to a person's family and private life, it will not automatically be protected by the courts: for instance the information may be of slight significance, generally expressed or anodyne in nature.".

109 *Prismall*, n 90, [72]. See also *ZC v Royal Free London NHS Foundation Trust* [2019] EWHC 2040 (QB); *Underwood v Bounty UK Ltd* [2022] EWHC 888 (QB).

110 *Underwood*, n 109, [53].

111 *Prismall*, n 90, [133].

112 Ibid.

113 *Prismall*, n 90, [78].

114 Ibid., [144].

115 *In re S (A Child) (Identification: Restrictions on Publication)* [2005] 1 AC 593 at [17].

116 *PJS*, n 73, especially [57–66]. Wragg has identified that public interest in disclosure of private information is often the key stage two consideration in the extant cases. See Paul Wragg, "Protecting Private Information of Public Interest: *Campbell*'s Great Promise, Unfulfilled", in Bennett and Mac Síthigh, n 5, 75–100, at 77.

117 The High Court decision in *Gulati v Mirror Group Newspapers Ltd* [2015] EWHC 1482 (Ch), and upheld by the Court of Appeal in [2015] EWCA Civ 1291, would seem to confirm this, as the High Court awarded MOPI damages for the activities of hacking and listening to voicemails, even though none of the information was published. See also NA Moreham, "Liability for Listening: Why Phone Hacking is an Actionable Breach of Privacy", in Thomas DC Bennett and Daithí Mac Síthigh, n 5, 6–20.

118 Contrast with *C v Chief Constable*, n 76, and Strasbourg court jurisprudence, which has recognized that privacy under Article 8 ECHR is not limited to protection of personal information and that is also concerns intrusion, and prior disclosure does not negate the right to privacy. See *Hajovsky v Slovakia* (App no 7796/16) 2021.

119 *Pryor*, n 75, [26].

120 [2015] EWCA Civ 1291.

121 [2018] EWHC 799 (QB).

122 *Pryor*, n 75, [27].

123 Compare the position in New Zealand, where in *C v Holland* [2012] NZHC 2155, the New Zealand High Court recognized a tort of intrusion into private space and awarded the claimant damages for being secretly filmed while she was showering. There was no evidence that the defendant published or showed the recordings to anyone else. Compare also the position in Belgium, where a "right of intimacy" is recognized in Article 10 of the Belgian Law of Patients' Rights as a full and independent patient right, affording a right to spatial privacy in examination and treatment rooms. See Thierry Vansweevelt, Nils Broeckx, and Filip Dewallens, "Privacy and Health in Belgium", in Thierry Vansweevelt and Nicola Glover-Thomas (eds), *Privacy and Medical Confidentiality in Healthcare: A Comparative Analysis* (Edward Elgar 2023), 5–23.

124 Although it is unclear if it would reach the threshold of unreasonable and oppressive persistent conduct, likely to cause the recipient alarm, fear, and distress.

125 [2015] EWCA Civ 1291.

126 There is not space in this chapter to describe *Gulati* in detail.

127 Moreham, "Liability for Listening", n 117, at 10.

128 Ibid., 17.

129 Ibid.
130 See n 57.
131 Moreham, "Liability for Listening", n 117, at 13.
132 Edward S Dove and Mark J Taylor, "Confidentiality, Privacy, and Data Protection" in Judith Laing and Jean McHale (eds), *Principles of Medical Law* (5th edn, Oxford University Press 2025), Chapter 12, at para 12.122.
133 See e.g. Robert Eiss, "We Must Dismantle the Barriers that GDPR Creates for Global Science" Financial Times (3 January 2023), available at: https://www.ft.com/content/622e8097-ef6b-4ec9-939e-5d95743532c1.
134 For arguments in favour of group privacy rights, see generally Linnet Taylor, Luciano Floridi, and Bart van der Sloot (eds), *Group Privacy: New Challenges of Data Technologies* (Springer 2017).
135 See e.g. *PJS*, n 73 (where the Supreme Court did not in fact definitively settle the issue, but instead only affirmed the relevance of third-party interests in MOPI claims); *Rocknroll v NGN Ltd* [2013] EWHC 24 (Ch); *CDE v MGN Ltd* [2010] EWHC 3308 (QB); and *K (formerly 'ETK') v News Group Newspapers Ltd* [2011] EWCA Civ 439, all of which concerned the interests of children affected by the interests of their parents' privacy. See also *ABC v St George's Healthcare NHS Foundation Trust* [2020] EWHC 455 (QB), in which Mrs Justice Yip of the High Court held that a daughter of a patient was owed a duty of care by one of the NHS Trusts (specifically, the family therapy team) to "balance her interest in being alerted the genetic risk against the interest of [the father] and the public interest in confidentiality" [166]. However, on the facts of this case, there was no breach of that duty. Unrelated to MOPI, this suggests that courts may allow lawful disclosure of confidential information on the grounds of public interest when a patient refuses to consent to such disclosure, where there are exceptional circumstances of danger or harm to others.
136 Bennett, n 11.
137 See e.g. *O v A* (also known as *Rhodes v OPO*) [2014] EWHC 2468 (QB), [2014] EWCA Civ 1277, [2015] UKSC 32, in which the High Court, Court of Appeal, and Supreme Court each held that an individual who is not themselves the subject of information, but whose psychological integrity would be harmed by its reputation, has no standing to bring a MOPI claim, but rather, only the subject of the private information has standing to bring a MOPI claim.
138 John Hartshorne, "*Gulati v Mirror Group Newspapers* (2015)", in Wragg and Coe, n 11, 281–300, at 297.
139 An open question is what the relevant legal test would be to establish such a tort. English courts may look to jurisdictions such as Ontario (Canada) for inspiration. There, the claimant must show that (1) the defendant's conduct was intentional or reckless, (2) the defendant invaded the plaintiff's privacy affairs or concerns without lawful justification, and (3) a reasonable person would regard the invasion as highly offensive, causing distress, humiliation, or anguish. See *Jones v Tsige*, 2012 ONCA 32 (Canada). This, of course, differs from the MOPI test, which does not require establishing intentional or reckless conduct by the defendant.

9

HACKERS AND HACKED

How does data breach notification law respond to and remedy health data breaches in the Asia-Pacific?

Megan Prictor

Introduction

Health data breaches—the unauthorized access to, disclosure, or loss of people's health information—are now ubiquitous. Their increasingly giant scale, driven both by poor cyber-security practices and highly skilled and resourced nefarious actors (including some that are state-sponsored[1]), can cause severe harm to individuals, groups, and data custodians. In recent years there have been massive health data breaches internationally, with thousands of health services and millions of patients affected. As an example, Medibank Private, Australia's largest private health insurer,[2] suffered a major hack by Russian cyber-criminals in 2022. Data of almost ten million current, former, and prospective customers were published on the dark web after the company refused to pay ransom demands. The data released included name, address, and date of birth, as well as health claims such as information about people's drug and alcohol treatment, pregnancy termination, and mental illness.[3] Significant media attention ensued,[4] with those affected expressing deep concern about the privacy breach and potential repercussions.[5]

Research has shown that the impacts of personal information breaches can be severe, increasing affected individuals' privacy concerns, reducing trust,[6] and engendering feelings of violation,[7] anger, sadness, and disgust.[8] Breaches of personal health-related data may be more distressing and less easily remedied than those of financial information or identity, causing anxiety around reputational impact and consequential effects on employment and business prospects.[9] Healthcare service delivery can also be impacted, for instance by ransomware attacks, leading to patient harm and even loss of life.[10]

DOI: 10.4324/9781003394518-12

Mandatory data breach notification is one of several regulatory tools for addressing data breaches (among others outlined below). Although they vary between jurisdictions, these notifiable data breach (NDB) statutory schemes have some common features. If a data breach meets a given threshold, data custodians must both report to a regulatory authority and notify affected individuals that their personal data have been subject to unauthorized access, disclosure, or loss, often within a specified timeframe. In certain cases, individual notification can be replaced with a general notice published online. Risk of harm caused by the breach may be a moderating factor, with effective remediation measures sometimes displacing the need to report or notify. Punitive provisions usually attach to a failure to report or notify when the law requires it. Generally, NDB schemes themselves do not extend to mandatory harm mitigation measures (the implementation of credit reporting on behalf of customers, the replacement of identity documentation, etc.) although other regulatory requirements may do so.

Since the first NDB scheme was introduced in California in 2002, laws requiring data breach notification to affected individuals and a regulatory body[11] have become increasingly common internationally. The EU General Data Protection Regulation (GDPR) introduced data breach notification on a wide scale in 2018, a few months after Australia's mandatory NDB scheme came into force through amendments to the Commonwealth Privacy Act 1988. Numerous countries in the Asia-Pacific region also have such schemes. The Asia-Pacific Economic Cooperation (APEC) and Organisation for Economic Co-operation and Development (OECD) support NDB laws in light of their capacity to improve data custodians' accountability and enable individuals to take protective action following a breach.[12] The OECD Privacy Framework states that NDB laws also assist in developing evidence for data protection policies "by generating information about the number, severity and causes of security breaches".[13]

In previous research focusing on Australian law, I identified numerous purposes of mandatory NDB schemes, including: harm minimization for and by data subjects who are victims; transparency; reduced identity fraud; and impetus for data custodians to enhance data security. I examined how well these aims were met, through the Australian NDB scheme, in the specific context of health data. This research suggested that mandatory NDB regimes, which have been principally designed to address problems arising from breaches of financial and identity information more broadly, are an imperfect fit with breaches of health data. This is particularly the case since (as noted earlier) the emotional harms of such a breach are not easily remedied. Notification itself may cause or intensify distress to an affected person.[14] I noted that other legal and policy measures may be needed to minimize harm, to improve transparency, and to motivate data custodians to improve data security.

This chapter will expand on that previous work, focusing here on large-scale, deliberate health data breaches, to compare and critically evaluate statutory data breach notification schemes across the Asia-Pacific. The chapter proceeds by: (i) briefly examining recent large-scale health data breaches in this region; (ii) situating NDB schemes within the broader regulatory environment; (iii) unpacking the aims and elements of NDB schemes; (iv) summarizing and comparing regional data breach notification schemes; and (v) critiquing these schemes and proposing future regulatory reform to address this substantial and growing issue in the region. It will argue that stronger alignment between NDB scheme aims and the design of legislation is needed, together with tailoring to the particular harms of health data breaches and new research on the effects of notification on affected individuals.

Health data breaches in the Asia-Pacific

Data form the core of healthcare. Since 2020, the urgent operational demands of the COVID-19 pandemic forced greater reliance on online health data processing,[15] including the large-scale collection of data from SARS-CoV-2 test results, infections, and vaccinations, and health-related location data in a time of restrictive public health measures. While small-scale breaches of health data through human error (for instance, information sent to the wrong recipient[16]) are commonplace, malicious or criminal attack is now behind at least half of health data breaches reported to the Australian regulator.[17] In 2020 the Australian Department of Foreign Affairs and Trade and the Australian Cyber Security Centre jointly stated that "malicious cyber actors are seeking to damage or impair the operation of hospitals, medical services and facilities".[18] These attacks, via ransomware, compromised credentials, and hacking, have the potential to impact millions of people.[19]

Cyber-incidents were recently ranked as the most important risk globally in a major industry report,[20] with the World Economic Forum noting that "Alongside a rise in cybercrime, attempts to disrupt critical technology-enabled resources and services will become more common".[21] Cyber-crime is big business, "with an entire illicit economy set up to support it with service providers, recruiters and financial services",[22] and generating income greater than that of many countries.[23] Ransomware-as-a-service has emerged as an increasingly professionalized domain of criminal activity,[24] offering expertise including software deployment, third-party negotiation and dispute resolution, and the facilitation of ransom payments.

Health data are particularly appealing to hackers. These data are voluminous and held within systems that have traditionally been poorly protected. System complexity and interoperability can make for an easier target,[25] which is somewhat ironic, given the push to increase health data interoperability and reduce siloing to improve patient care. Further, data privacy is highly valued, and the disclosure of sensitive information can be deeply harmful—highly embarrassing, distressing, and stigmatizing—to individuals. As the very functionality of healthcare systems can be impeded by a ransomware attack, posing a serious threat to people's health and lives, the locked or stolen data function as lucrative bargaining chips. Hackers often use "double extortion", seeking a fee to release data back to the organization as well as to avoid its publication online.[26]

Multiple large-scale malicious breaches involving health data have taken place across the Asia-Pacific region. As well as the Medibank hack, in 2023 Australian pathology company TissuPath was hacked by a Russian cyber-gang, who published 735,000 files, which included clinical data.[27] In 2018 "Whitefly" hackers used custom malware to attack Singapore's SingHealth system over a ten-month period, obtaining personal information of 1.5 million patients, including the country's prime minister.[28] One industry leader reported recently that more than three quarters of medical devices in the Philippines (closely followed by Bangladesh and Thailand) were infected with malicious code.[29] Beyond the multifaceted impacts of health data breaches on individuals, the average global cost to healthcare entities of managing each data breach is now over US$10 million.[30] It is pertinent, therefore, to explore the regulatory response to this problem.

Health data breaches: Regulatory responses

While NDB schemes are the focus of this chapter, it is important to understand these within the broader regulatory environment that applies to cyber-security. Despite governments presenting data breach notification as a solution to the problem of data breaches,[31] notification, by itself, arguably does very little directly to improve data security or to remediate harm. Other statutory mechanisms are, therefore, important, but these are also complex and overlapping (particularly in federal systems). Regulation to prevent, manage, punish, and remedy data breaches tends to be situated in both privacy and critical infrastructure legislation. However, it can encompass a variety of instruments: voluntary or prescriptive standards for data protection and cyber-security; criminal laws addressing hacking; and post-breach remedial measures under privacy law, contract, tort, equity, consumer, and corporations law. In Australia, a 2021 discussion paper identified at least 51 national or state and territory laws with potential to create obligations on businesses in relation to data breaches.[32]

A recent and novel development is the emergence of class actions by both shareholders and affected individuals against companies that have suffered large-scale data breaches. For instance, Medibank investors who acquired shares around the time of the cyber-attack referenced above are pursuing the company for an alleged breach of its corporate continuous disclosure obligations as well as for misleading or deceptive conduct under Australian consumer law.[33] Additionally, Medibank customers affected by the attack have launched separate class actions with the national privacy regulator for a breach of privacy legislation, and with the Federal Court for a breach of consumer law.[34] The group of people affected by a breach who are notified under an NDB scheme could be identified as an obvious "class" able to pursue legal remedies.[35] In this way, breach notification can act as a gateway to the deployment of other regulatory mechanisms to remedy harm.

The aims and elements of NDB schemes

Within this constellation of legal possibilities, mandatory NDB schemes seem logical and straightforward: they require certain actions of a data custodian following a sufficiently serious ("notifiable") data breach. The aims underpinning these requirements are, however, diverse, and range from the individual to the system and societal level. Previous research has described the following aims of NDB schemes overall (with jurisdictions usually focusing on a selection of these):[36]

1 To enable individual harm mitigation and access to compensation, assuming that once individuals are aware their data have been subject to a breach, they will take steps to protect their interests (e.g. initiate credit monitoring, update identity documents) and seek a remedy.
2 To motivate data custodians to make pre-emptive investments in and improvements to data security, through the fear of being subject to a data breach that, were it to occur, would necessitate notification (with its flow-on impacts).
3 To promote transparency (for purposes including accountability, the public interest, and epistemic rights ((or the "right to know"[37])).
4 To overcome the lack of market incentives for notification. This aim assumes that since markets punish entities that are known to have incurred a data breach, data custodians would not self-disclose in the absence of a legislative requirement to do so.
5 To enable vicarious punishment of the data custodian (through imposition of notification costs and post-notification measures, and raising the risk of reputational damage, adverse media attention, and market chastisement).
6 To reduce overall identity fraud (because individual harm mitigation and pre-emptive cyber security measures will reduce overall business costs).
7 To facilitate system-wide learnings (since transparent information about data breaches can yield new insights, applicable across whole systems, into the causes and impacts of, and effective measures against, data breaches).

How do NDB schemes pursue these aims?

In this chapter, I selected key elements of the NDB statutory schemes in order to make a systematic comparison across jurisdictions. First, I considered how NDB schemes are typically constructed to achieve their diverse aims, outlined above. Based on a high-level review of selected laws, I propose that there are five important constituent elements within statutes that can be logically expected and/or are typically present, by which the above aims can be realized. A comprehensive model statutory scheme would include all five elements, to meet the broadest set of aims, but in practice there will be variation in what schemes include. The five elements are as follows (and summarized in Figure 9.1). The first is a requirement that the data custodian suffering or suspecting a data breach must notify a regulatory authority; and the second is a requirement to also notify affected individuals. Third, these notification requirements are backed up by financial penalties for non-compliance. Fourth is a requirement or expectation placed on the regulator to publicly report a de-identified aggregate summary of notified data breaches, and fifth, to publicly report in a way that discloses identifiable information about the breached entity.

Each of these elements can vary in degree: for example, in the time limit for reporting to the regulator and notification to individuals; the amount of the penalty for failure to report/notify; and the level of detail in public reporting. Even robust schemes may exclude certain elements, or not legislate them directly. For instance, anonymised/aggregated reporting, where it occurs, is rarely required by the statute itself but rather appears in legislative instruments or policies, while the identifiable public reporting element, as suggested by Greenleaf,[38] is almost entirely absent in practice. Nonetheless, public reporting is included here since it aids in delivering on the overarching aims of NDB schemes.

These five elements of NDB schemes could be combined and tailored in different ways to support the seven overarching scheme aims, as noted in Figure 9.2. For instance, making the scheme as onerous as possible (e.g.

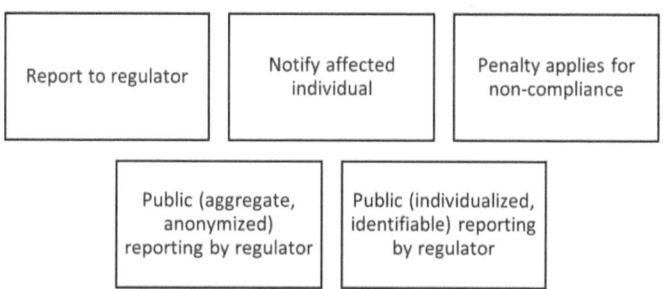

FIGURE 9.1   Key elements of NDB schemes.

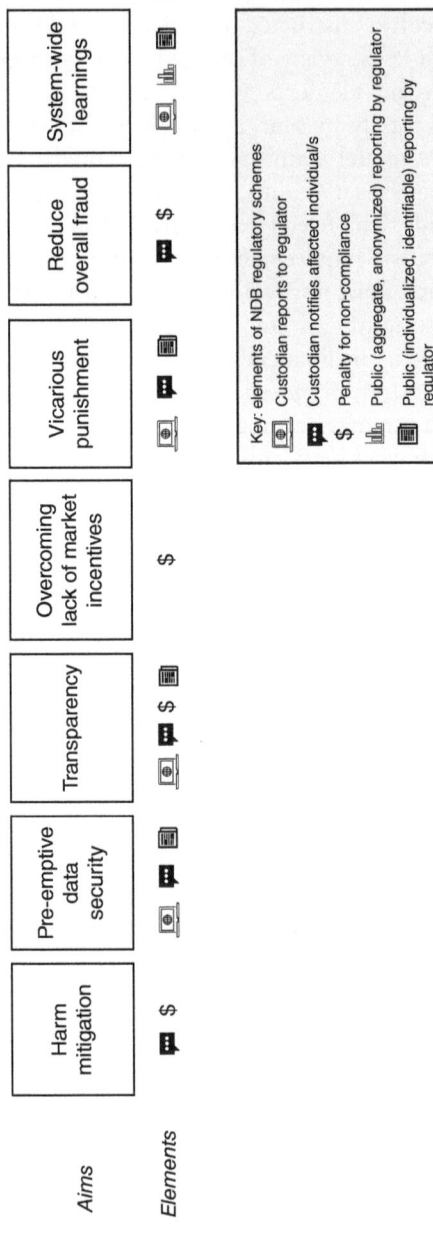

FIGURE 9.2 NDB scheme aims and key regulatory elements.

giving a very short time to report to the regulator and notify affected parties) and requiring identifiable public reporting can mean a scheme is optimized to both motivate data custodians to invest pre-emptively cyber-security measures, and to ensure vicarious punishment[39] if a breach does occur. A requirement for prompt notification to affected individuals, with a penalty for non-compliance with notification requirements, can help people to more effectively mitigate the harm a breach may cause. System-wide learnings are optimized through rapid notification to the regulator and detailed public reporting requirements to aid widespread awareness and understanding of a breach's cause, effects, and effective remediation actions.

This schema, as reflected in Figure 9.2, can facilitate a systematic comparative analysis of NDB laws across jurisdictions. While a model scheme would incorporate all five elements, different jurisdictions may reasonably focus their attention on fewer, or other, aims, and accordingly incorporate fewer (or different) elements.

In the next section, I present a high-level summary of NDB laws in selected jurisdictions across the Asia-Pacific. It must be noted that while the coverage of NDB requirements *within* each jurisdiction varies significantly, gaps in coverage are not considered in detail here. For instance, in Australia, state and territory authorities (including public hospitals) and small business are largely exempt from the national scheme at present,[40] and the Singaporean scheme does not apply to public agencies.[41]

Selected NDB schemes across the Asia-Pacific

Between September and November 2023, NDB schemes in selected jurisdictions within the Asia-Pacific region were reviewed (updated January 2024). The schemes were selected pragmatically based on the accessibility of the legislation (or reliable secondary sources) in English, and location within the region, to provide a broad indication of regulatory trends. Primary sources were prioritized where available. The EU GDPR was also included due to its role as an international quasi-benchmark.[42] Table 9.1 summarizes the 17 selected data breach notification schemes, addressing the five regulatory elements identified above.[43]

It is important to note that numerous countries in the region have no mandatory NDB scheme, including Cambodia,[44] Timor Leste,[45] Lao People's Democratic Republic,[46] Myanmar,[47] and Papua New Guinea.[48]

Critical reflection and considerations for reform

When considered at the macro level, legislation and guidelines for data breach notification in the Asia-Pacific region are reasonably common, albeit often very recent. Several countries (China, India, Indonesia, Malaysia, Sri Lanka)

TABLE 9.1 Data breach notification schemes: GDPR and Asia-Pacific region

Jurisdiction	Key legislation or normative instrument	Data breach definition	Threshold for notification 🖥	Report to regulator: timing	Notification to individuals: timing 💬	Exceptions to notification	Penalty: [failure to notify $	Public reporting
European Union/ European Economic Area	General Data Protection Regulation[49] and Guidelines on Personal Data Breach Notification under GDPR[50]	"a breach of security leading to the accidental or unlawful destruction, loss, alteration, unauthorised disclosure of, or access to, personal data transmitted, stored or otherwise processed".[51]	To the individual: where the breach "is likely to result in a high risk to the rights and freedoms of the natural person in order to allow him or her to take the necessary precautions".[52]	72 hours[53]	"without undue delay"[54]	Notification to individuals not required if the breach "is unlikely to result in a risk to the rights and freedoms of natural persons".[55]	< €10 million [£8.6 million] or 2% of annual global turnover in previous financial year–whichever is greater.[56]	Not stipulated in GDPR. National supervisory authorities may publish information.

| Australia | Privacy Act 1988[57] | "there is unauthorised access to, or unauthorised disclosure of, the information[58] or 'the information is lost in circumstances where… unauthorised access to, or unauthorised disclosure of, the information is likely to occur"[59] | "a reasonable person would conclude that the access or disclosure would be likely to result in serious harm to any of the individuals to whom the information relates".[60] The entity must consider: the kind of information, its sensitivity, who might obtain it, any security measures and the likelihood that they could be overcome, the nature of the harm and 'any other relevant matters".[61] Notification not required where the entity "takes action in relation to the access or disclosure" before it "results in serious harm" and "as a result of the action, a reasonable person would conclude that the access or disclosure would not be likely to result in serious harm…".[62] | "a reasonable and expeditious assessment" within 30 days after becoming aware that there may have been a notifiable data breach,[63] and notification to the regulator "as soon as practicable" after becoming aware.[64] NOTE: The Australian Government has announced in-principle agreement to amending the reporting period to 72 hours "but will further explore appropriate timeframes with stakeholders and alignment with other relevant reporting frameworks".[65] | "as soon as practicable after the completion of the preparation of the statement" [to the regulator][66] | Public notice permitted if individual notification not practicable.[67] Notification not required if the entity believes on reasonable grounds that it would: prejudice an enforcement-related activity;[68] be inconsistent with a Commonwealth secrecy provision.[69] The Commissioner can extend the reporting and notification period.[70] | <A$2.5M [£1.3M] for a person other than a body corporate and for a body corporate < the greater of $50M [£26.1M], or three times the value of the benefit reasonably attributable to the conduct, or 30% of the adjusted turnover during the period.[71] | "[T]he Commissioner will regularly publish de-identified statistical information about data breaches notified under the scheme".[72] |

(Continued)

TABLE 9.1 (Continued)

Jurisdiction	Key legislation or normative instrument	Data breach definition	Threshold for notification 🖥	Report to regulator: timing	Notification to individuals: timing 📱	Exceptions to notification	Penalty: failure to notify $	Public reporting 🖥
China	Personal Information Protection Law of the People's Republic of China 2021, and Draft Regulations on Network Data Security Management ("Draft Regulations")[73]	Notification is required for "any leakage of, tampering with, or loss of personal information".[74]	There is a harm threshold for individuals (see Exceptions).	The Draft Regulations were released for public comment in November 2021. If implemented, they would require initial notification to the regulator within 8 hours of a data security incident involving important data or the personal information of more than 100,000 people. [75]	The Draft Regulations require an interested party to be notified of a security incident that has caused harm to an individual or organisation within three business days.[76]	May not have to notify an individual if "measures to effectively avoid harm caused" can be taken.[77] The authorities may require individual notification if they believe "harm may be caused to the individual".[78] Under the Draft Regulations, a public announcement can be made if the interested party "cannot be reached".[79] Where such a notification is not required according to a statutory provision, that provision will prevail.	Under the Draft Regulations, if a correction is not made or serious consequences are caused, a fine of 0.5M to 2M RMB [£55,792 to £223,170] can be imposed "and they may be ordered to stop relevant operations, suspend operations for rectification, and have relevant business permits or licenses cancelled".[80] Directly responsible personnel can be fined 50,000 to 200,000 RMB [£5,579 to £22,317].[81]	Not specified

Hong Kong	Guidance on Data Breach Handling and Data Breach Notifications ("Guidance Note")[82]	"[A] suspected or actual breach of the security of personal data held by a data user, which exposes the personal data of data subject(s) to the risk of unauthorized or accidental access, processing, erasure, loss or use".[83]	No statutory requirement to report data breaches. Voluntary reporting is encouraged by the Guidance Note, especially where "the data breach is likely to result in a real risk of harm to those affected data subjects".[84]	"As soon as practicable after becoming aware of the data breach".[85]	N/A	"As soon as practicable after becoming aware of the data breach".[86]	N/A	Not specified. A general summary of data breach notifications is published in the Office of the Privacy Commissioner for Personal Data's annual report.[87]
India	Digital Personal Data Protection Act 2023 ("DPDP Act"),[88] and CERT—In directions[89]	"any unauthorised processing of personal data or accidental disclosure, acquisition, sharing, use, alteration, destruction or loss of access to personal data, that compromises the confidentiality, integrity or availability of personal data"[90] Includes diverse incidents including data breach, leak, unauthorised access, malicious code attacks, unauthorised access to social media accounts, identity theft, spoofing and phishing attacks.[91]	None specified.	DPDP Act: Not yet prescribed. CERT-In directions: within 6 hours of noticing cyber-incidents or being brought to notice about them.[92]	None specified.	DPDP Act: Not yet prescribed. CERT-In directions: None.	DPDP Act: Up to 2B rupees [£18.97M].[93] Cert-IN directions: Imprisonment for up to 1 year or a fine of up to 100,000 rupees [£948] or both.[94]	Not stipulated in the Act. The Data Protection Board has not been established at the date of writing.[95]

(Continued)

TABLE 9.1 (Continued)

Jurisdiction	Key legislation or normative instrument	Data breach definition	Threshold for notification	Report to regulator: timing	Notification to individuals: timing	Exceptions to notification	Penalty: failure to notify $	Public reporting
Indonesia	Personal Data Protection Law 2022 ("PDPL"), and Draft Government Regulation Implementing the Personal Data Protection Law[96] ("Draft Regulation")	Defined by the PDPL as "any failure in protecting a person's personal data in terms of confidentiality, integrity, and availability of the personal data, including security breaches, whether intentional or unintentional, which lead to the unlawful destruction, loss, alteration, unauthorised disclosure of, or access to, personal data transmitted, stored or processed".[97]	No threshold for notifying the regulator and data subjects. Public notification is also required if there is a disruption to the provision of public services or a serious impact on the public interest.[98]	72 hours[99]	72 hours[100]	If implemented, the Draft Regulation would provide an exemption for public notification requirements if a breach has not led to the disclosure of personal data.[101]	Administrative sanctions may include a written warning, temporary suspension of personal data processing activities, deletion or destruction of personal data, and/or administrative fines.[102]	A separate institution is being formed. The Draft Regulation provides it with supervisory powers, the outcomes of which are to be published in a manner accessible to the public.[103]
Japan	Act on the Protection of Personal Information 2003, and Personal Information Protection Commission Guidelines	"[A] leak, loss or damage and other situation concerning the security of the personal information".[104]	Notification to the regulator and affected data subjects is required if individual rights and interests are likely to be harmed.[105] The Personal Information Protection Commission has specified that notification is required for breaches that involve (or are likely to involve) sensitive personal information, personal information likely to cause financial damage, a wrongful purpose and/or more than 1,000 data subjects.[106]	Immediately (generally within 3 to 5 days).[107]	Promptly.[108]	Notification to the regulator is not required where personal information was not actually accessible to third parties (e.g. if it was encrypted).[109] Notification to an individual is not required if it is practically difficult to make, and if other measures (e.g. publication on a business website) are taken.[110]	Failure to comply with an order of the regulator is punishable by a fine of up to JPY 1M [£5,348] or one year in prison.[111]	The Commission may request reports from administrative entities on the Act's enforcement and if so, must compile these reports and publish a summary.[112] Statistics on reported personal data breaches have been published.[113]

Malaysia	Personal Data Protection Act 2010, Public Consultation Paper No 1/2018, and Public Consultation Paper No 1/2020	Not defined	There is no legislative requirement to make a notification. A data leakage notification form can be downloaded from the Department of Personal Data Protection's website. It can be used to report a personal data breach "in circumstances where the breach presents a risk to the affected data subjects".[114] Authorities previously issued two public consultation papers. The Minister of Communications and Digital indicated an intention to present a draft amendment bill to the Personal Data Protection Act 2010 by the end of 2023.[115]	Public Consultation Paper No 1/2018 suggested 72 hours.[116]	N/A	N/A	N/A	Not specified. The Personal Data Protection Commissioner is "to promote awareness and dissemination of information to the public" about the operation of the Act.[117]

(Continued)

TABLE 9.1 (Continued)

Jurisdiction	Key legislation or normative instrument	Data breach definition	Threshold for notification 🖥	Report to regulator: timing	Notification to individuals: timing 🔲	Exceptions to notification	Penalty: failure to notify $	Public reporting 📊
Mongolia	Law of Mongolia on Personal Data Protection 2021	"Any violations identified during data collection and processing" are subject to notification requirements.[118]	No threshold for Data Processor notifying Data Controller.[119] If the violation causes damage to the rights and legitimate interest of a Data Owner (i.e. the data subject), the Data Controller (not the Data Processor) must notify them.[120] Only annual reporting to the regulator is required.[121]	Annual reporting in January (or on request) to the National Human Rights Commission of Mongolia.[122]	'Immediately.'[123]	None specified.	A person or legal entity that violates the law is subject to liability specified in the Criminal Code or the Law on Violations.[124] Under the latter, individuals can be fined 500,000 to 2M MNT [£114 to £458] and legal entities 5M to 20M MNT [£1,144 to £4,576].[125]	The National Human Rights Commission is to "specify data... violations... in the report on the situation of human rights and freedoms in Mongolia".[126]

| New Zealand | Privacy Act 2020 | "(i) unauthorised or accidental access to, or disclosure, alteration, loss, or destruction of, the personal information; or (ii) an action that prevents the agency from accessing the information on either a temporary or permanent basis".[127]

"a privacy breach that it is reasonable to believe has caused serious harm to an affected individual or individuals or is likely to do so".[128]

In assessing the breach against the threshold, the agency must consider "(a) any action taken by the agency to reduce the risk of harm following the breach: (b) whether the personal information is sensitive in nature: (c) the nature of the harm that may be caused to affected individuals: (d) the person or body that has obtained or may obtain personal information as a result of the breach (if known): (e) whether the personal information is protected by a security measure: (f) any other relevant matters".[129] | "as soon as practicable after becoming aware that a notifiable privacy breach has occurred"[130] (Guideline states "our expectation is that a breach notification should be made to our Office no later than 72 hours after agencies are aware of a notifiable privacy breach"[131]).

"as soon as practicable after becoming aware that a notifiable privacy breach has occurred", with exceptions.[132] | Public notice permitted if individual notification not "reasonably practicable".[133] Notification not required if the agency believes on reasonable grounds that it would: endanger a person's safety; reveal a trade secret; prejudice security, defence, international relations or the maintenance of the law;[134] if the person is under 16 years and notification would be contrary to their interests; or after consulting with the individual's health practitioner the agency reasonably believes that the notification would be likely to prejudice the person's health.[135] | <NZ$10,000 [£4,893]. | The Commissioner may publish the identity of an agency that has reported a data breach a) with consent or b) in the public interest. The Commissioner may publish de-identified to inform "the public about the extent and nature of privacy breaches".[136] |

(Continued)

TABLE 9.1 (Continued)

Jurisdiction	Key legislation or normative instrument	Data breach definition	Threshold for notification	Report to regulator: timing	Notification to individuals: timing	Exceptions to notification	Penalty: failure to notify $	Public reporting
The Philippines	Data Privacy Act 2012, National Privacy Commission Circular 16-03 (15 December 2016), and Implementing Rules and Regulations of Republic Act No. 10173 (IRR)	"a breach of security leading to the accidental or unlawful destruction, loss, alteration, unauthorized disclosure of, or access to, personal data… [This may be]: 1. An availability breach resulting from loss, accidental or unlawful destruction of personal data; 2. Integrity breach resulting from alteration of personal data; and/or 3. A confidentiality breach resulting from the unauthorized disclosure of or access to personal data".[137]	Information that may, "under the circumstances, be used to enable identity fraud are reasonably believed to have been acquired by an unauthorized person, and the personal information controller or the commission believes that such unauthorized acquisition is likely to give rise to a real risk of serious harm to any affected data subject".[138] Threshold further stipulated as knowledge or reasonable belief that a breach requiring notification has occurred: of "sensitive personal information" or "other information", including financial data; usernames, passwords; biometric data; identification documents or identifiers; where the information may have been acquired by an unauthorized person and this is likely to generate "a real risk of serious harm to any affected data subject".[139]	Within 72 hours.[140] "Notification may be delayed only to the extent necessary to determine the scope of the breach, to prevent further disclosures, or to restore reasonable integrity to the information and communications system".[141] No delay permitted if the breach involves >100 data subjects or the disclosure of sensitive personal information would harm the data subject.[142]	Within 72 hours.[143] An exemption or delay may be sought from the regulator.[144] "Notification may be delayed only to the extent necessary to determine the scope of the breach, to prevent further disclosures, or to restore reasonable integrity to the information and communications system".[145]	"(1) In evaluating if notification is unwarranted, the Commission may take into account compliance by the personal information controller with this section and existence of good faith in the acquisition of personal information.(2) The Commission may exempt a personal information controller from notification where, in its reasonable judgment, such notification would not be in the public interest or in the interests of the affected data subjects.(3) The Commission may authorize postponement of notification where it may hinder the progress of a criminal investigation related to a serious breach".[146]	Imprisonment for 1.5 to 5 years and a fine of Php 0.5M to 1M [£7,116 to £14,232] for a person who knows of a security breach and the obligation to notify the Commissioner, and "intentionally or by omission conceals the fact of such security breach".[147]	General summary in the annual report of the National Privacy Commission.

| Singapore | Personal Data Protection Act 2012 | "(a) the unauthorised access, collection, use, disclosure, copying, modification or disposal of personal data; or (b) the loss of any storage medium or device on which personal data is stored in circumstances where the unauthorised access, collection, use, disclosure, copying, modification or disposal of the personal data is likely to occur".[148] | If the data breach "(a) results in, or is likely to result in, significant harm to an affected individual; or (b) is, or is likely to be, of a significant scale".[149] A notifiable breach includes a breach of name or identification number coupled with information about a sexually transmitted disease, HIV, schizophrenia, substance abuse and addiction, contraceptive care, organ donation or removal, pregnancy termination, suicide or attempted suicide, or abuse.[150] Significant harm includes "physical, psychological, emotional, economic and financial harm, as well as harm to reputation and other forms of harms that a reasonable person would identify as a possible outcome of a data breach".[151] A significant scale is >500 people.[152] | An organisation with a reasonable belief that a data breach has occurred must conduct an assessment "in a reasonable and expeditious manner".[153] Notification to the regulator is required as soon as is practicable, but not more than 3 calendar days after this assessment.[154] The assessment and notification process should generally be complete within 30 calendar days.[155] | "on or after notifying the Commission".[156] | A breach within an organisation is excluded.[157] Notification to affected individuals not permitted if the Commission or a law enforcement agency directs otherwise. Notification not required when the data custodian takes steps to make it unlikely that the data breach would result in significant harm to the individual.[158] | For intentional or negligent contravention, up to 10% of annual turnover (of over $10 million [£5.92M]) in Singapore; or in any other case $1 million [£591,855].[159] | Not specified. |

(Continued)

TABLE 9.1 (Continued)

Jurisdiction	Key legislation or normative instrument	Data breach definition	Threshold for notification	Report to regulator: timing	Notification to individuals: timing	Exceptions to notification	Penalty: failure to notify $	Public reporting
South Korea	Personal Information Protection Act 2020, and Enforcement Decree of the Personal Information Protection Act 2023[160]	"[W]hen the personal information controller becomes aware [data subjects'] personal information has been divulged".[161] Described in the Enforcement Decree as "loss, theft, or divulgence".[162]	Data controllers are required to notify affected individuals, but not the regulator unless >1000 people have been affected, the information involved is sensitive or personally identifiable, or personal information has been divulged "due to illegal external access to personal information processing systems or information technology equipment used by personal handlers for processing personal information".[163]	72 hours[164]	72 hours[165]	An individual notification can be made outside the 72-hour period if urgent measures need to be taken to prevent widespread/ further divulgence and/or a natural disaster or "any other unavoidable cause" makes it impractical.[166] The report to the regulator can also be delayed if a natural disaster "or any other unavoidable cause" makes it impractical. If "the possibility of infringing on the rights and interests of data subjects is substantially reduced… and measures are taken such as the recovery and deletion of the personal information… the personal information controller need not file a report".[167] If the contact information of an individual is not known, "or if any other good cause exits", a personal information controller can post the required information on its website (for at least 30 days) in lieu of giving a notification.[168]	Failure to notify or file a report will attract an administrative fine not exceeding 30M won [£182].[169]	An annual report detailing the "infringement on the rights of data subjects" must be submitted by the Personal Information Protection Commission to the National Assembly.[170] It details measures taken to respond to personal data breaches, including the number of cases involving personal information exposed in images and posts.[171]

Sri Lanka	Personal Data Protection Act 2022 ("PDPA")	"[A]ny act or omission that results in accidental or unlawful destruction, loss, alternation, unauthorized disclosure of, or access to, personal data transmitted, stored or otherwise processed".[172]	To be established. The PDPA provides the Personal Data Protection Authority with the power to determine the circumstances where it will be notified of a personal data breach.[173] The Authority is still in the process of being created and plans to implement policy frameworks and regulations following public consultations.[174]	Not yet specified	Not yet specified	Not yet specified	A penalty not exceeding 10M rupees [£24,084] may be applied if there is a failure to comply with a directive of the Authority.[175]	Not specified. The Authority will submit an annual report of its activities to the relevant minister, who will then present the report to Parliament.[176]
Taiwan	Personal Data Protection Act 1995, and Enforcement Rules of the Personal Data Protection Act 1996	A notification is required where "any personal data is stolen, disclosed, altered, or otherwise infringed upon due to a violation of the PDPA by a government or non-government agency".[177]	No threshold for notifying individuals. Only have to notify the regulator if sector-specific regulations require this. The Regulations Governing the Production and Issuance of the National Health Insurance IC Card and Data Storage do not specify any additional notification requirements.	"In a prompt manner"[178] after the relevant facts have been clarified.[179]	N/A	None specified.	A fine of NT $20,000 to $200,000 [£505 to £5,046] shall be imposed on a non-government agency for each violation.[180]	Not specified. The National Development Council's Personal Data Protection Office does not appear to publish data. A new independent agency—the Personal Data Protection Commission—is being established to strengthen enforcement of the Act.[181]

TABLE 9.1 (Continued)

Jurisdiction	Key legislation or normative instrument	Data breach definition	Threshold for notification	Report to regulator: timing	Notification to individuals: timing	Exceptions to notification	Penalty: failure to notify $	Public reporting
Thailand	Personal Data Protection Act 2019, and Notification of the PDPC on Rules and Methods of Personal Data Breach Notification 2022	Defined as "any breach of security measures resulting in unauthorized or unlawful loss, access to, use, alteration, correction, or disclosure of personal data whether caused by intent, wilfulness, negligence, or an unauthorized or unlawful act, a computer crime, a cyber threat, an error or accident, or any other cause".[182]	Must notify the regulator unless the breach "is unlikely to result in a risk to the rights and freedoms" of persons.[183] Only have to notify individuals if the breach "is likely to result in a high risk to the rights and freedoms" of persons.[184]	"Without delay" and, "where feasible, within 72 hours".[185]	"Without delay".[186]	If there is a reasonable cause, can request the fine for failing to notify on-time be waived, but only within 15 days of becoming aware of the breach.[187]	Up to 3M Baht [£67,312].[188]	Not specified. An annual operation report of the Office of Personal Data Protection Committee is to be publicly disseminated.[189]
Vietnam	Decree No. 13/2023/ND—CP on Personal Data Protection	"a violation against regulations on protection of personal data".[190]	Not stated	72 hours[191]	Not required.	Reasons for delay must be provided if notice is given outside the 72-hour window.[192]	Not specified (disciplinary action, administrative penalties, or criminal prosecution).[193]	None specified

have a scheme either in draft form, partially developed, or in force but still requiring the enactment of subordinate legislation to fully specify NDB requirements. As noted earlier, numerous countries in the region still have no such schemes, and not all existing schemes apply uniformly across a jurisdiction. The NDB schemes discussed here show partial consistency, aligning more in some elements than in others. A summary of findings in relation to the five key elements follows.

Reporting to regulatory authorities

Most of the 17 assessed NDB schemes require entities affected by a data breach to report this to a national regulator. However, reporting is voluntary in Hong Kong and Malaysia; it is not required in Taiwan unless sector-specific regulations require it; and it is only required annually in Mongolia (to the National Human Rights Commission, rather than a privacy regulator). The threshold for reporting varies, with several jurisdictions applying some form of risk, harm, or scale threshold. For instance, in Japan the regulator must be informed of a breach if individual rights and interests are likely to be harmed, but not where personal information was not actually accessible to third parties (e.g. if encrypted). In Australia, a breach must be reported to the Office of the Australian Information Commissioner if it is likely to result in serious harm to at least one person and the risk cannot be prevented through remedial action.

Almost all of the jurisdictions considered here that mandate reporting breaches to a regulator stipulate a timeframe of 72 hours to do so after awareness of the breach arises, mirroring the GDPR provision. Some set an even shorter timeframe for high level reporting of basic information: 6 hours under India's CERT-IN directions, and in China a proposed 8 hours for incidents involving the data of more than 100,000 people, or involving "important" data (data whose use may harm national security or the public interest, including a wide range of data types specified in the draft regulation). Australia is an outlier with a 30-day grace period for assessment, although it is considering reducing this to align with the 72-hour limit (see Table 9.1). Only a handful of jurisdictions merely require reporting to be "as soon as practicable after becoming aware" of a breach (e.g. Hong Kong, which has voluntary reporting).

A short timeframe for alerting the regulator should enhance NDB schemes' ability to meet at least four key aims: to motivate pre-emptive data security improvements, promote transparency, enable vicarious punishment of the data custodian, and facilitate system-wide learnings. It should also enable data custodians affected by a breach to quickly access advice and support from the regulator on other harm minimization and regulatory compliance steps.

Notification to affected individuals

Individual notification of those affected by a breach is not always required. In many jurisdictions such notification is conditional, based on a risk or harm threshold (e.g. EU GDPR, Australia, New Zealand, the Philippines, Singapore, Thailand). Others (e.g. South Korea, Taiwan) stipulate unconditional notification to affected individuals. Timeframes are often more generous for notifying individuals than they are for advising the regulator of a breach. For instance, Australia, Hong Kong, and New Zealand adopt "'as soon as practicable" individual notification requirements, similar to the EU GDPR's "without undue delay" and Thailand's "without delay". A few countries stipulate a 72-hour period to notify both the regulator and affected individuals (e.g. Indonesia, the Philippines, South Korea).

Flexibility in notification timing may be useful: to accommodate diverse breach circumstances; to prioritize investigation and harm mitigation by the data custodian; and to ensure that notification proceeds in an orderly manner. However undue delays in notification may negate several regulatory aims, most obviously the mitigation of individual harm by the data subject, as well as the transparency aim. Achieving transparency through rapid notification may be especially important for individuals affected by health data breaches, who are likely to prioritize their "right to know" even when harm mitigation is not easy or possible.

Penalties for failure to report/notify

All NDB schemes that currently mandate reporting and/or notification incorporate penalties for non-compliance. While these vary, they can be surprisingly large. For instance, in Singapore fines may be up to 10% of annual turnover; under the GDPR, up to €10M [£8.6M] or 2% of annual global turnover, and in Australia, more than AUS$50M [£26.1M]. Imprisonment for breaching NDB requirements is a potential punishment in India, Japan, and the Philippines.

Strong penalties are important in overcoming companies' natural reticence to hide cyber-attacks, and in encouraging transparency (with flow-on benefits such as individual harm mitigation). They should, however, be balanced with recognition that the data custodian may itself have suffered a major data breach through others' criminal activities, and that in the context of a rapidly developing cyber-attack threatening privacy, commercial interests, and even physical well-being (e.g. during hospital ransomware attacks), attention may be properly focused on repelling the attack or negotiating with hackers for release of data, rather than primarily on regulatory disclosure obligations.

Public reporting (aggregate/identifiable)

Only two of the jurisdictions analysed here (Mongolia and South Korea) included a legislated requirement that the regulator publish information about reported data breaches. New Zealand's Privacy Act 2020 is unique among the reviewed schemes in permitting the regulator to publish both de-identified information and identified information about a breach (the latter with the consent of the breached entity, or if the Commissioner is satisfied that doing so is in the public interest). Other jurisdictions either make no reference to public reporting, or undertake it as a procedural rather than a statutory step (e.g. Australia, Hong Kong, Japan, the Philippines). Given the relevance of public reporting for promoting NDB scheme aims of transparency (in particular), as well as vicarious punishment and stimulating pre-emptive investment in data security measures, this is an element ripe for strengthening. Further research should examine the case for regulators' public reporting of data breaches in more detail, and consider its most useful format in light of the specific aims being pursued. Preventing and responding to breaches of health data, in particular, focuses attention on the NDB scheme aims of pre-emptive investment in data security, transparency, and system-wide learnings, all of which can be supported by public reporting measures.

Considerations for reform

NDB regulation is evolving dynamically in the Asia-Pacific region, with numerous countries soon to introduce, recently introducing, reforming, or planning reform of their statutory schemes. In all instances, law- and policy-makers should critically reflect on the principal aims of the scheme within their jurisdiction, and select and fashion specific regulatory elements to best achieve those aims. Although such a statement may seem a truism, this analysis reveals that there is often a mismatch between NDB scheme aims (as broadly identified in scholarly literature) and legislative design. For instance, individual harm mitigation is often touted as justification for data breach notification schemes, but achieving this goal could be undermined in jurisdictions where reporting to a regulatory authority is prioritized over notification to individuals, and when the timing of such notification is permissive. Promoting transparency—another important aim—is undermined by lack of, or minimalist, public reporting rules and practices. Very short notification timeframes and severe penalties for non-compliance may, in some instances, be unduly punitive when often there is little a data custodian could have done to prevent a breach (given the level of sophistication of attacks and resourcing of attackers).

To solidify general expectations of how NDB schemes operate, and to streamline obligations upon transnational organizations, broad alignment between national schemes is desirable, and seems to be occurring. What is generally absent, however, is fundamental recognition that data breach notification as a regulated practice arose primarily to serve needs relating to financial and identity data loss, some two decades ago. At that time, health information was mainly held in paper records. Now, electronic health data constitutes approximately 30% of the world's data, and this proportion is growing rapidly.[194] Arguably, a statutory requirement to notify people about breaches, including of health data, yet which currently treats health data the same as bank account numbers and email addresses, needs thorough reconsideration. Notification schemes that are generically configured will fail to address the unique distress and other harms flowing from a breach of potentially stigmatizing health information. Moreover, some of the schemes reviewed here prioritize reporting data breaches to a national regulator over notifying those affected, and omit notification unless there is a risk of "significant harm". However, "significant harm" under the statute, even if construed broadly, may not consistently cover the risk of dignitary harm from simply knowing that one's health data have been breached.[195] There appears to be a risk that data custodians, in jurisdictions with these conditional notification requirements, may judge that if a breach generates no risk of identity theft or pecuniary loss, there is no need to notify those affected. This warrants legislative reconsideration of the conditional elements of breach notification with a view to more nuanced identification of, and remedial measures for, the personal harms of health data breaches specifically.

Further research on the effects and effectiveness of NDB schemes, and specifically, the act of notification itself, is overdue. This should disaggregate effects by data type and industry sector. Qualitative research with individuals who are notified about a breach should carefully examine the impact of notification separately from the effects of the breach itself. The Singaporean scheme would be particularly fruitful to examine given its explicit focus on sensitive health information. Conducting research across different types of information breaches will help to address the question of whether notification should be more closely tailored according to data type. Further, and as indicated earlier, detailed examination of optimal requirements for public reporting by regulators is also warranted. The operation and impact of the New Zealand scheme, which details both aggregate and identifiable reporting within the statute itself, would be a useful starting point. Regulators should be involved in jointly reflecting on how best to communicate to the public about reported data breaches, in ways aligned with the overarching aims of NDB schemes discussed here.

Conclusion

Analysing NDB schemes across the Asia-Pacific region sheds light on regulators' efforts to grapple urgently with preventing and mitigating the harms caused by an onslaught of major cyber-attacks involving individuals' personal information. There is rapid growth of such schemes and increasing, and welcome, alignment around GDPR-like provisions, particularly in relation to reporting timeframes. However, the schemes considered here struggle to adequately address the particular problems caused by breaches of health data. Emphasizing the precautionary steps individuals should take after a breach which focus on identity theft and financial risk; delays in notification; and absent or vague public reporting requirements all limit NDB schemes' ability to aid those who find their most personal data have been wrongly accessed, and perhaps stolen or published. The ever-greater sophistication of cyber-attacks on personal data in general, and health data in particular, demands an NDB framework across the region whose design is more strongly connected to its underpinning aims, with more robust harm mitigation measures that accommodate diverse types of breached data, and based upon greater evidence of the impacts of notification on those affected.

Acknowledgements

I thank Melbourne Law School Librarian Carole Hinchcliff and research assistant Ms Nicola Ziaris for their help with (respectively) locating sources and collecting information about data breach notification schemes.

Notes

1 Adam Vincent, "State-Sponsored Hackers: The New Normal for Business" (2017) 2017 *Network Security* 10.
2 "Operations of Private Health Insurers Annual Report | APRA", available at: https://www.apra.gov.au/operations-of-private-health-insurers-annual-report.
3 Josh Taylor, "Medibank Hackers Announce 'Case Closed' and Dump Huge Data File on Dark Web" *The Guardian* (1 December 2022), available at: https://www.theguardian.com/australia-news/2022/dec/01/medibank-hackers-announce-case-closed-and-dump-huge-data-file-on-dark-web.
4 Colin Biggs and Tim Kruger, "$US1 per Customer: Alleged Medibank Hackers Reveal Ransom Demands" *The Age* (Melbourne, 9 November 2022), available at: https://www.theage.com.au/business/companies/suspected-medibank-hackers-reveal-ransom-demands-20221110-p5bx10.html; Hilary Whiteman, "Medibank Data Breach: Australia Blames Cyber Criminals in Russia for Attack" *CNN Business* (11 November 2022), available at: https://edition.cnn.com/2022/11/11/tech/medibank-australia-ransomware-attack-intl-hnk/index.html; Taylor, n 3.
5 Aleisha Orr and Wei Wang, "Elaine's Data was Stolen in the Medibank Hack. She Says 'sorry' Isn't Enough" *SBS News* (12 November 2022), available at: https://www.sbs.com.au/news/article/elaines-data-was-stolen-in-the-medibank-hack-she-says-sorry-isnt-enough/4c7ktafnx.
6 Javad K Pool and others, "Causes and Impacts of Personal Health Information (PHI) Breaches: A Scoping Review and Thematic Analysis" (2019), available at: https://papers.ssrn.com/abstract=3584865.
7 Frederic Schlackl, Nico Link, and Hartmut Hoehle, "Antecedents and Consequences of Data Breaches: A Systematic Review" (2022) 59 *Information & Management* 103638.

8 Romilla Syed, "Enterprise Reputation Threats on Social Media: A Case of Data Breach Framing" (2019) 28 *The Journal of Strategic Information Systems* 257.

9 Ravi Pilla, Taiwo Oseni, and Andrew Stranieri, "A Study Into the Impact of Data Breaches of Electronic Health Records", *Proceedings of the 2023 Australasian Computer Science Week (Association for Computing Machinery 2023)*, available at: https://doi.org/10.1145/3579375.3579415.

10 Alexis Zacharakos, "Studies Show Ransomware Has Already Caused Patient Deaths" *TechTarget* (May 2023), available at: https://www. techtarget.com/searchsecurity/feature/Studies-show-ransomware-has-already-caused-patient-deaths.

11 In Europe these regulatory bodies are the Data Protection Authorities, while titles vary elsewhere. For instance, Australia has the Office of the Australian Information Commissioner (OAIC), Japan and South Korea have a Personal Information Protection Commission, and in Malaysia the Personal Data Protection Department is the relevant body.

12 APEC, *APEC Privacy Framework* (APEC Secretariat 2015) 10–11, 28; OECD, *OECD Privacy Framework* (OECD 2013) 26, available at: https://www.oecd. org/sti/ieconomy/oecd_privacy_framework.pdf.

13 OECD, n 12, 26.

14 Megan Prictor, "Mandatory Data Breach Notification Laws and Australian Health Data Privacy: Fragments and Fault Lines" (2021) 47 *Monash University Law Review* 21.

15 European Union Agency for Cybersecurity (ENISA), "ENISA Threat Landscape: Health Sector (January 2021 to March 2023)" (ENISA 2023) Report/Study 3, available at: https://www.enisa.europa.eu/publications/health-threat-landscape.

16 OAIC, "Notifiable Data Breaches Report: January to June 2023", *OAIC* (5 September 2023) 35, available at: https://www.oaic.gov.au/privacy/notifiable-data-breaches/notifiable-data-breaches-publications/notifiable-data-breaches-report-january-to-june-2023.

17 Ibid., 32.

18 "Unacceptable Malicious Cyber Activity", Australian Government Department of Foreign Affairs and Trade (20 May 2020), available at: https://www.dfat.gov. au/news/news/unacceptable-malicious-cyber-activity.

19 OAIC, "Notifiable Data Breaches Report", n 16, 11.

20 "Allianz Risk Barometer 2023" (2023) 7, available at: https://www.allianz.com. au/about-us/media-hub/allianz-risk-barometer-2023.html.

21 World Economic Forum, "The Global Risks Report 2023" (18th edn, World Economic Forum 2023) 8.

22 "IOCTA 2023: Forget Hackers in a Hoodie, Cybercrime Has Become a Big Business" (*Europol*), available at: https://www.europol.europa.eu/media-press/newsroom/news/iocta-2023-forget-hackers-in-hoodie-cybercrime-has-become-big-business.

23 "Cybercrime: The Next Entrepreneurial Growth Business?"|WIRED, available at: https://www.wired.com/insights/2014/10/cybercrime-growth-business/.

24 Australian Signals Directorate, "ACSC Annual Cyber Threat Report" (2021) 45, available at: https://www.cyber.gov.au/about-us/reports-and-statistics/acsc-annual-cyber-threat-report-july-2021-june-2022.

25 Sung J Choi, Min Chen, and Xuan Tan, "Assessing the Impact of Health Information Exchange on Hospital Data Breach Risk" (2023) 177 *International Journal of Medical Informatics* 105149; Elizabeth Averill Samaras and George Michael Samaras, "Confronting Systemic Challenges in Interoperable Medical Device Safety, Security & Usability" (2016) 63 *Journal of Biomedical Informatics* 226.

26 Mohiuddin Ahmed and Paul Haskell-Dowland, "Why Health Data Hacks Keep Happening", *NewsGP* (9 May 2023), available at: https://www1.racgp.org.au/newsgp/professional/why-health-data-hacks-keep-happening.

27 LaFrenz and Max Mason, "Hackers Steal 10 Years of Patient Forms from TPG Asia-Backed TissuPath" *Australian Financial Review* (6 September 2023), available at: https://www.afr.com/companies/healthcare-and-fitness/tpg-asia-backed-tissupath-tangled-in-data-breach-20230906-p5e2fl.

28 Eileen Yu, "Firms Fined $1M for SingHealth Data Security Breach", *ZDNET* (15 January 2019), available at: https://www.zdnet.com/article/firms-fined-1m-for-singhealth-data-security-breach/.

29 Victor Barriero, Jr, "76% of Devices in Healthcare Facilities in PH Infected by Malicious Code", *Rappler* (14 September 2019), available at: https://www.rappler.com/technology/features/240084-medical-devices-philippines-malicious-infections-kaspersky-cybersecurity-weekend/.

30 IBM Security, "Cost of a Data Breach Report 2023" (2023) 8, available at: https://www.ibm.com/reports/data-breach.

31 See e.g. "Second Reading Speech, Privacy Amendment (Notifiable Data Breaches) Bill 2016 (Mr Keenan)", available at: https://parlinfo.aph.gov.au/parlInfo/search/display/display.w3p;query=Id%3A%22chamber%2Fhansardr%2Fbb53e009-91c0-438a-af01-a60fc481fdbf%2F0013%22.

32 Commonwealth of Australia, "Strengthening Australia's Cyber Security Regulations and Incentives—A Call for Views" (2021) 12, available at: https://www.homeaffairs.gov.au/reports-and-publications/submissions-and-discussion-papers/cyber-security-regulations-incentives.

33 "Cybercrime – Shareholder Class Action", *Medibank Newsroom*, available at: https://www.medibank.com.au/livebetter/newsroom/post/cybercrime-shareholder-classaction.

34 Laurel Henning, "Data Breaches Usher in a New Era for Australian Class Actions", available at: https://www.lexisnexis.com.au/en/insights-and-analysis/practice-intelligence/2023/data-breaches-usher-in-a-new-era-for-australian-class-actions.

35 John Emmerig, "Data Breach Class Actions in Australia: White Paper" (Jones Day 2019) 2, available at: https://www.jonesday.com/en/insights/2019/05/data-breach-class-actions-in-australia.

36 Prictor, n 14; Burkhard Schafer, "Speaking Truth to/as Victims—A Jurisprudential Analysis of Data Breach Notification Laws" in Mariarosaria Taddeo and Luciano Floridi (eds), *The Responsibilities of Online Service Providers* (Springer International Publishing 2017), available at: https://doi.org/10.1007/978-3-319-47852-4_5; Angela Daly, "The Introduction of Data Breach Notification Legislation in Australia: A Comparative View" (2018) 34 *Computer Law & Security Review* 477; Mark Burdon, "Contextualizing the Tensions and Weaknesses of Information Privacy and Data Breach Notification Laws" (2010) 27 *Santa Clara Computer & High Technology Law Journal* 63.

37 Lani Watson, *The Right to Know: Epistemic Rights and Why We Need Them* (Routledge 2021).

38 Graham Greenleaf, "Australia's Data Breach Notification Bill: Transparency Deficits" [2016] UNSWLRS 54, 3.

39 Roy Shapira, "When Does Corporate Shaming Translate into Reputational Fallouts?", *The Legal Aspects of Shaming: An Ancient Sanction in the Modern World* (Edward Elgar 2023) 79, available at: <https://www.elgaronline.com/edcollchap/book/9781800880221/book-part-9781800880221-11.xml.

40 OAIC, "Part 4: Notifiable Data Breach (NDB) Scheme", *OAIC* (10 March 2023), available at: https://www.oaic.gov.au/privacy/privacy-guidance-

for-organisations-and-government-agencies/preventing-preparing-for-and-responding-to-data-breaches/data-breach-preparation-and-response/part-4-notifiable-data-breach-ndb-scheme.

41 Personal Data Protection Act 2012 (Singapore) 2012 (Singapore), s 4(1)(c).

42 Vibhushinie Bentotahewa, Chaminda Hewage, and Jason Williams, "The Normative Power of the GDPR: A Case Study of Data Protection Laws of South Asian Countries" (2022) 3 SN *Computer Science* 183.

43 Penalty amounts are provided in their original currency and in GBP (£) as at 1 December 2023.

44 "Law in Cambodia—DLA Piper Global Data Protection Laws of the World", available at: https://www.dlapiperdataprotection.com/index.html?t=law&c=KH.

45 "Timor Leste—Data Protection Overview", *DataGuidance* (7 July 2021), available at: https://www.dataguidance.com/notes/timor-leste-data-protection-overview.

46 "Lao PDR—Data Protection Overview", *DataGuidance* (28 November 2022), available at: https://www.dataguidance.com/notes/lao-pdr-data-protection-overview.

47 "Myanmar—Data Protection Overview", *DataGuidance* (31 August 2023), available at: https://www.dataguidance.com/notes/myanmar-data-protection-overview.

48 Deloitte, "Unity in Diversity: The Asia Pacific Privacy Guide" (2019) 68, available at: https://www2.deloitte.com/content/dam/Deloitte/nz/Documents/risk/apac-privacy-guide-interactive.pdf.

49 Regulation (EU) 2016/679 of the European Parliament and of the Council of 27 April 2016 on the protection of natural persons with regard to the processing of personal data and on the free movement of such data, and repealing Directive 95/46/EC (General Data Protection Regulation), OJ 2016 L 119/1. Other NDB legislation includes Directive (EU) 2016/1148 concerning measures for a high common level of security of network and information systems across the Union (NIS Directive) and Regulation (EU) 910/2014 on electronic identification and trust services for electronic transactions in the internal market (eIDAS Regulation).

50 European Data Protection Board, "Guidelines 9/2022 on Personal Data Breach Notification under GDPR (Version 2.0)".

51 EU General Data Protection Regulation (GDPR), Art 4(12).

52 Ibid., Recital 86(1).

53 Ibid., Art 33(1).

54 Ibid., Recital 86(1).

55 Ibid., Art 33(1).

56 Ibid., Art 83(4)(a).

57 There are additional NDB requirements under other laws, e.g. *My Health Records Act 2012* (Cth), *National Cancer Screening Register Act 2016* (Cth), *Privacy and Personal Information Protection Act 1998* (NSW), and cyber-security incident reporting under the *Security of Critical Infrastructure Act 2018* (Cth).

58 Privacy Act 1988 (Cth [Australia]), s 26WF(2)(a)(i).

59 Ibid., s 26WF(2)(b)(i).

60 Ibid., s 26WF(2)(a)(ii), (b)(ii).

61 Ibid., s 26WG(c)-(j).

62 Ibid., s 26WF(1).

63 Ibid., s 26WH(2).

64 Ibid., s 26WK(1),(2).

65 Attorney-General's Department, "Government Response—Privacy Act Review Report" (2023) 9, available at: https://www.ag.gov.au/rights-and-protections/publications/government-response-privacy-act-review-report.

66 Privacy Act, s 26WL(3).
67 Ibid., s 26WL(2)(c).
68 Ibid., s 26WN.
69 Ibid., s 26WP.
70 Ibid., s 26WQ.
71 OAIC, "Chapter 7: Civil Penalties—Serious or Repeated Interference with Privacy and Other Penalty Provisions", *OAIC* (10 March 2023), available at: https://www.oaic.gov.au/about-the-OAIC/our-regulatory-approach/guide-to-privacy-regulatory-action/chapter-7-privacy-assessments.
72 OAIC, "Part 4", n 39.
73 "Circular of the Cyberspace Administration of China on Seeking Public Comments on the Regulations on Network Data Security Management (Draft for Comment)"; see also Cybersecurity Law of the People's Republic of China 2016; Data Security Law of the People's Republic of China 2021.
74 Personal Information Protection Law of the People's Republic of China 2021, Art 57.
75 Draft Regulations on Network Data Security Management (China), Art 11.
76 Ibid.
77 Personal Information Protection Law of the People's Republic of China, Art 57.
78 Ibid.
79 Draft Regulations on Network Data Security Management (China), Art 11.
80 Ibid., Art 60.
81 Ibid.
82 Office of the Privacy Commissioner for Personal Data, Hong Kong, "Guidance on Data Breach Handling and Data Breach Notifications", available at: https://www.pcpd.org.hk/english/resources_centre/publications/guidance/guidance.html.
83 Ibid., 1.
84 Ibid., 6.
85 Ibid.
86 Ibid.
87 See Office of the Privacy Commissioner for Personal Data, Hong Kong, "Protecting Personal Data Privacy for a Smart Hong Kong: Annual Report 2022–23" 57–8, available at: https://www.pcpd.org.hk/english/resources_centre/publications/annual_report/annualreport2023.html.
88 This Act is not in operation at the date of writing.
89 Directions under sub-section (6) of section 70B of the Information Technology Act, 2000 (Indian Computer Emergency Response Team (CERT-In)).
90 Digital Personal Data Protection Act 2023 (India), s 2(u).
91 Directions under sub-section (6) of section 70B of the Information Technology Act, 2000 Annexure 1.
92 Ibid., 2.
93 Digital Personal Data Protection Act 2023 (India), Schedule.
94 Information Technology Act 2000 (India), s 70B(7).
95 P Suraksha, "Will Notify Data Protection Board, Rules Soon: MoS IT Rajeev Chandrasekhar", *The Economic Times* (21 August 2023), available at: https://economictimes.indiatimes.com/tech/technology/will-notify-data-protection-board-rules-soon-mos-it-rajeev-chandrasekhar/articleshow/102880460.cms?from=mdr.
96 The regulation is expected to come into force in October 2024; see Luciana Fransiska, "A Closer Look at Indonesia's Government Regulation Draft on the Implementation of Personal Data Protection Law (Indonesia)" (2023) 72 *NO&T Asia Legal Review* 1, 1.

97 "Breach Notification in Indonesia—DLA Piper Global Data Protection Laws of the World", available at: https://www.dlapiperdataprotection.com/index.html?t=breach-notification&c=ID; see also "General Data Security Breach Notification Requirements | Indonesia | Global Data Privacy & Security Handbook | Baker McKenzie Resource Hub", available at: https://resourcehub.bakermckenzie.com/en/resources/data-privacy-security/asia-pacific/indonesia/topics/general-data-security-breach-notification-requirements.

98 Indrawan Dwi Yuriutomo, "Indonesia—Data Protection Overview", *DataGuidance* (13 October 2023) para 7.6, available at: https://www.dataguidance.com/notes/indonesia-data-protection-overview; "Breach Notification in Indonesia—DLA Piper Global Data Protection Laws of the World", n 96; "General Data Security Breach Notification Requirements" | Indonesia | Global Data Privacy & Security Handbook | Baker McKenzie Resource Hub', n 96.

99 Yuriutomo, n 97.

100 Ibid.

101 Ibid.

102 Ibid.; "Enforcement in Indonesia—DLA Piper Global Data Protection Laws of the World", available at: https://www.dlapiperdataprotection.com/index.html?t=enforcement&c=ID.

103 Yuriutomo, n 98, at para 3.2.

104 Act on the Protection of Personal Information 2003 (Japan), Art 68(1).

105 Ibid., Art 26.

106 "General Data Security Breach Notification Requirements" | Japan | Global Data Privacy & Security Handbook | Baker McKenzie Resource Hub, available at: https://resourcehub.bakermckenzie.com/en/resources/data-privacy-security/asia-pacific/japan/topics/general-data-security-breach-notification-requirements; "Breach Notification in Japan"—DLA Piper Global Data Protection Laws of the World, available at: https://www.dlapiperdataprotection.com/index.html?t=breach-notification&c=JP.

107 "General Data Security Breach Notification Requirements" | Japan | Global Data Privacy & Security Handbook | Baker McKenzie Resource Hub, n 105; Takahiro Nonaka, "Important Changes to Japan's Privacy Law Take Effect April 1, 2022: Is Your Business Ready?", *Morrison Foerster*, available at: https://www.mofo.com/resources/insights/220329-important-changes-japans-privacy-law-take-effect.

108 "General Data Security Breach Notification Requirements" | Japan | Global Data Privacy & Security Handbook | Baker McKenzie Resource Hub, n 105; Nonaka, n 106.

109 "Breach Notification in Japan"—DLA Piper Global Data Protection Laws of the World, n 105.

110 Act on the Protection of Personal Information 2003 (Japan), Art 26(2); Nonaka, n 106; Hiromi Hayashi and Masaki Yukawa, "Data Protection Laws and Regulations Japan 2023", *International Comparative Legal Guides International Business Reports*, available at: https://iclg.com/practice-areas/data-protection-laws-and-regulations/japan.

111 Act on the Protection of Personal Information 2003 (Japan), Art 178.

112 Ibid., Art 165.

113 "Japan: PPC Releases Data Breach Statistics for First Half of 2022", *DataGuidance* (15 November 2022), available at: https://www.dataguidance.com/news/japan-ppc-releases-data-breach-statistics-first-half.

114 Department of Personal Data Protection, "Data Leakage Notification Form", available at: https://www.pdp.gov.my/jpdpv2/download-form-document/?lang=en.

115 See "Malaysia: 90 Days under Malaysia Madani—Personal Data Protection Redux", available at: https://insightplus.bakermckenzie.com/bm/data-technology/malaysia-90-days-under-malaysia-madani-personal-data-protection-redux.

116 "General Data Security Breach Notification Requirements" | Malaysia | Global Data Privacy & Security Handbook | Baker McKenzie Resource Hub, available at: https://resourcehub.bakermckenzie.com/en/resources/data-privacy-security/asia-pacific/malaysia/topics/general-data-security-breach-notification-requirements.

117 Personal Data Protection Act 2010 (Malaysia), s 48(h).

118 Law of Mongolia on Personal Data Protection 2021, Art 22.1.

119 Ibid.

120 Ibid.

121 Graham Greenleaf and Tamar Kaldani, "Mongolia's Unique Data Privacy Law Completes Coverage of Central Asia" (2022) 178 *Privacy Laws and Business International Report* 25.

122 Law of Mongolia on Personal Data Protection, Art 22.6.

123 Ibid., Art 22.2.

124 Ibid., Art 30.2.

125 Chris Melville, "Mongolia—Data Protection Overview", *DataGuidance* (14 June 2023), available at: https://www.dataguidance.com/notes/mongolia-data-protection-overview.

126 Law of Mongolia on Personal Data Protection, Art 24.1.6.

127 Privacy Act 2020 (New Zealand), s 112(1) definition of "privacy breach" (a).

128 Ibid., s 112(1) definition of "notifiable privacy breach".

129 Ibid.; s 113.

130 Ibid., s 114.

131 "Office of the Privacy Commissioner | Privacy Breaches", available at: https://www.privacy.org.nz/responsibilities/privacy-breaches/.

132 Privacy Act, s 115(1).

133 Ibid., s 115(2).

134 Ibid., s 116(1).

135 Ibid., s 116(2).

136 Ibid., s 122(2).

137 National Privacy Commission Circular 16-03—Personal Data Breach Management (Philippines) 2016, s 3(F).

138 Data Privacy Act 2012 (Philippines), s 20(f).

139 National Privacy Commission Circular 16-03—Personal Data Breach Management (Philippines), s 11.

140 Ibid., s 17(A).

141 Data Privacy Act, s 20(f).

142 National Privacy Commission Circular 16-03—Personal Data Breach Management (Philippines), s 17(C).

143 Ibid., s 18(A).

144 Ibid., s 18(B).

145 Data Privacy Act, s 20(f).

146 Ibid., s 20(f).

147 Ibid., s 30.

148 Personal Data Protection Act 2012 (Singapore), s 26A (definition of "data breach").

149 Ibid., s 26B(1).

150 Personal Data Protection (Notification of Data Breaches) Regulations 2021 (Singapore), Reg 3 (Sch 1).

151 Personal Data Protection Commission Singapore, "Guide on Managing and Notifying Data Breaches Under the PDPA" 23, available at: https://www.pdpc.gov.sg/Help-and-Resources/2021/01/Data-Breach-Management-Guide.

152 Personal Data Protection (Notification of Data Breaches) Regulations 2021 (Singapore), Reg 4.

153 Personal Data Protection Act 2012 (Singapore), s 26C(2).

154 Ibid., s 26D(1).

155 Personal Data Protection Commission, Singapore, "Advisory Guidelines on Key Concepts in the PDPA", s 20.4.

156 Personal Data Protection Act 2012 (Singapore), s 26D(2).

157 Ibid., s 26B(4).

158 Ibid., s 26D(5).

159 Ibid., s 48J(1), (3).

160 As amended by "Presidential Decree No. 33723, Sep. 12, 2023".

161 Personal Information Protection Act 2020 (South Korea), Art 34(1).

162 Enforcement Decree of the Personal Information Protection Act (South Korea) 2023, Art 39(1).

163 Personal Information Protection Act, Art 34(3); Enforcement Decree of the Personal Information Protection Act (South Korea), Art 40(1).

164 Enforcement Decree of the Personal Information Protection Act (South Korea), Art 40(1).

165 Ibid., Art 39(1).

166 Ibid.

167 Ibid., Art 40(1).

168 Ibid., Art 39(3).

169 Personal Information Protection Act, Art 75(2).

170 Ibid., Art 67.

171 Personal Information Protection Commission (South Korea), "Personal Information Protection Annual Report 2021" 106.

172 Personal Data Protection Act 2022 (Sri Lanka), s 56.

173 Ibid., s 23(2)(a).

174 The board of directors was only appointed in October 2023; see "Sri Lanka's Personal Data Protection Authority Progresses with Board of Directors Appointment—Presidential Secretariat of Sri Lanka", available at: https://www.presidentsoffice.gov.lk/index.php/2023/10/09/sri-lankas-personal-data-protection-authority-progresses-with-board-of-directors-appointment/.

175 Personal Data Protection Act 2022 (Sri Lanka), s 38(1).

176 Ibid., s 48.

177 Personal Data Protection Act 1995 (Taiwan), Art 12.

178 Enforcement Rules of the Personal Data Protection Act 1996 (Taiwan), Art 22.

179 Personal Data Protection Act 1995 (Taiwan), Art 12.

180 Ibid., Art 48.

181 Grace Shao and Sean JC Shih, "Taiwan: Amendment to the Taiwan Personal Data Protection Act", *Global Compliance News* (1 June 2023), available at: https://www.globalcompliancenews.com/2023/06/01/https-insightplus-bakermckenzie-com-bm-data-technology-taiwan-amendment-to-the-taiwan-personal-data-protection-act-increased-fines-for-data-breaches-and-establishment-of-the-personal-data-protection/.

182 Dhirapol Suwanprateep, "Thailand—Data Protection Overview", *DataGuidance* (18 October 2022), available at: https://www.dataguidance.com/notes/thailand-data-protection-overview; "General Data Security Breach Notification Requirements" | Thailand | Global Data Privacy & Security Handbook | Baker McKenzie Resource Hub, available at: https://resourcehub.bakermckenzie.com/en/resources/data-privacy-security/asia-pacific/thailand/topics/general-data-security-breach-notification-requirements.

183 Personal Data Protection Act 2019 (Thailand), s 37(4).
184 Ibid.
185 Ibid.
186 Ibid.
187 Provided in the PDPC Notification. See "Breach Notification in Thailand"—DLA Piper Global Data Protection Laws of the World, available at: https://www.dlapiperdataprotection.com/index.html?t=breach-notification&c=TH; "PDPA Update—Thailand's New Legislation on Personal Data Breach Notification", *Data Notes* (21 December 2022), available at: https://hsfnotes.com/data/2022/12/21/pdpa-update-thailands-new-legislation-on-personal-data-breach-notification/.
188 Personal Data Protection Act 2019 (Thailand), s 83.
189 Ibid., s 70.
190 Decree No. 13/2023/ND-CP on Personal Data Protection 2023 (Vietnam), Art 23(1).
191 Ibid.
192 Ibid.
193 Decree No. 13/2023/ND-CP on Personal Data Protection art 4.
194 RBC Capital Markets, "The Healthcare Data Explosion", available at: https://www.rbccm.com/en/gib/healthcare/story.page.
195 Grayson Wells, "What's the Harm? Federalism, the Separation of Powers, and Standing in Data Breach Litigation" (2021) 96 *Indiana Law Journal* 937, 966.

PART III

Acute challenges

10
CHALLENGES AND OPPORTUNITIES FOR DATA TRUSTS FOR HEALTH RESEARCH

Jessica Bell

Introduction

As the scale and variety of health research data grow, so too do the questions around information governance and how to protect and promote privacy and data protection. Studies persistently show concerns among publics over large-scale data collections, but as the COVID-19 pandemic has also shown, these are needed more than ever. In this changing and rapidly developing technological environment, designing data governance approaches is an iterative endeavour—there is no one-size-fits-all model that will work in every scenario, and it is necessary to constantly revisit and evaluate existing approaches to strive for trustworthy and fit-for-purpose data practices.

A trend that seems to be increasingly prevalent in many countries is that of data intermediaries.[1] Calls for "independent" decision-making in governance have intensified, partly in recognition of the increasingly blurring boundaries around health data that can be gathered and used for research, and data collected across different contexts such as across the public and private sector. There is also a well-established and ongoing academic and policy debate around data governance models with the potential to move beyond traditional broad consent models that leave significant discretion to researchers and research funders, towards more participatory, possibly collective, approaches. These include data commons, data collaboratives and data marketplaces, data cooperatives, and data trusts. These models are being used in different sectors for negotiating and facilitating data access and have also been proposed as governance models that can empower data subjects by facilitating increased involvement in governance decisions and collective bargaining power.

DOI: 10.4324/9781003394518-14

As noted above, one model is the data trust. While the concept of data trusts is evolving, and steps are currently being taken to move the concept from theory to practice with respect to health research, there already exist a few examples of legal structures for data access based on principles and mechanisms associated with trust law. As such, this chapter will set out some of the challenges and opportunities associated with the use of data trusts for health research. In so doing, it draws on some existing examples that can be used as a template for building new data trusts in this sphere. Rather than reinvent the wheel, these can provide some insights into how principles and mechanisms associated with data trusts could be developed to help address some of the continuing challenges associated with data use for health research.

The chapter will first provide a brief overview of the definitional challenges associated with data trusts, the parameters for consideration in the health research context, and the possibilities for where a data trust might "fit" in the existing health data governance landscape. Next, and with a focus on the UK context, some of the key opportunities presented by data trusts to pressing challenges for health research are outlined, including: (i) enriching and streamlining research access to health data through increased data linkage and data sharing opportunities, especially in terms of data that is not currently readily available for research, such as data from wearables/smartphones; (ii) improved and informed exercise of data subject rights under the UK General Data Protection Regulation (GDPR) to further protect participant interests in health data use; (iii) additional safeguards derived from trust law, including fiduciary duties to act in the best interests of data subjects; and (iv) opportunities in relation to children's data and engagement of children in data governance.

To build on the literature that has thus far noted conceptual and legal challenges associated with data trusts, and to move these discussions forward in the health research space, the challenges discussed herein largely relate to the operationalization of data trusts on the ground and highlight outstanding legal issues to be addressed in the future. Overall, it will be suggested that data trusts do hold significant promise, but much work remains to be done if data trusts are to be operationalized for health data governance.

Data intermediaries and defining data trusts

Recent controversies concerning health data, as well as the COVID-19 pandemic, have demonstrated the importance of trustworthy health data sharing for scientific and public benefit.[2] Numerous "safe" infrastructures have been proposed with the aim of facilitating lawful and fair data sharing that inspires trust and confidence in the use of that data. The EU's Data Governance Act[3] advocates for a broad category of "data intermediaries", which are providers of data sharing services and services to support individuals to exercise their data rights. The UK Government explicitly referred to data intermediaries in their response to a public consultation on reforms to the UK's data protection regime,[4] suggesting that data intermediaries may also be part of the future UK data landscape. Currently, different models of "data intermediaries" are being considered internationally, and data trusts are one example of intermediaries that increasingly focus on more participatory governance approaches.

Despite (or perhaps because of) decades of discussion, there is no single definition or conceptualization of a data trust. Rather, several conceptions have been explored in both academic and policy spheres, ranging from broader definitions loosely based on the concept of a trust, to narrower models that take the specific legal framework of trust law and apply it to data governance. Early ideas for this model can be traced back to 2003, when Winickoff and Winickoff proposed a charitable trust model for the governance of genomic biobanks,[5] and 2004, when Edwards, in the early days of internet shopping, proposed a data trust to redress inadequacies of the US and EU approaches to data protection and privacy online.[6] Some broader approaches take the language of a trust and apply it loosely to data governance, while more narrow conceptions take the specific legal framework of a trust model and apply that to the management of data and data rights. Generally, though, conceptions of a data trust share the common aim of creating a trustworthy environment for data sharing and rebalancing power asymmetries in data exchanges.[7]

Different approaches have been suggested as to how to achieve this, and again, these vary depending on whether a literal or metaphorical conception of the model is taken. For example, Delacroix and Lawrence propose that those who provide data (referred to herein as data subjects) are "empowered" to pool their data and data rights into an independent organization (the trust) and play an active role in setting the terms of data use and providing a platform for collective negotiation.[8]

One of the early notable policy proposals for data trusts emerged in the UK in relation to AI. The Hall-Pesenti Report, conducted on request by the Business Secretary and Culture Secretary of the UK Government in 2017, recommended data trusts as a model for improving simplicity, trust security, and mutual benefits in data sharing.[9] The Report refers to data trusts not as legal entities or institutions, but as "a set of relationships underpinned by a repeatable framework [of standard terms and mechanisms], compliant with parties' obligation, to share data in a fair, safe and equitable way".[10] Subsequently, in the Canadian context, Paprica and colleagues have suggested that this "repeatable framework" neither requires nor precludes data trusts taking the form of a legal entity or independent institution.[11] The authors modified the Hall-Pesenti definition and, drawing on first-hand experience of Canadian data infrastructures (including public sector health data) and the relevant literature, developed the working definition that "a data trust is a repeatable mechanism or approach to sharing data in a timely, fair, safe and equitable way" which neither requires nor precludes the data trust taking the form of a legal entity or independent institution. This informed twelve "minimum specification requirements" for data trusts, with the aim of "understanding the essential requirements for data trusts, irrespective of the form that a data trust may take".[12] Most recently, the UK-based Data Trust Initiative (DTI) has defined data trusts as "a mechanism for individuals to take the data rights that are set out in the law and pool these into an organisation (a trust) in which trustees make decisions about data use on their behalf".[13] Broader definitions include those adopted by the Open Data Institute (ODI), which views data trusts as an application of the concept of legal trusts to data and defines the data trust as "a legal structure that provides independent stewardship of data".[14]

Considering these varying conceptualizations, this chapter draws particularly on the approach adopted by the DTI and puts forward a working definition of a data trust as "an institution that uses trust law as a framework for data governance". This definition encapsulates the aim of facilitating data sharing in a way that addresses current power imbalances between data subjects and those using data, but also seeks to make use of the specific legal mechanisms offered by the trust structure. This is deliberate. Adopting a narrower construction of a data trust that examines the specific trust law framework and the resulting mechanisms facilitates an exploration and deeper understanding of the value added of this legal form in what is arguably already a well-populated health research governance landscape.

It is clear from the richness of definitional and conceptual approaches to data trusts that momentum has intensified since the Hall-Pesenti Report in 2017. Much has now been written about some of the key legal and governance considerations,[15] as well as academic critique of the nature of the trust and whether data subject rights[16] are the subject of the trust. Relatedly, there have been debates as to whether information is necessarily "property" if it is to be able to be held on trust.[17] Since these debates have been well documented elsewhere, they will not be explored in this chapter. Instead, the focus will be on how some of the key principles and mechanisms associated with data trusts may interact with, and possibly enhance, privacy and data protection in health data and health research governance.

Data trusts as a mechanism for increased informational control

Of particular interest are the opportunities for increased accessibility and uptake of data subject rights under the UK GDPR, and, relatedly, increased *informational control* by data subjects. This conceptualization of privacy-as-control is widely attributed to Westin's 1967 account of privacy[18] and some of the earliest data protection laws seen in the German state of Hesse, which recognized the right to self-determination.[19] Since then, the creation of a right to data protection in the Charter of Fundamental Rights of the European Union[20] has prompted rigorous debate among privacy scholars as to the substantive nature and distinction of this additional right from the longer-standing right to respect for private and family life,[21] reflected in the Charter and the older European Convention on Human Rights. Space does not permit a recap here, but one argument can be found in leading scholarship from Lynskey, who states that "Data protection is distinct from the right to privacy as it grants individuals more rights over more types of personal data than the right to privacy, or enhanced control over personal data".[22] Also relevant for our purposes is the fact that Article 16 of the Treaty on the Functioning of the European Union (TFEU) obliges the EU to lay down data protection rules for the processing of personal data. It therefore puts the protection of fundamental rights and freedoms on an equal footing with the internal market objectives. Importantly, Article 16 TFEU is the legal basis of the EU's GDPR. Together, it could be argued that this legal basis has founded and facilitated stronger data subject rights in the GDPR.[23]

Against this backdrop, it can be argued that GDPR data subject rights are instrumental to the realization of the right to data protection and, debatably, privacy. As will be shown in this chapter, this is one of the key mechanisms of data protection law that can help enhance individual engagement with uses of their data. However, data subject rights have been subject to intense criticism on the grounds of lack of enforcement on the part of data controllers,[24] and understanding among data subjects in terms of how to use them. For example, Tzanou critiques:

> The meaningful exercise of these rights in the context of big data is considered both unrealistic and deeply paradoxical. How are individuals expected to monitor all this data deluge every day and have control of how their information is imputed in databases, aggregated and used in order to be able to effectively exercise their access, rectification and erasure rights? Even if they are aware of this information, big data and its multiple lifecycles are notoriously antithetical to the very rationale and ways of exercising these rights. Against which controller should individuals turn, on the basis of which jurisdiction and regulatory framework, when and how?[25]

It is with this in mind that the opportunity for data trusts to act as a vehicle for increased accessibility and uptake will be explored. Before undertaking this exploration, it is necessary to contextualize data trusts in the context of health research specifically and set out where these structures might "fit" in the existing landscape. Only by understanding their interaction with existing approaches can we evaluate their relative merits (and challenges) and ensure data trusts do not reinvent the wheel.

Designing data trusts for health research

In brief, a "trust" creates a relationship between a "trustee" (someone who holds property for someone else) and a beneficiary (who "owns" and benefits from the property that is held on their behalf). A trustee is a person or group of persons who are required by law, as "fiduciaries", to look after the property according to terms agreed by a settlor that are set out in the governing document for the trust—the trust instrument. A trust instrument will typically describe the ways in which the object of the trust can be used, and the powers and responsibilities of trustees in the administration of the trust assets. The relationship between a settlor, trustee, and beneficiary is one of trust and confidence, known as a "fiduciary relationship". In the data context, trusts can either be purpose-based, such as charitable trusts, where the general public are beneficiaries, or private trusts, where individual data subjects from whom the data is derived are the beneficiaries and where no purpose is specified.[26]

There are currently no examples of data trusts for health research that adopt the trust law framework. However, there are existing examples in the health research arena that showcase some of the key features of data trusts. One example is the UK Biobank (a longitudinal population study of 500,000 participants), which was set up in 2006 as a charitable company limited by guarantee. The consequence of this choice of legal structure is that the biobank is governed by a board of directors, who are "trustees" in law and make decisions about data access on behalf of participants for the benefit of the public subject to fiduciary obligations. UK Biobank could therefore be seen as an exemplar for data trusts in the health research context, as explored further below.

A similar example can be found in the Michigan BioTrust for Health, which is a Michigan Department of Health and Human Services (MDHHS) programme that oversees the research use of stored blood spots and allows participants to play a part in research. The BioTrust was established in 2008 using the charitable trust model in keeping with the charitable trust model proposed by Winickoff and Winickoff.[27]

In traditional approaches to health research, there are generally no binding legal duties that require governance decision-makers to act in the best interests of research participants, as fiduciaries are legally obliged to do under trust law. Instead, there may be non-binding project policies or guidelines that guide how decisions around data access should be made, such as including that access is only provided to "bona fide" researchers for research with scientific merit and for public benefit, and these requirements are broadly seen to protect the interests of those participating in the project. In the next section of this chapter, some of the principal opportunities for data trusts to improve existing approaches will be outlined, including the potential for an additional layer of safeguarding through well-established trust law mechanisms, opportunities for researchers to access wider categories of data, and opportunities for participants to be more involved in information governance should they wish.

Different potential forms

Before exploring these opportunities in more depth, it is helpful to consider the contexts in which a data trust might operate in relation to health data collected for research.[28] One approach could be to structure health research projects as legally constituted data trusts at the set-up phase, before any data is collected and when ethics approval is sought. Early decisions would need to be made about the form of the trust—for example, charitable or non-charitable—as well as the appointment of trustees who would owe fiduciary and statutory duties.[29] This could involve, for example, adapting traditional governance mechanisms such as data access committees by enhancing legal duties that are owed by those making decisions about data access to include duties of undivided loyalty and duties to avoid conflicts of interest, and obligations to make data access decisions based on a trust instrument that had been co-designed by those providing their data at the set-up stage. Participants would join the data trust and provide broad consent to research, subject to the terms of this trust instrument.

Alternatively, a different approach would involve "outsourcing" data access decisions to data trustees—who would be responsible for making the same decisions about data access but from an impartial, independent standpoint and restricted by duties as fiduciaries to avoid any conflicts of interest. In this "ancillary" model, concerns about the vested interests of researchers in research taking place are arguably ameliorated, and the potential for conflicts of interest between parents and children (or between parents of children)[30] could be handed to trustees as independent adjudicators and negotiators of the data access requests, bound always by a duty of loyalty to the terms of the trust instrument agreed by participants. Participants would be informed of this approach before participation and provide broad consent on the basis that the data trustees would decide matters of data access, such as to new categories of data use in line with the trusts purpose over time. This would in effect allow the birth cohort study researchers to be "researchers", while entrusting data access decisions to a group separate from the project.

Another iteration of a data trust that holds promise and could add value to existing approaches could involve the development of supplementary datasets, governed by a trust model, which could facilitate access to a wider pool of data for linkage to existing data sets. This model could supplement and enrich existing health research projects. There is considerable potential to move existing approaches forward through the use of data derived from wearables and smartphones, etc., which, at present, is not routinely gathered by health research projects. This potential is largely currently untapped in the public sector, in both health and administrative contexts. Comparative examples from the private sector include Apple ResearchKit[31] and Google Health Studies.[32]

A further iteration could be more indirect, whereby data access decisions are still be made within a health research project by relevant committees in line with traditional approaches, but there is an ancillary data trust oversight for participant preferences and data subject rights. With the cooperation of, for example, data access committees, trustees could be responsible for scrutinizing such data access decisions to ensure that they are being made in accordance with the expectations and preferences of data trust beneficiaries, as set out in the trust instrument and developed with the study participants. This additional oversight could also potentially facilitate the exercise of certain rights where decisions are found to be outside a participant's reasonable expectations, such as rights to information under the UK GDPR.

This final approach shares similarities with the UK Biobank Ethics and Governance Council (EGC) (as it was previously formed), with an additional layer of safeguards provided by trust law. The EGC was originally established in 2007 as a kind of "critical friend" to UK Biobank Ltd and with a commitment to ensuring that UK Biobank Ltd was run in the public interest. In March 2018, it was announced that the EGC had been superseded by an Ethics Advisory Committee (EAC),[33] whose function is to advise and make recommendations to the Board on ethical issues that relate to the resource. Parallels can be drawn here—as result of the legal structure of a charitable company, members of the UK Biobank Board of Directors are also trustees under charity law. This means they owe fiduciary duties to the public. My prior research has investigated the scale and scope of these duties in UK Biobank, which will be explored further below.[34]

With these approaches in mind, this chapter will now explore some of the opportunities and challenges that may be associated with the operationalization of data trusts in these contexts, to understand the added value, if any, of a legal trust model for health data governance.

Opportunities offered by health research data trusts

Increased data sharing

Many health datasets are siloed and under the control of individual groups or institutions, following the more traditional one-institution, one-PI model of research.[35] One of the clearest opportunities for new governance approaches is finding ways to free up access to new kinds of data, including new data linkages between projects to "link up and learn from each other, ideally on a global scale".[36] It is also the case that there is significant untapped potential in the collection and access to previously unattainable data for research purposes. Previously mentioned examples from the private sector, such as Apple Research Kit and Google Health Services, although not currently available in the UK or EU, enable iOS and Android users to allow researchers access to their personal device data. The benefits of the collection of such "happenstance" data, i.e. "data that is created as a by-product of individuals pursuing daily activities, rather than that which is collected through formal surveys or other methods" for research, have been noted in relation to behavioural science research.[37] There are also health research projects under development specifically with the aim of collecting data from smartphones and wearables to investigate research questions related to, for example, environmental exposures such as UV exposure and pollution and their impact on pregnancy health.[38]

Data trusts could help develop supplementary datasets, and research projects could apply to an independent source to grant access to these datasets, thereby facilitating a wider, richer pool of data. As is the case with any governance model, to do so they would need to inspire trust and confidence in the collection of the data, and those with the discretion to make decisions about which researchers and organizations could access data collected and for what purpose (i.e. the trustees) would need to be demonstrably trustworthy and accountable. This may be achieved through the additional safeguards provided by trust law, which are explored below.

Improving respect for data subject rights

As mentioned in the earlier part of this chapter, privacy can be conceived as informational control. Arguably, one of the key consequences of the shift in the EU treaty basis from the EU Data Protection Directive to the GDPR is a strengthening of the individual rights of data subjects as embodied by Chapter III's data subject rights. However, it is not always easy for data subjects to scrutinize data processing and ensure compliance with data subject rights, particularly as data processing becomes increasingly multifaceted and complex.[39] The knowledge and capacity required to do so is likely beyond a "lay" data subject's capacity and arguably even beyond that of regulators, especially in the face of resourcing concerns.[40] This may be seen as a missed opportunity for more individual (and collective) control over how our data is used. Admittedly, the rights may be significantly curtailed in the research context,[41] but rights such as the right to be informed about how one's data is used are unaffected by research exemptions and have the potential to supplement participant and patient information provided in health research projects.

Data trusts aim to empower data subjects to have more control over uses of data, balancing power asymmetries that persist and may be exacerbated in the digital age. The opportunity to do so through data subject rights has been recently noted by Delacroix and Montgomery:

> The provisions set out in the GDPR give individuals rights over how data about them is collected and processed. By setting standards around the processing of information about individuals by organisations, the GDPR creates protections for individual privacy and routes through which individuals can exert agency over how data about them is used... However, despite this progress, there remain significant weaknesses or power asymmetries in the governance environment that influence the extent to which individuals are able to assert these rights. Fundamental to most current data exchanges is consent. In such governance arrangements, parties entering into a data sharing arrangement agree their rights and responsibilities to each other and, both understanding and consenting to these terms, agree to the exchange of data voluntarily. As patterns of data use and re-use change, however, the limitations of consent as a foundation for data governance are becoming increasingly apparent.[42]

Indeed, data subject rights could be used to provide a platform for research participants to ask questions about how health data gathered about them is used, particularly in contexts where broad consent has been given. This raises important questions for health research governance in terms of data access requests and disclosure of clinically relevant, additional, or incidental findings in the course of research. Some organizations, like Genomics England, provide "individual rights request forms"[43] for participants to request a copy of data about them, including whole genome sequence data, with the proviso: "Please note that because we're not your doctors, we can't tell you what it means for your health."[44] In and of itself, this raw data may not be useful to individuals, but if, for example, a group of rare disease patients wanted to obtain more information to take to another research project or healthcare provider, data subject rights could be a useful vehicle to do so.

Collectivizing rights in this way is something that is envisaged by the data trust model—but how it can be achieved in practice remains to be seen in the health context. One of the key questions facing data trusts is whether the rights of a data subject can be lawfully mandated to trustees to exercise on their behalf. While explicitly providing for data intermediation services,[45] the EU's Data Governance Act states that data subject rights under the GDPR can only be exercised by each respective individual and cannot be conferred or delegated, for example in the context of a cooperative.[46] Giannopoulou and others have distinguished between the transfer of rights (not permitted) and a mandate granted to "data rights intermediaries" to exercise rights on one's behalf, concluding that there is no reason to suggest that the latter should be prohibited given the explicit aim of the GDPR to facilitate the exercise of data subject rights.[47]

Arguably, if trustees were appointed as intermediaries, with expertise in data protection, this could provide a beneficial means for those data subjects who would be unlikely to exercise their rights due to lack of sufficient information or understanding to maximize the use of their data subject rights; it could thereby also redress power asymmetries widely acknowledged between those holding data and those from whom data are derived. However, the enforcement of data rights under the GDPR often depends on an individual making a decision to exercise their rights and this decision is very specific to an individual's circumstances. It could therefore be difficult for the trustees to pre-empt when beneficiaries want to exercise their GDPR rights and how. As such, one of the key issues to be tackled by the trust instrument is agreeing and establishing a pathway for data subjects to set terms and preferences in relation to data subject rights, and to communicate with trustees over the exercising of these rights. This raises a question regarding the scope and substance of trustee duties in the health research context, and how trustees may be held accountable, which will now be explored.

Additional safeguards (i): Trustees

Under trust law, trustees are fiduciaries with both statutory and common law duties and powers. As a fiduciary, trustees owe a duty of undivided loyalty to beneficiaries, which means they must only act with the beneficiaries in mind and in the best interest of the beneficiaries. Trustees must consider their fiduciary duties when deciding whether to act and have a minimum duty to act honestly and in good faith for the benefit of the beneficiaries. This means that a trustee must administer the trust property solely for the interest of the beneficiary and must not be influenced by third parties or by motives other than to accomplish the purposes of the trust. Under the Trustee Act 2000, trustees owe a separate, statutory duty of skill and care.[48] When performing their duties, the general standard of care and skill required of a trustee is that of the "prudent man of business acting in the management of his own affairs".[49]

The additional benefits of these fiduciary responsibilities have been well-debated since Balkin's proposal for information fiduciaries in 2016.[50] In the US context, the benefits of a move towards recognition of a duty of loyalty for privacy protection have also been explored.[51] Taking UK Biobank as an example, I have previously explored some of the implications of such fiduciary responsibilities which can be instructive for the health research context more broadly. Unless a charitable trust is created (where discretion will be limited to the public benefit purposes in day-to-day activities), a trust instrument will set the parameters for whether trustees have more or less discretion in how their powers are exercised. The fiduciary duty of a trustee of a private trust requires them to exercise their powers and duties in line with the trust instrument. For example, a key implication of the charity company structure of UK Biobank Ltd means that implementation of its Access Procedures Policy and decisions regarding data access are directly linked to the public benefit purposes of the charity. I have argued, therefore, that as fiduciaries, it is plausible that members of a charity with purposes to provide access to data for public interest research should draft and amend their charity's constitution in a way that protects against risks associated with data access and provides mechanisms to promote public benefit data access.

In non-charitable trusts, the importance of the trust instrument is again brought to the fore. It will be important to construct and settle the trust on grounds that those providing the data subscribe to, with direction and transparency as to the uses for which data may be put and the terms on which access to data may be granted, as well as the degree of discretion afforded to trustees to make decisions on the boundary.

Another important question will be the appointment of trustees, and whether there are any skills or expertise that those forming the trust wish the trustees to possess. Trustees may be individuals or a corporation. A settlor will usually appoint the first trustees—they then lose this right but may reserve the power to appoint trustees in the future by being named in the trust. Otherwise, the power of appointment should be carefully considered, given the central role trustees will play in decision-making, especially where significant discretionary powers are granted. If no one is appointed, the trustees have the power to appoint trustees. In the present context, a settlor could, for example, be a university (if the health research takes place in a university setting) or a corporation (if the project is set up as a separate legal entity).

When appointing trustees, it will be important to ensure that decisions, for example about data access, are made by those who have the appropriate authority to do so. When setting up a data trust, this will also need to be agreed and set out in the trust instrument. It is important to note that fiduciary responsibilities and a duty of undivided loyalty do not mean that trustees cannot be remunerated; also, professional trustees can be appointed where specialist skills or knowledge are important.[52] To appoint a professional or corporate trustee, the trust document must contain a "charging clause" to allow a trustee to be paid. In highly complex and emerging trusts such as data trusts, it might be preferable to appoint an individual professional trustee who works alongside lay trustees (who will act without payment), as there are not yet any companies that would be able to specialize in the management of a data trust. With individual trustees, there are practical problems if they die or lose capacity and in consequence, these risks should be considered and addressed.

In the health data context, we may therefore want the trustees to have the following expertise:

- data protection knowledge;
- understanding of health research; and
- knowledge and experience of managing a large trust.

These skills could help protect against misuse of personal data in the running of a data trust. Arguably, a trustee's duty of care and skill could be interpreted to extend to responsibilities to manage risks and the requirements of data protection law. These risks emphasize the importance of the composition of a board that may be expected to have requisite expertise regarding information governance to meet the standard of care required if they are a professional trustee.

Given the aims of a data trust as a mechanism for increased empowerment of data subjects, it would also be beneficial to consult participants on who they would want to manage the data trust for them. "Trusted" entities in this context may include healthcare professionals, lawyers, teachers, and so on, and may also include representatives of the data subjects themselves. Although the dangers of representation in health data governance have been well debated elsewhere,[53] there are arguably opportunities for multi-stakeholder approaches here. Particularly important, though, is that trustees must not be conflicted between their personal interests and their duties as trustees, and so aims for self-realization and representation must be carefully balanced with caution about independence and undivided loyalty. For this reason, it may be preferable to opt for a mix of lay and professional trustees in a data trust in the health context.

Crucially, a trustee's core obligation—to perform trusts honestly and in good faith for the benefit of beneficiaries—cannot be excluded.[54] Beneficiaries have a personal claim against trustees who have acted in breach of trust, and, if found liable, trustees must replace any consequent loss to the trust funds. Because of this, trustees will typically expect appropriate clauses in the trust document exempting them from liability or excluding certain duties, or both.

However, this raises the question of value, and the unanswered question of the value of the data trust against which these costs could be offset, and the associated difficulties with quantifying the monetary value of data and data rights. Bearing in mind examples from other health research projects, a fee recovery model could be built into the trust model, for example, by charging standard data access fees and using the funds for the administration of the trust. This arguably relies on the trust being highly scalable and funds to remunerate or indemnify trustees, who will be personally liable for any breach, could be very high. The question of quantifying data trusts' assets is complex, and as such, an evaluation of different approaches is needed to help drive the operationalization of trusts from theory to practice.

Additional safeguards (ii): Trustee accountability

Given the extensive responsibilities of trustees set out above, a major hurdle for data trusts is finding unpaid volunteers or professional volunteers who will require payment, the funds for which will need to be raised. Acting as a trustee of a data trust is likely to be time consuming and specialized, and a high degree of trust will be placed in someone in the role. This sets a high bar and could understandably put off volunteers. Indeed, a trustee who breaches the trust document or fails to live up to the standard expected of them will be guilty of acting in breach of trust.[55] That said, a trustee who is honest and reasonably competent will not be held responsible for a mere error of judgement, and a trustee will not be liable merely because their decision is wrong or results in a "loss" to the trust.[56]

What would a breach look like for data trusts for health research? In *Armitage v Nurse*,[57] misappropriation or misapplication of trust property was highlighted as a potential breach. Arguably, in the present context this could mean that any data access that was granted outside the permissions set out in the trust instrument could constitute misapplication. For example, if the terms of the trust instrument specifically prohibited commercial access, then trustees could reasonably be expected to forbid granting access to an exclusively commercial entity. However, where boundary questions arise, for example where a private organization partners with a public body such as the NHS, it could be a matter for the trustees' discretion to decide whether the application is in line with the best interests of the beneficiaries and to their benefit.

Therefore, a few things to consider when setting up the trust and drafting the trust instrument will be:

- Will the trustees be acting with their discretion (i.e. do they have a choice whether to act in a certain way)?
- What decisions will trustees need to make within a health research context?
- Will the duties of trustees need to change over time?
- Will additional processing purposes be added and what implications will this have for the trust and/or privacy policy/governance documents?
- How will trustees avoid personal liability?
- How much should lay and professional trustees be remunerated, and how will these costs be covered?

Discussion until now has proceeded on the basis that data trust beneficiaries are adults, and there is a wealth of questions that need to be answered before the added value of data trusts to existing models is convincing. However, the final section of this chapter will explore some of the particularly valuable opportunities associated with data trusts in terms of the prospect of greater representation of children in relation to uses of their health data in research projects.

Data trusts for children in health research

A complex ethical and legal landscape for health research applies to health research projects involving children, such as longitudinal studies and birth cohort studies. Typically, consent will govern the collection and storage of data and tissue samples from participants over decades. In this paradigm, the parent or guardian will consent to be involved in the research project on behalf of the child. In view of the long-term and potentially multi-generational commitment to involvement in health research, data trusts offer promise for increasing involvement and engagement of parents and children, including via respective data subject rights, in longitudinal health research projects like birth cohort studies. Perhaps most significantly, data trusts may offer a vehicle for researchers to meet their legal obligations to act in the child's best interests in the running of a health research project. These opportunities will now be explored in more detail.

The child's data subject rights

Although children may not be empowered to consent to certain forms of processing under the GDPR,[58] they possess all the same data subject rights as adults. Children will be able to exercise these rights if they are found to have capacity to do so, and where a child is not considered to have the requisite capacity, an adult with parental responsibility will usually exercise the child's data protection rights on their behalf.

Currently, the position of children in health research, particularly in terms of their consenting age, is a grey area that is largely informed by case law from the medical treatment context. The latter is often based (at least in English law) on the "Gillick competence" test[59]—used in healthcare law to assess whether a child is mature enough to consent to treatment. The test provides that where a child has attained sufficient maturity "to understand the nature and consequences of a proposed intervention, and it is in their best interest to do so, then they can provide a valid legal consent on their own behalf".[60] If relying on consent, to be compliant, health research projects must make sure that the child understands what they are consenting to, and be sure not to exploit any imbalance of power in the relationship between the child providing the data and the person collecting and using it. This is a high bar, particularly in circumstances where there may be low levels of digital literacy and engagement around uses of health data for research.[61] Individual consent may be particularly difficult in longitudinal studies that would need to continually review and assess the capacity of their cohort for new data uses.

In many cases, children will not be considered competent to exercise their own data subject rights, or to make decisions more generally in relation to research participation. It is in these circumstances that the role of a trustee, acting in the best interests of the child, has significant potential to enhance the rights of the child and operationalize best interest decision-making in health research.

Best interests of the child

Perhaps most significantly, data trusts have the potential to help address a growing challenge in health research: making research data processing decisions in the best interests of the child. This may be particularly compelling in relation to projects where children are born into health research projects that continue throughout their lifetime. In this context, most choices about the processing of children's data will be made by adults exercising parental responsibility. However, situations may arise where researchers are concerned that a parent's decision is in conflict with the wishes of their child (notwithstanding the child being too young to make the decision on their own) or, more significantly, that the decision may negatively impact the current or future welfare of the child.

For example, a parent or guardian might request that a child's genetic data is deleted from a research database, removing the opportunity for identification of harmful genetic variants the child may possess as scientific knowledge develops, and consequently preventing measures that could be taken to reduce or mitigate harm. This may particularly be the case where researchers have already identified variants potentially relating to a serious disease but where the evidence has yet to fully develop and confirm a link between the condition and genetic indicator. Such scenarios may become increasingly frequent as population-scale genomic research initiatives develop,[62] and in health research more widely as multidimensional—even AI-driven—data processing develops new insights and meaningful predictions of future health outcomes. Although a parent or guardian's decisions are likely to be followed in most circumstances, the legal framework does not necessarily require data controllers to uphold those decisions where they are not in the best interests of the child.

The concept of best interests derives from the 1989 United Nations Convention on the Rights of the Child, which states that, "in all actions concerning children, whether undertaken by public or private social welfare institutions, courts of law, administrative authorities or legislative bodies, the best interests of the child shall be a primary consideration".[63] As the UK's Information Commissioner's Office (ICO) acknowledges, although the

Convention has not been made part of UK domestic law, it should be taken into consideration by law-makers, courts, and regulators when making decisions that affect children.[64]

Moreover, as Taylor and colleagues discuss, the relatively well-developed body of law governing healthcare and treatment decisions may considerably influence the approach taken by courts and regulators in other areas, such as data protection.[65] This is important as the position in cases of dispute or concern about parental decisions regarding the treatment of minors is clear: a court is empowered to substitute its judgment for that of the parents (or healthcare team) on the basis of what is in the best interests of the child.

If data controllers are required to have regard to the best interests of the child (as the ICO already advises in the context of online services using children's data[66]) when processing data for health research purposes, including in cases of dispute or concern surrounding the welfare implications for a child, this presents a complex and significant challenge. A best-interests assessment requires careful consideration of the relevant benefits and harms at stake as well as a range of other factors such as the following:

- the views of the child or young person, so far as they can express them, including any previously expressed preferences;
- the views of parents;
- the views of others close to the child or young person;
- the cultural, religious, or other beliefs and values of the child or parents;
- the views of other healthcare professionals involved in providing care to the child or young person, and of any other professionals who have an interest in their welfare; and
- which choice, if there is more than one, will least restrict the child or young person's future options.[67]

On the whole, health research data controllers are unlikely to possess the skills, experience, and resources to perform such an assessment alone. This is where the potential support of a data trust could be important.

Introducing an independent trustee with legal responsibility to act in the best interests of the beneficiaries, i.e. children in the data trust, could present an opportunity to represent young people independently from their family and the research team, helping resolve disputes and facilitating decisions in the best interests of children. A particular advantage of data trustees could be a specific role in building a relationship with young people and ensuring that their data subject rights and best interests are being protected throughout the project. A trustee could also more generally keep them informed about the research process and enable them to have a say in how their data are collected, stored, and used. This could be achieved through regular meetings with beneficiaries (including those that are young people) to explain and review data uses or communicate when there were changes to the use of their data as the birth cohort study progresses.

Considering earlier points about the expertise of trustees, it could be that experience of working with children would be particularly valuable expertise for a data trustee to possess for a data trust concerning children's data. Trustworthiness may mean something different to young people, and it is important to understand their views and preferences around data if data trusts are to inspire willingness to engage in research projects that use data trusts and help children understand how their data rights are being protected through the data trust. Steps could be put in place to ensure young people will be sufficiently informed about their data rights, ability to provide informed consent themselves, and their right to withdraw from a birth cohort study.

Conclusion

Overall, there are considerable opportunities associated with data trusts in the health research context that make them worthy of interrogation and further testing moving forward. The concept of a data trust is still novel, and introducing the trust model into the health research setting is complex. Participation will not be effective where there are knowledge gaps about the concept, utility, and operationality of the data trust. There need to be very clear parameters at the outset and, ideally, co-design with those involved. The dangers of lapsing into tokenistic engagement within data trusts have been well-noted by the leading public participation charity, Involve.[68] Indeed, data trusts have much to learn from the health governance landscape in terms of participatory approaches to data governance,[69] and should not risk jeopardizing existing trust and confidence in models that are working well.

Much more needs to be done if data trusts are to realize some of these opportunities in practice. For example, for data trusts to help further empowerment and informational control through more information about, and informed use of, data subject rights, there will need to be meaningful channels of engagement between data subjects and trustees. This relationship will need to be articulated at the outset and embodied in the trust instrument if trustees are to be truly accountable to beneficiaries over the course of a project.

Another major challenge is overcomplicating the existing health research space. The aim of the examples provided in this chapter is to showcase some of the ways in which a data trust might *add value to existing approaches*. If done in a trustworthy manner, the potential to compete with private organizations, such as Apple ResearchKit, by providing an independent and accountable organization responsible for acting solely in the best interests of beneficiaries while also facilitating access to new types of data, is noteworthy. Equally promising is the potential for increased engagement with young people and protection of their rights and interests through independent data trustees with legal obligations to act in their best interests.

But trustworthiness will depend on open and transparent practices, and robust institutional checks and balances. For example, calls have been made for professionalization of the role of trustees for increased standardization, oversight, and trustworthy decision-making,[70] and these require further consideration and learning from existing approaches so as not to reinvent the wheel. Institutional checks and balances for health research such as ethics committees and data access committees have not just appeared overnight. They have been carefully curated over decades,[71] and there may be reluctance to embrace new approaches. Institutional readiness, as well as population readiness, will take time and will require clarity before there is reason to have confidence in the new models. The previously discussed work from Involve draws on the British Academy and Royal Society's *Report on Data Governance*[72] and identifies points for clarification and consideration on a case-by-case basis prior to establishing a data trust. These include setting parameters around the decisions that the trust will make, including:

- the terms for data access and the kinds of data that will be available and to whom;
- the objectives of the trust that will govern these decisions, particularly the benefits to be prioritized and the rights to be protected;
- the key stakeholders of the trust and how trade-offs should be navigated between interests;
- the values underpinning the trust and the policies and mechanisms to pursue these values; and
- the accountability mechanisms that will help demonstrate trustworthiness, protect stakeholders' interests, and manage risks.[73]

Although not a "Panglossian solution"[74] for health data governance, there are a number of possibilities for data trusts to add value to existing approaches that would benefit both those seeking to use health data and those being asked to provide it. Since much of the literature in relation to data trusts is still theoretical, only with worked up examples can we properly evaluate their relative strengths and weaknesses. As such, pilot projects currently underway that seek to move data trusts from theory to practice will provide valuable insights into whether the benefits are realizable and shed light on some of the outstanding issues to be addressed. Most important will be ensuring that these examples are given ample time to develop robust, trustworthy practices, rather than falling into the trap of an idea for which rhetoric overshadows reality.

Notes

1 Regulation (EU) 2022/868 of the European parliament and of the Council on European data governance (EU Data Governance Act). The EU Data Governance Act provides a framework for data intermediation services (Chapter III).
2 Julia Powles and Hal Hudson, "Google DeepMind and Healthcare in an Age of Algorithms" (2017) 7 *Health and Technology* 351; Department of Health and Social Care, "Data Saves Lives: Reshaping Health and Social Care with Data" (2022), available at: https://www.gov.uk/government/publications/data-saves-lives-reshaping-health-and-social-care-with-data/data-saves-lives-reshaping-health-and-social-care-with-data.
3 EU Data Governance Act, n 1.
4 Department for Digital, Culture, Media 7 Sport, "Consultation Outcome—Data: A New Direction" (2021), available at: https://www.gov.uk/government/consultations/data-a-new-direction.
5 David E Winickoff and Richard N Winickoff, "The Charitable Trust as a Model for Genomic Biobanks" (2003) 349 *New England Journal of Medicine* 1180.
6 Lilian Edwards, "The Problem with Privacy" (2004) 18 *International Review of Law, Computers & Technology* 263.
7 Open Data Institute, "Data Trusts: Why we are Interested" (2018), available at: https://theodi.org/article/how-were-exploring-the-definition-of-a-data-trust.
8 Sylvie Delacroix and Neil D Lawrence, "Bottom-Up Data Trusts: Disturbing the 'One Size Fits All' Approach to Data Governance" (2019) 9 *International Data Privacy Law* 236. For a literal example of a data trust, see "LifeCycle", a pilot data trust in Jersey, available at: https://www.lifecycle.je/about.
9 Wendy Hall and Jérôme Pesenti, "Growing the Artificial Intelligence Industry in the UK" (2017), available at: https://assets.publishing.service.gov.uk/government/uploads/system/uploads/attachment_data/file/652097/Growing_the_artificial_intelligence_industry_in_the_UK.pdf, Recommendation 1, 46.
10 Ibid. It is notable that the Hall-Pesenti recommendations have not yet been implemented by the UK Government.
11 P Alison Paprica and others, "Essential Requirements for Establishing and Operating Data Trusts: Practical Guidance Based on a Working Meeting of Fifteen Canadian Organizations and Initiatives" (2020) 5 *International Journal of Population Data Science* 1, 1–2.
12 Ibid., at 1:

> The foundational min spec is that data trusts must meet all legal requirements, including legal authority to collect, hold or share data. In addition, there was agreement that data trusts must have (i) an accountable governing body which ensures the data trust advances its stated purpose and is transparent, (ii) comprehensive data management including responsible parties and clear processes for the collection, storage, access, disclosure and use of data, (iii) training and accountability requirements for all data users and (iv) ongoing public and stakeholder engagement.

13 Data Trust Initiative (2022), available at: https://datatrusts.uk/about.
14 Open Data Institute, "Defining a Data Trust" (2018), available at: https://theodi.org/insights/explainers/defining-a-data-trust/.
15 BPE Solicitors, Pinsent Mason, and QMUL, "Data Trusts: Legal and Governance Considerations" (2019), available at: https://www.theodi.org/wp-content/uploads/2019/04/General-legal-report-on-data-trust.pdf.
16 Alexandra Giannopoulou and others, "Intermediating Data Rights Exercises: The Role of Legal Mandates" (2022) 12 *International Data Privacy Law* 316.

17 Ben McFarlane, "Data Trusts and Defining Property" (2019), available at: https://blogs.law.ox.ac.uk/research-and-subject-groups/property-law/blog/2019/10/data-trusts-and-defining-property.

18 Alan F Westin, *Privacy and Freedom* (Atheneum 1967).

19 The German state of Hesse enacted the world's first Data Protection Act in 1970. This was followed by Federal data protection laws in Sweden (1973), Germany (1977)—the German Federal Data Protection Act 1977 (Bundesdatenschutzgesetz or "BDSG")—and France (1978). See Hendrik Mildebrath, "Understanding EU Data Protection Policy" (2023) European Parliament Research Services—EU policies—Insights 2, available at: https://www.europarl.europa.eu/RegData/etudes/BRIE/2022/698898/EPRS_BRI(2022)698898_EN.pdf.

20 Charter of Fundamental Rights of the European Union (2000/C 364/01), Article 8.

21 Ibid., Article 7.

22 Orla Lynskey, *The Foundations of EU Data Protection Law* (Oxford University Press 2015), 131.

23 Giulia Gentile and Orla Lynskey, "Deficient by Design? The Transnational Enforcement of the GDPR" (2022) 71 *International & Comparative Law Quarterly* 799, 828–829: "Although Article 16(2) TFEU does not refer explicitly to procedural rules, this Article could constitute the legal basis to introduce procedures aimed at protecting individual rights connected to data processing".

24 Jef Ausloos, Michael Veale, and René Mahieu, "Getting Data Subject Rights Right" (2019) 10 *Journal of Intellectual Property, Information Technology and E-Commerce Law* 283, 309. The authors raise questions about accommodation of data subject rights and argue that the interpretation and accommodation of data subject rights should follow established CJEU case law, requiring an "effective and complete protection of the fundamental rights and freedoms" of data subjects and the "efficient and timely protection" of their rights. The authors argue that it is therefore critical that data controllers consider data rights as part of their overarching transparency and fairness obligations, as well as broader obligations under Article 47 Charter (right to an effective remedy), and that they do not ignore, but instead develop, ways to facilitate the exercise of such rights.

25 Maria Tzanou, *Health Data Privacy under the GDPR: Big Data Challenges and Regulatory Responses* (Routledge 2021), 114.

26 Jeremiah Lau, James Penner, and Benjamin Wong, "The Basics of Private and Public Data Trusts" (2019) NUS Law Working Paper 2019/019, available at: https://law.nus.edu.sg/ewbclb/wp-content/uploads/sites/6/2020/04/019_2019_JeremiahJamesBenjamin.pdf.

27 Winickoff and Winickoff, n 5, 1182–1184.

28 This context was originally developed by the author for a bi-national workshop held in September 2021. The workshop was co-led by the author and brought together participants from multidisciplinary backgrounds in the UK and Australia to discuss the suitability and desirability of a data trust model of governance for health research, especially in the population birth cohort context. The outcome of the workshop is being developed into a research article: Jessica Bell and others, "Data Trusts for Health Research: Emperor's New Clothes or Model for Increased Participation in Birth Cohort Studies?" (article in preparation).

29 Trustee Act 2000.

30 And analogously, to legal guardians of adults lacking capacity under the Mental Capacity Act 2005.

31 Apple, "ResearchKit and CareKit: Empowering Medical Researchers, Doctors, And You", available at: https://www.apple.com/uk/researchkit/.

32 Google Health, "Participate in research with Google Health Studies", available at: https://health.google/consumers/health-studies/.
33 UK Biobank, "The Ethics Advisory Committee (EAC)", available at: https://www.ukbiobank.ac.uk/learn-more-about-uk-biobank/governance/ethics-advisory-committee.
34 Jessica Bell, "Governing Commercial Access to Health Data for Public Benefit: Charity Law Solutions" (2020) 28 *Medical Law Review* 247.
35 Timothy Kariotis and others, "Emerging Health Data Platforms: from Individual Control to Collective Data Governance" (2020) *Data & Policy* 2, E13.
36 Graeme Laurie, "Reflexive Governance in Biobanking: On the Value of Policy Led Approaches and the Need to Recognise the Limits of Law" (2011) 130 *Human Genetics* 347, 349; Mark Walport and Paul Brest, "Sharing Research Data to Improve Public Health" (2011) 377 *The Lancet* 537; Anne Cambon-Thomsen, Emmanuelle Rial-Sebbag, and Bartha M Knoppers, "Trends in Ethical and Legal Frameworks for the Use of Human Biobanks" (2007) 30 *European Respiratory Journal* 373.
37 Sylvie Delacroix and Jessica Montgomery, "From Research Data Ethics Principles to Practice: Data Trusts as a Governance Tool" (November 23, 2020), in Ganna Pogrebna and Thomas Hills (eds), *Handbook of Behavioural Data Science* (Cambridge University Press forthcoming), available at: http://doi.org/10.2139/ssrn.3736090; Neil Lawrence, "Machine Learning and Data Science: Data First Design" (2019), available at: https://inverseprobability.com/talks/notes/machine-learning-and-data-science.html.
38 The Born in Scotland birth cohort study (BIS) is an example of such research project: University of Edinburgh, "Born in Scotland", available at: https://www.ed.ac.uk/cardiovascular-science/born-in-scotland/join. The DiPPy Baby project provides another example of how smartphone data can help discover links between environmental factors and health in pregnancy: The Edinburgh Pregnancy Research Team, "DiPPy Baby", available at: https://www.ed.ac.uk/edinburgh-pregnancy-research/current-studies/dippybaby.
39 Tzanou, n 25.
40 Michael Veale, Reuben Binns, and Jef Ausloos, "When Data Protection by Design and Data Subject Rights Clash" (2018) 8 *International Data Privacy Law* 105.
41 GDPR, Article 5(1)(e), Article 89(1 and 2), and Recital 33; Regulation (EU) 2016/679 on the protection of natural persons with regard to the processing of personal data and on the free movement of such data, and repealing Directive 95/46/EC (United Kingdom General Data Protection Regulation) (Text with EEA relevance) (Retained EU Legislation) Sch 2 pt 6.
42 Delacroix and Montgomery, n 37, 4.
43 Genomics England, "Participant Data Requests Under the GDPR and Data Protection Act 2018", available at: https://www.genomicsengland.co.uk/patients-participants/data/participant-data-requests.
44 Ibid.
45 EU Data Governance Act (n 1), Article 12.
46 Ibid., Recital 31:

> Data cooperatives seek to achieve a number of objectives, in particular to strengthen the position of individuals in making informed choices before consenting to data use, influencing the terms and conditions of data user organizations attached to data use in a manner that gives better choices to the individual members of the group or potentially finding solutions to conflicting positions of individual members of a group on how data can be used where such data relates to several data subjects within that group. In that context it is important to acknowledge that the rights under Regulation

(EU) 2016/679 are personal rights of the data subject and that data subjects cannot waive such rights. Data cooperatives could also provide a useful means for one-person undertakings and SMEs which, in terms of knowledge of data sharing, are often comparable to individuals.

47 Alexandra Giannopoulou and others, n 16, 323:

> Data rights in particular are specifically designed as intent-agnostic tools aimed at empowering data subjects in any situation where the processing of personal data may affect any of their interests, rights or freedoms. In light of the legislator's explicit aim to facilitate the exercise of these rights, that exercise cannot a priori be considered to be constrained to specific purposes or contexts only.

48 Trustee Act 2000, s 1.
49 *Speight* v *Gaunt* [1883] 9 App Cas 1 (HL), 19.
50 Jack M Balkin, "Information Fiduciaries and the First Amendment" (2016) 49 *UC Davis Law Review* 1183.
51 Neil M Richards and Woodrow Hartzog, "A Duty of Loyalty for Privacy Law" (2021) 99 *Washington University Law Review* 961.
52 For example, in the digital era, we are witnessing the emergence of "digital trustees". See Jenny Lowthrop, "How to Recruit the Right Digital Trustee" (2022), available at: https://charitydigital.org.uk/topics/topics/how-to-recruit-the-right-digital-trustee-10388.
53 David E Winickoff, "Partnership in UK Biobank: A Third Way for Genomic Property?" (2007) 35 *Journal of Law, Medicine & Ethics* 440, 449; Kathryn G Hunter and Graeme T Laurie, "Involving Publics in Biobank Governance: Moving Beyond Existing Approaches" in Heather Widdows and Caroline Mullen, *The Governance of Genetic Information: Who Decides?* (Cambridge University Press 2009) 151–177, 174.
54 *Armitage* v *Nurse* [1997] 2 All ER 705, 710.
55 Ibid.
56 *Bartlett* v *Barclays Bank Trust Co Ltd (No.1)* [1980] Ch 515, 531.
57 [1997] 2 All ER 705, 710.
58 For example, children under age 13 cannot consent to an offer of information society services. See Article 8, GDPR.
59 *Gillick* v *West Norfolk and Wisbech AHA* [1986] AC 112 (HL).
60 Mark J Taylor and others, "When Can the Child Speak for Herself? The Limits of Parental Consent in Data Protection Law for Health Research" (2018) 26 *Medical Law Review* 369, 372.
61 Although noting efforts to increase engagement and understanding from organizations such as the Association for Young People's Health (AYPH): https://ayph.org.uk/.
62 For example, Genomics England are piloting a Newborn Genomes Programme which could lead to the lifelong storage and use of individuals' whole genome for both research and healthcare purposes. See https://www.genomicsengland.co.uk/initiatives/newborns.
63 Article 3(1), United Nations Convention on the Rights of the Child 1989.
64 ICO, "Best Interests of the Child", available at: https://ico.org.uk/for-organisations/uk-gdpr-guidance-and-resources/childrens-information/childrens-code-guidance-and-resources/age-appropriate-design-a-code-of-practice-for-online-services/1-best-interests-of-the-child/.
65 Taylor and others, n 60, 372.
66 ICO, "Best Interests of the Child Self-Assessment", available at: https://ico.org.uk/for-organisations/uk-gdpr-guidance-and-resources/childrens-information/childrens-code-guidance-and-resources/best-interests-self-assessment/.

67 General Medical Council, "Assessing Best Interests", available at: https://www.gmc-uk.org/ethical-guidance/ethical-guidance-for-doctors/0-18-years/assessing-best-interests.

68 Mark Bunting and Suzannah Lansdell, "Designing Decision Making Processes for Data Trusts Lessons from Three Pilots" (2019) 5, available at: https://involve.org.uk/resource/designing-decision-making-processes-data-trusts-lessons-three-pilots: "A data trust is not a 'quick fix' to complex governance issues. Developing the right decision-making process requires resources, commitment and time".

69 Richard Milne, Annie Sorbie, and Mary Dixon-Woods, "What Can Data Trusts for Health Research Learn from Participatory Governance in Biobanks?" (2022) 48 *Journal of Medical Ethics* 323.

70 Sylvie Delacroix, "Professional Responsibility: Conceptual Rescue and Plea for Reform" (2022) 42 *Oxford Journal of Legal Studies* 1.

71 World Medical Association, "WMA Declaration of Helsinki—Ethical Principles for Medical Research Involving Human Subjects" (2013), available at: https://www.wma.net/policies-post/wma-declaration-of-helsinki-ethical-principles-for-medical-research-involving-human-subjects/.

72 According to the British Academy and Royal Society, the system of data governance should "protect individual and collective rights and interests; ensure that trade-offs affected by data management and data use are made transparently, accountably and inclusively; seek out good practices and learn from success and failure; enhance existing democratic governance". See British Academy and the Royal Society, "Data Management and Use: Governance in the 21st Century" (2017) 9, available at: https://royalsociety.org/-/media/policy/projects/data-governance/data-management-governance.pdf.

73 Bunting and Lansdell, n 68.

74 Sean McDonald, "Reclaiming Data Trusts" (2020), available at: https://www.cigionline.org/articles/reclaiming-data-trusts, as cited in Kathleen Liddell and others, "Patient data Ownership: Who Owns your Health?" (2021) 8 *Journal of Law and the Biosciences* 1, 42.

11

HUMAN ORGANOIDS

Things or data?

Heidi Beate Bentzen

Introduction

Time magazine declared human embryo models as one of the 200 best inventions of 2023, changing how we live.[1] Such models can be used to study early human development and aspects of women's health, including fertility and miscarriages that are currently scientific black boxes due to regulatory restraints on real human embryo research in many jurisdictions.

Human embryo models are based on pluripotent stem cells, meaning stem cells that can give rise to all cells of the tissues of the body. The models vary in completeness. Some models, for instance blastoids, very closely resemble real human embryos and are often referred to as integrated models as they contain the relevant embryonic and extra-embryonic structures needed for further integrated development.[2] Other models, for instance gastruloids, are partial or non-integrated as they recapitulate only some aspects of a real embryo.[3]

Blastoids and gastruloids are examples of organoids, which the International Society of Stem Cell Research (ISSCR) defines as a "tissue culture-derived structure growing in 3D and derived from stem cells that recapitulate the cell composition and a subset of the physiological functions of an organ through principles of self-organization".[4] Organoids can be used for basic science and a range of medical applications, such as drug development, toxicology screening, disease modelling, and personalized medicine. The US Congress recently approved the FDA Modernization Act 2.0, breaking the 1938 FDA mandate requiring all new drugs to be tested on animals and paving the way to replace research on animals with more relevant and accurate models such as organoids and organ-on-chip—microfabricated devices resembling in vivo microenvironments that support cell culture and often include microfluidic flow.[5] In January 2024 this was followed by the US National Institutes of Health (NIH) Council of Councils approving the concept of the NIH Common Fund's Complement Animal Research In

DOI: 10.4324/9781003394518-15

Experimentation (Complement-ARIE) Program to speed up the development, standardization, validation, and use of human-based New Approach Methodologies (NAM).[6] NAM are "lab or computer-based research approaches intended to more accurately model human biology, and complement, or in some cases, replace traditional research models".[7] Millions of animal lives can potentially be spared by animal experiments being replaced by organoid experiments.

When organoids are used for personalized medicine, cells from the patient in question are used to generate the organoids. The organoids are created to be a useful data source that can mimic the patient and give information on how the patient will react to various treatments, making it possible to test many treatments at once to find the most effective one as quickly as possible, while shielding the patient from side-effects and less or non-effective treatment. Thus, the purpose of the organoid is pure information provision.

Organoids face regulatory uncertainty, as they may be covered by overlapping regulatory frameworks pertaining both to human biological samples and data protection. This may in part be due to conceptual or ontological uncertainty, as it is unclear how we should conceive of entities that cannot be categorized as either things or data. This disrupts the familiar boundaries, and, as elaborated below, to a larger degree than human biological samples traditionally have done.

Furthermore, the pluripotent stem cell lines the organoids are based on are typically obtained commercially, often from the United States or a European country, and imported to the laboratory where the organoid will be created. This entails transfer of stem cell lines across jurisdictions—in other words, transfer of human material. If the organoid is to provide information about a specified individual, as in the case of personalized treatment, the stem cells will be obtained from that person and transported to the laboratory that will create the organoids, which may also entail international transfer. From a data protection point of view, this raises legal questions pertaining both to personal data flow within the European Union (EU) and personal data transfers to third countries or international organizations. But it also raises a more fundamental question relating to the definition of personal data as such—whether the organoid is or can be personal data or not—and data identifiability. And if individuals are identifiable, this not only has consequences related to data protection law, but also to confidentiality.

Thus, in the following part of this chapter, focus will first be on the legal classification of organoids as things or data, drawing in particular on data protection legislation, jurisprudence, and literature. I argue that organoids are not personal data. However, the potential for identifiability from data generated from stem cells and organoids has, in conjunction with developments in genetic sequencing technology, increased drastically in the last decades. This challenges the notion that the donors are anonymous, a promise that donors have frequently been given when consenting to generation of stem cell lines. Hence, privacy and confidentiality aspects will be explored in relation to the stem cell donors. This does not solve the question of what organoids are, though. I argue that they are currently human biological material and carriers of information, but that we may soon need to start considering them "legal hybrids".

The journal *Nature Methods* declared human embryo models the "model of the year" for 2023, and the scientific advancements move at lightning speed.[8] Therefore, I finally consider by means of legal analysis the consequences of the legal classification of organoids for international collaborations in this emerging biotechnology field, predominantly from a data protection law point of view. I argue that legal obstacles to third country personal data transfers, and particularly obstacles to scientific collaboration between the EU and major research funders and institutions, such as in the United States, must be addressed, and I suggest how. Throughout, discourse analysis will be used to identify the legal issues and legal doctrinal methodology will be applied for the analysis.

The legal starting point

Biological samples

The first question that arises is whether biological samples are data. And if they are not, the question arises whether there is anything special about organoids that make them more likely than (other) biological samples to be considered data.

Traditionally, human biological samples are considered carriers of information in data protection law, and not data or information in and of themselves.[9] For instance, a blood sample will be considered a carrier of information in the same manner as a USB stick. But the information obtained from an analysis of the blood sample, or the information stored on the USB stick, will be considered data. Hence, carriers of information are typically seen as material vessels for immaterial data or information.

A case from the Privacy Appeals Board in Norway from 2002 can be illustrative.[10] It regarded the transfer to a former scientific employee of 400 blood samples and associated data used for cholesterol research at a hospital. The Norwegian Data Protection Authority (DPA) considered that biological samples that are directly or indirectly identifiable always will be classified as personal data and regulated by data protection legislation. Given this, the DPA mandated the hospital to transfer the blood samples to the former employee. The hospital appealed this decision to the Privacy Appeals Board, arguing that the DPA lacked a legal basis for their decision as human biological samples are not within the scope of data protection legislation. The Board asked a Professor of Law (Lee A. Bygrave of the University of Oslo) to write a legal consideration on the relationship between biological samples and personal data, and the Board stated that this was meant to cast light on the issue in general irrespective of the concrete case being decided.[11] The majority of the Board voted in favour of the conceptual approach favoured in the legal consideration of Prof Bygrave, distinguishing carriers of information from the information itself, though noting that this requires coordinated regulation of human biological samples and personal data.

Such coordination can be found, for example, in Denmark, where the Danish Act on Data Protection and the EU General Data Protection Regulation (GDPR) also apply to human biological samples because this is considered practical.[12] During the national Danish implementation of the previous EU Data Protection Directive 95/46, the Danish Ministry of Health asked the Danish DPA whether a biobank should be considered a registry. The DPA found not only the data, but also the tissue collection itself to constitute a registry under the previous Danish Act on Processing of Personal Data (Act no. 429 of 31/05/2000).[13] The DPA stated that it considered the conclusion reasonable, it would strengthen the protection and legal certainty for data subjects, and ensure uniform regulation of biobanks across sectors.[14] Following the replacement of the Directive by the GDPR, the Danish Personal Data Act was also revised. The current Act on Data Protection does not specifically state that biological samples are personal data, but it provides a rule regarding biological samples, implying that biological samples are still to be covered by the data protection rules, as they were under the previous Danish Act on Processing of Personal Data.[15] This lack of clarity in the law pertaining to such an important national derogation is problematic.

Furthermore, coordination creates problems of another nature, if one goes as far as to consider human biological samples personal data, irrespective of whether they are part of a biobank. The wording of the GDPR does not fit well with the ontology of biological samples. It can therefore lead to some rather strange data processing situations, such as the hairdresser having personal data strewn across the floor.[16] Where is the information security according to Article 32 of the GDPR in such a setting? Or consider, for instance, data protection regulation pertaining to "erasure" in Article 17 of the GDPR. How does the hairdresser intend to erase the hair strewn across the floor? By mopping up the hair/personal data and throwing it in the bin? Is that a common understanding of the term "erasure"?

Returning to the above example in Norway, the minority of the Privacy Appeals Board argued that it did not make sense to distinguish between human biological samples and personal data when the reason to process biological samples is to obtain information from them, adding that more personal identification than what is found in a blood sample is hard to imagine. A similar argumentation has since been made by Hallinan and De Hert. They argue that "many have it wrong—samples do contain personal data", concluding that therefore, human biological samples are personal data.[17] Written before the GDPR entered into force, their argument was that the EU legislative framework relating to samples was inadequate and the GDPR could fix that, and they viewed the argument that samples are not data as flawed as samples contain data, hence the GDPR should apply.[18] But the discussion has never been whether the samples are carriers of information—to that all can agree—but rather whether the samples as physical objects are to be considered personal data. This distinction between samples carrying personal data and being personal data can admittedly be difficult to make in light of technological developments where technical systems directly utilize, say, retina scans for biometric identification.

On an EU level, the Article 29 Working Party—the predecessor to today's European Data Protection Board—commented on the issue in 2007 in relation to the now appealed EU Data Protection Directive 95/46:

> Human tissue samples (like a blood sample) are themselves sources out of which biometric data are extracted, but they are not biometric data themselves (as for instance a pattern of fingerprints is biometric data, but the finger itself is not). Therefore the extraction of information from the samples is collection of personal data, to which the rules of the Directive apply. The collection, storage and use of tissue samples themselves may be subject to separate sets of rules.[19]

Though not legally binding, unanimous opinions by the EU Member State DPAs carry significant weight when a legal situation is otherwise uncertain. But on a Council of Europe level, this uncertainty did not last long. In relation to the Council of Europe's 1981 Convention for the Protection of Individuals with regard to Automatic Processing of Personal Data (Convention 108), in 2008 the European Court of Human Rights found cell samples to constitute personal data in the case of *S and Marper v United Kingdom*:

> The Court notes at the outset that all three categories of the personal information retained by the authorities in the present case, namely fingerprints, DNA profiles and cellular samples, constitute personal data within the meaning of the Data Protection Convention as they relate to identified or identifiable individuals.[20]

This decision was heavily criticized in the legal literature, and it was noted that although the view of European Court of Human Rights carries substantial weight, it is not legally binding for the interpretation of Directive 95/46—a similar view would apply as well to the GDPR.[21]

It was therefore interesting when another decision by the Norwegian DPA relating to whether biological samples are personal data was appealed to the Privacy Appeals Board in 2013.[22] Following an inspection by the DPA, Rettsmedisinsk Institutt (the Forensic Institute) processing data for DNA analyses and forensic pathology examinations was required to delete data. The Forensic Institute stored a significant number of biological samples in biobanks. The DPA, with reference to the 2002 case, based their decision on the samples not being personal data, but characterized the legal situation as unclear.

Of particular concern was Article 8 of the European Convention on Human Rights, as the DPA speculated that it may be mandatory to have a law in place regulating such extensive processing of biological samples, and Norway did not have a law regulating biobanks outside the healthcare and health research context. Norwegian law must be interpreted in conformity with international law. This could be an argument for interpreting the data protection legislation in a manner that includes biological samples within its scope, in cases where specific legislation does not exist. It was furthermore noted that the part of the processing of biological samples that was on behalf of law enforcement would soon be subject to a specific law—the Police Registry Act—where personal data was defined to also include biological samples provided that the material is analysed or otherwise identified.[23]

The Board agreed that there was a clear need for regulation of forensic biobanks, but unanimously did not consider this need sufficient reason to define human biological samples as personal data. In the legal literature, Urgessa has argued that including biological samples in the concept of personal data can fill regulatory gaps in biobank legislation.[24] Though undoubtedly true, in general I agree with the Privacy Appeals Board that a regulatory gap in biobank law is insufficient reason to define samples as data.

Under the previous EU Directive 95/46, this question was interpreted differently across the EU Member States: similarly to Denmark, Bulgaria, Estonia, Latvia, Romania, and Slovenia considered human biological samples as personal data. In contrast, Belgium, Germany, Portugal, and Spain drew a distinction between the two.[25] With the advent of the GDPR, this was one of the issues expected to be clarified and carved in stone. That was, after all, one of the main reasons to replace the Directive, which left it up to each Member State to determine the choice of form and methods to achieve the results, with a Regulation which has direct and general application in its entirety in all Member States.[26]

In the European Commission's proposal for the GDPR, Recital 26 touched directly on this issue:[27]

> Personal data relating to health should include in particular all data pertaining to the health status of a data subject; information about the registration of the individual for the provision of health services; information about payments or eligibility for healthcare with respect to the individual; a number, symbol or particular assigned to an individual to uniquely identify the individual for health purposes; any information about the individual collected in the course of the provision of health services to the individual; *information derived from the testing or examination of a body part or bodily substance, including biological samples*; identification of a person as provider of healthcare to the individual; or any information on e.g. a disease, disability, disease risk, medical history, clinical treatment, or the actual physiological or biomedical state of the data subject independent of its source, such as e.g. from a physician or other health professional, a hospital, a medical device, or an in vitro diagnostic test.
>
> *(emphasis added)*

The proposed text was, unfortunately, not very clearly formulated and ambiguous in several of the regulation proposal's official language versions. Elsewhere, I checked the English, French, German, Swedish, and Danish language versions of the proposed text, and concluded that the choice of wording, combined with grammatical rules and comma rules, indicated that the most proximate interpretation was *not* to consider human biological samples as personal data in relation to the proposed text.[28] Normally in EU law, the purpose can be used as guidance for the interpretation, but the purpose could here support both interpretations, and thus did not provide further guidance. But there was reason to believe that the European Commission would not diverge from the Article 29 Working Party Opinion 4/2007, at least not without unambiguously stating that biological samples are personal data. Though valuable interpretive tools, under EU law recitals are not legally binding, so a divergence from established practice would furthermore be expected to be dealt with in an Article.[29] For instance, in *Puppinck and Others* v *Commission*, the Court of Justice of the European Union in Grand Chamber stated that

> the preamble to an EU act has no binding legal force and cannot be relied on as a ground either for derogating from the actual provisions of the act in question or for interpreting those provisions in a manner that is clearly contrary to their wording.[30]

Recital 26 was rephrased, and the current Recital 35 of the GDPR now reads:

> Personal data concerning health should include all data pertaining to the health status of a data subject which reveal information relating to the past, current or future physical or mental health status of the data subject. This includes information about the natural person collected in the course of the registration for, or the provision of, health care services as referred to in Directive 2011/24/EU of the European Parliament and of the Council to that natural person; a number, symbol or particular assigned to a natural person to uniquely identify the natural person for health purposes; *information derived from the testing or examination of a body part or bodily substance, including from genetic data and biological samples*; and any information on, for example, a disease, disability, disease risk, medical history, clinical treatment or the physiological or biomedical state of the data subject independent of its source, for example from a physician or other health professional, a hospital, a medical device or an in vitro diagnostic test.
>
> *(emphasis added)*

Thus, it is now mentioned that both information derived from data and information derived from samples are personal data. Article 4(13) and Recital 34, respectively, provide more clarity:

> "*genetic data*" means personal data relating to the inherited or acquired genetic characteristics of a natural person which give *unique information* about the physiology or the health of that natural person and *which result, in particular, from an analysis of a biological sample* from the natural person in question
>
> Genetic data should be defined as *personal data* relating to the inherited or acquired genetic characteristics of a natural person *which result from the analysis of a biological sample* from the natural person in question, in particular chromosomal, deoxyribonucleic acid (DNA) or ribonucleic acid (RNA) analysis, or from the analysis of another element enabling equivalent information to be obtained.
>
> *(emphasis added)*

Article 4(13) is clear in that information results from analysis of a biological sample. As the Court of Justice of the European Union repeated in *Mowi ASA* v *European Commission*,

> the preamble to an EU act has no binding legal force and cannot be validly relied on either as a ground for derogating from the actual provisions of the act in question or for interpreting those provisions in a manner clearly contrary to their wording.[31]

Hence, the wording of Recital 34 should be read in light of Article 4(13).

The wording in Recital 34 would not make sense if biological samples were also per se to be considered personal data, as the sentence would then be circular: personal data which results from the analysis of personal data. Therefore, the distinction should instead be drawn between data and information as described in both Article 4(13) and Recital 35, where information is not used synonymously with data, but as something that can be derived from either data or samples. Bygrave has described this as a distinction between data as a formalized representation of objects or processes, and information as comprising a cognitive element involving comprehension of the representation.[32]

Purtova and van Maanen further divide information into three categories: semantic information, which is data plus meaning; syntactic, where meaning is irrelevant, but also where information for instance can be seen as belonging to the natural world, expressed in biological structures; and functional, which reconciles syntactic and semantic approaches defining information by what it does.[33] Purtova and van Maanen's approach is useful in that it allows genetic data to both be regarded as semantic and syntactic information, an approach that can shed further light on the Recitals mentioned. However, even though DNA information can also be syntactic, only the semantic DNA information should be subject to data protection legislation.

In 2020, in the case of *Trajkovski and Chipovski* v *North Macedonia*, the European Court of Human Rights again referred to samples as personal data.[34] However, contrary to the much-criticized *Marper* judgment, this time the Court simply noted that it was not disputed by the Government that DNA material is personal data. As such, it the Court did not itself analyse the question. And in *P.N.* v *Germany*, later in 2020, the Court stated that:

> In its assessment of the proportionality of the impugned measure, the Court further considers it an important element that the collection and retention of the identification data here at issue—photographs, fingerprints and palm prints and a description of the person—constitute a less intrusive interference with the applicant's right to respect for his private life notably than the collection of *cellular samples and* the retention of *DNA profiles, which contain* considerably more sensitive *information*.[35]
>
> *(emphasis added)*

In this statement, the Court refers to biological samples and DNA profiles as *containing* information, in other words, as them being carriers of information. The Court does not state that the samples and profiles *are* information. In *P.N.* v *Germany*, the European Court of Human Rights referred to the Council of Europe's Convention 108, which is currently being modernized as "Convention 108+".[36] Though not explicitly referring to the GDPR, the Court's wording can now be seen to have been brought in line with

Article 4(13) of the GDPR and even more clearly with Recital 35 of the GDPR: "Personal data concerning health should include (...) information derived from the testing or examination of a body part or bodily substance, including from genetic data and biological samples."[37]

Though discussions in the legal literature regarding the European Court of Human Right's jurisprudence are likely to continue, under EU data protection law, the current *de lege lata* is that human biological samples are not personal data per se.[38] A distinction is drawn between the biological samples and the personal data one can obtain through an analysis of the samples. The biological samples are considered carriers of information, and these samples are not personal data. However, such samples function as carriers of information from which one can generate personal data through analysis. The data resulting from the analysis of the samples or accompanying the samples *are* personal data.

For organoids that are based on stem cells, it is clear that the stem cell lines are not personal data per se. Whether that makes them a mere thing, is however, questionable. Once an organoid has been created from the stem cell line, the question arises whether there is anything special about organoids that make them more likely than the stem cells to be considered data.

One distinction that can be drawn between the stem cells and the organoids is that the stem cells are obtained from organic material, whereas organoids are biotechnological artefacts solely created to be information providers. Unlike blood, for example, organoids have no function in this world apart from being models. The purpose of the creation of the organoids can therefore be seen to tilt the interpretation of whether they constitute personal data in favour of including them under the scope of data protection law. Practically, this will create problems when stem cells are not considered personal data, and functional concerns can be reason to consider organoids, at least for the time being, as carriers of information, and not data or information in and of themselves. This places the organoids as such outside the scope of EU data protection law.

Organoids and other emerging biotechnologies may in time push the current boundaries to a stage where it may become necessary to consider a hybrid category spanning traditional classifications and distinctions between human biological samples, things, persons, and personal data.[39] For the most advanced models—the complete integrated embryo models—the distinction between a real embryo and the embryo model may become increasingly blurred. The long-term aim of some organoid research is to develop full-size organs suitable for being transplanted into human beings. In such cases, the distinction between human biological samples and personal data no longer remains the most crucial one to ascertain, but rather the challenge to the classical Roman legal distinction between things and persons. The same applies to the development of neural organoids, particularly if these in the future are developed to a stage where they develop consciousness and become sentient. Questions of legal personhood will arise.[40] All these situations share the commonality of the current legal categories being unsatisfactory for adequately capturing the correct nature of organoids, and thereby adequately capturing the issues that ought to be subject to legal regulation. If for instance organoids develop consciousness, it will be difficult to treat them as mere things. The question then arises as to their protection and the legal rights they should have and to which extent: should they be treated like animals, human foetuses, born human beings, or something else? I return with some recommendations towards the end of the chapter.

Personal data

If the organoid is not personal data, the question is whether the data resulting from an analysis of the organoid constitutes personal data.

The pluripotent stem cells used for creation of human organoids can be of two types: human-induced pluripotent stem cells or human embryonic stem cells.

Human-induced pluripotent stem cells (hiPSCs) are stem cells obtained from a living individual that undergo a process to become pluripotent. One can, for instance, take skin or liver cells from an individual and put the cells through a process that brings them back into a more naïve state where they have the potential to become any type of tissue cell.

Research on organoids typically involves one or more genetic analyses. When hiPSCs or the organoids created from the hiPSCs are DNA or RNA sequenced, personal data are revealed about the individual from which the cells used for creating hiPSCs were obtained from. Thus, this data must be processed in accordance with data protection law. Other legislation pertaining to the processing of this data must also be observed, such as the Council of Europe's Oviedo Convention Additional Protocol on Biomedical Research, which requires findings of relevance to the current or future health or quality of life of a research participant to be fed back to them in a context where the right to know and the right not to know is respected.[41]

Human embryonic stem cells (hESCs) are typically obtained from embryos. The embryos can be superfluous embryos stemming from IVF treatments, or they can be aborted embryos. As the GDPR only applies to living individuals (Recital 27), genetic analyses performed on hESCs cannot be considered personal data about the embryo protected under EU data protection law. However, the genetic data may constitute personal data about the family members. This data can be particularly sensitive in jurisdictions where abortions are illegal or carry a stigma. Yet, it is not common in the stem cell research field to consider genetic data stemming from hESC analyses as personal data, so these data are usually shared openly. The worst-case scenario is that someone links the genetic data with data from other sources and manages to identify the individuals who had abortions. The consequences for these individuals can in such a scenario be dire. However, this biomedical research field is not currently set up for large-scale processing of health and genetic data in compliance with EU data protection law. Doing so would necessitate substantial financial investments as new secure servers would be needed. It would also require a shift in the manner the researchers conduct their work.

Many of the most used hESCs for organoid creation were donated decades ago. For instance, H1 and H9 were both derived in the 1990s. This was prior to the mapping of the human genome, in a time when anonymization was routinely promised to the donors. Confidentiality owed by researchers to donors was realistic and achievable as both the hESC and the data generated from analysing it was anonymous. Furthermore, as hESCs are not generated from living individuals, there was an expectation that the parents would remain anonymous. There was therefore also a tradition for making any data obtained from the analysis of the hESCs openly available, and there were no concerns related to this as no one was identifiable with the tools available at that time. The anonymity of the parents would ensure professional secrecy and guarantee the confidentiality of their IVF treatment or abortion.

Since then, things have changed drastically. Genetic sequencing is mainstream in scientific research, and the re-identification literature shows examples of how individuals can be identified on the basis of a genetic sequence. With hESCs, there is no individual having been born from the embryo to identify, but there is a theoretical possibility that women who have had an abortion can be identified on the basis of the genetic data that are made openly available through organoid research and stem cell research more generally. This has implications in that a release-and-forget strategy for the data processing may no longer be responsible, as we may be nearing the tipping point in Article 4(1) and Recital 26 of the GDPR where the genetic data obtained from analysis of hESCs should be considered data on identifiable individuals and processed in accordance with the GDPR.

Consequences

Based on the above analysis, I conclude that organoids are subject to legislation pertaining both to human biological samples and to protection of personal data.

As these laws are often not harmonized, organoid research may be subject to conflicting requirements. Complying with one law may mean breaching another. This problem is further exacerbated by human biological sample legislation not being harmonized within the EU.

In jurisdictions such as Denmark, where the GDPR applies also to the processing of human biological samples, there may be regulatory gaps or legislation not very suitable for the matter at hand. For instance, human biological samples are a finite resource, whereas data, being immaterial, have the ability to be shared indefinitely. Continuous or immortal cell lines, such as HeLa, have the potential to be propagated and grown indefinitely. But typically, there is a limit to the free movement and the number of transfers of human material that can be achieved.

As mentioned above, some data protection terminology also does not translate well to biological samples. "Information security" of personal data does not translate well to availability, authenticity, integrity, and confidentiality of organoids. For organoids, protection against loss or damage would entail specific wet lab procedures, for instance having sufficient culture medium with the appropriate nutrients available. What would indeed have been appropriate security for organoids is not described or mandated. One is left with legislation that will need to be further specified through guidelines or interpretations, which can lead to a lack of harmonization.

Finally, there may be an emerging need for a legal classification of organoids and related biotechnologies which do not fit into the existing categories, but rather are hybrid in nature, spanning not only the categories of human biological samples and personal data, but also the classic "things versus persons" distinction. One could for instance imagine that organoids be viewed similarly to foetuses, and gradually achieve more protection and (human) rights. One tipping point in this regard could be the level of consciousness and sentience developed. However, the problem with such a solution is that we do not currently know enough about consciousness or sentience to determine its progression with certainty. Another relevant aspect is the ability for viable implementation in a human uterus. If an organoid lacks the potential to develop into a self-sustaining organism, it may—depending on level of development—be more appropriate to view it akin to either a biotechnological artefact or an animal. Currently, the science is at a stage where organoids will most often be viewed as biotechnological artefacts. But it will likely not remain this way.

It can be argued that law tends to be designed to be technology neutral, and the GDPR is a prime example in that regard. This tends to make such laws remain relevant over time. But we also witness technology-specific regulations emerging, such as in the artificial intelligence field. This creates legal complexity that is not necessarily beneficial and may make the law more inaccessible to those it aims to reach. However, it may also create more suitable legislation for the specific field being regulated. Organoid research may be a field in which the hybrid dimensions both along the samples-data axis and the things-persons axis will become so pronounced that field-specific legislation may be appropriate and necessary to ensure a harmonized legal collaboration environment across jurisdictions.

International collaboration

Stem cell research is subject to highly diverse legislation across jurisdictions, and often very strict legislation, making international collaboration challenging. The hybrid nature of the stem cell derived organoids further complicates the scientific research endeavour.

Within the European Economic Area

The European Economic Area (EEA) comprises the 27 EU Member States plus Iceland, Liechtenstein, and Norway. Within the EEA, the data protection legislation is quite harmonized. We have the GDPR, and it is a Regulation, so in principle, general application in its entirety is ensured across Member States. However, the GDPR is not a typical Regulation in that it leaves considerable room for each Member State to supplement with domestic rules. And even where the text is harmonized, the interpretations of the GDPR and the day-to-day practices vary between the countries.

The aim, not only of the GDPR (which has numerous concessions for data processing for scientific purposes), but also of the functioning of the EU, where one of the aims is to create a competitive research and innovation area with free movement of data, is thus challenged by each Member State's not necessarily very well thought through domestic rules.[42] For instance, I already noted above that the GDPR applies to living individuals. But Denmark has decided that it will also apply to deceased individuals until ten years after their death.[43] Given that Denmark also considers biological samples as personal data, this means that samples on deceased individuals are subject to the GDPR until ten years after their death. This makes it more difficult to collaborate scientifically with Denmark as its rules diverge from those of its main international collaborators. Rules such as these can be seen to run counter to the aim of the EU of a research and innovation area with free movement of data.

In conjunction with the proposed establishment of a European Health Data Space, research has been conducted on the rules for processing of health data in the various Member States. It has been found that the domestic rules supplementing the GDPR provides significant challenges to data sharing within the EEA.[44] It has also been found that the diverging interpretations and day-to-day practices cause data sharing obstacles.[45] Simply repealing the supplementary domestic provisions may ease data sharing within the EEA. Measures to ensure unified interpretation are already described in the GDPR in the form of codes of conduct within specified fields. A code of conduct for health and genetic data sharing in scientific research may serve to further ease such data sharing within the EEA, though efforts to make such a general code have not come to fruition to date.

In contrast, legislation pertaining to human biological samples is not harmonized across the EEA. The EU does have some legislation on blood, tissues, and cells. Following an evaluation and an impact assessment, a Regulation on substances of human origin will repeal Directive 2002/98/EC on safety and quality of human blood and blood components and Directive 2004/23/EC on safety and quality of human tissues and cells and their implementing acts, thus concluding the revision of EU's legal framework for blood, tissues, and cells. The new Regulation, once adopted, will apply from 2027.[46]

The Regulation on substances of human origin will also have an effect in the stem cell field, where, for instance, it will apply to stem cell transplants for blood cancers. It is furthermore likely that organoids in time will be implanted into humans. However, organoids not intended for clinical application will not be subject to the new Regulation, unless classified as medical devices, in which case some, but not all, of the rules will apply.

The legislation pertaining to stem cells is not harmonized across the EEA. This in particular relates to human embryonic stem cell research, where the divergences are considerable. Some countries, such as Malta and Lithuania, are very restrictive, whereas other countries, such as some of the northwestern countries in the EEA, are more liberal. This is a contentious issue, and the prospect of harmonized legislation across the EEA is not good.

The legislation pertaining to human biological samples, and even more so specifically for stem cells, is therefore mostly not harmonized across EEA borders, creating inefficiency and additional regulatory burden when collaborating internationally. Organoid researchers have expressed a wish for a standard Material Transfer Agreement (MTA) template to be used within the EU/EEA to reduce the time it currently takes to draft these.[47] Risk aversion and varying legal interpretations across research institutions increase the drafting time. However, the lack of harmonized legislation on an EU level in this field makes it challenging to make a standard contract. Furthermore, a standard MTA would not fix issues relating to diverging domestic rules, interpretations, and day-to-day practices. A standard MTA could at best function as a plaster, but it is not a cure.

Beyond the EEA

Globally, neither data protection legislation nor legislation pertaining to human biological samples is harmonized. This has negative consequences for organoid researchers.

It can be difficult to use stem cell lines in the EEA obtained from other countries. This particularly relates to older stem cell lines, such as stem cell lines derived before the millennium which are commercially available from a non-EEA country. This is challenging because the consent obtained at the time of derivation was both obtained at a time where the data could usually be considered anonymous, and consent was obtained under another jurisdiction, typically with more lenient data protection rules. This can now leave us with "old consents", which likely do not fulfil the GDPR requirements for a valid consent for data processing. The consents may not even be valid as consents to research participation for all applications of the stem cell lines feasible now or in the future. Stem cell lines can, for instance, be used to create neural organoids. Some donors may not be comfortable with such use, and the closer one gets to clinical applications, the more likely it is that some donors would have objected to certain uses. But as these applications were not imaginable at the time of donation, they were not described to the donors. A few of the donors may turn out to be so-called "super donors", where their cells can be implanted into many humans—work is currently underway to build super donor biobanks to achieve this purpose. Situations similar to what we witnessed with Henrietta Lacks can then emerge, where the individual donors themselves and/or their family members feel exploited, unless new and properly informed consents are obtained.[48]

There is also a strong and justified hope that organoid models may reduce the number of animal experiments. The United States is, regulatorily speaking, ahead of the EU in this field, with the approval of the above-mentioned FDA Modernization Act 2.0 which paves the way for animal experiments to be replaced by organoids and organs-on-chip. This may also entail a need to transfer personal data, for instance genetic sequencing data of iPSCs for personalized medicine. But, unfortunately, the FDA is one of the most difficult institutions for EEA researchers to transfer personal data to.[49] This is because US federal institutions, including the FDA, are protected by sovereign immunity, meaning they cannot be sued. There is a sovereign immunity waiver in the US Privacy Act for US citizens and permanent residents, but it does not apply to Europeans.[50] This means that a data transfer mechanism pursuant to Article 46 of the GDPR cannot be established for data transfers from the EEA to the FDA as the legal requirement that "enforceable data subject rights and effective legal remedies for data subjects are available" cannot be fulfilled.[51] Only in specific situations where derogations apply can personal data transfers from the EEA to FDA take place.[52]

Potential solutions for eased international collaboration

The main issue causing trouble for international collaboration in organoid research is the contentious nature of its source material: hESCs or hiPSCs. Particularly when working with hESCs, the scrutiny of the funder, the research institution, the ethics committees, and the public is immense. There is no easy way around this, but it certainly helps to include team members with expertise in ethical, legal, and social issues (ELSI), who continuously help assess these issues and how best to address them.

Informed consent to organoid research participation can be challenging to obtain in a fast-moving field where the future developments are yet unknown and difficult to foresee. Modes for keeping research participants sufficiently informed should therefore be considered. Additionally, a lawful basis for data processing is required. In health research, many researchers in EU Member States rely on consent also as the lawful basis for data processing. Retaining consent validity is difficult when a scientific field moves as fast as organoid research does. Newer consent models designed for more continuous information provision to fulfil the requirements for a valid consent in accordance with the GDPR should, therefore, be considered.[53] Alternatively, and often more appropriately, one can rely on other lawful bases for data processing, such as processing for the performance of a task carried out in the public interest (Article 6(1)(e)), and in the case of special category personal data processing (e.g. genetic data and health data), additionally rely on the scientific research exemption of Article 9(1)(j). However, relying on Article 6(1)(e) requires a supplementary basis in Union or Member State law, but there are divergences between Member States as to whether they have such a supplementary basis in domestic law and whether they want to use it. This is an example of how Member States create obstacles to issues the GDPR aimed to solve. Whenever organoids are used for clinical trials, however, some personal data will need to be processed for safety purposes, and in those cases, law can function as the lawful basis for data processing, as the processing will be necessary for compliance with a legal obligation to which the controller is subject (Article 6(1)(c)), and the processing is necessary for reasons of public interest in the area of public health, such as (...) ensuring high standards of quality and safety of healthcare and of medicinal products or medical devices (Article 9(2)(i)). In fact, using consent as the lawful basis for data processing in such cases would not be legally feasible as there is no reality to a consent when the data nevertheless must be processed for safety purposes.[54]

International collaboration requires further legal considerations. In the absence of harmonized legislation pertaining to human biological samples, and a standard MTA template, an option to be considered could be suggested standard provisions and sections that could be adapted according to the countries involved in the transfer. Relevant actors to draft such a template could potentially be the ISSCR in collaboration with the relevant bodies in the European Commission that work on data transfers and human biological samples, such as DG CONNECT and DG SANTE. This could ease scientific collaboration within the EEA.

Furthermore, as colleagues and I have suggested elsewhere, an expansion of the sovereign immunity waiver in the US Privacy Act to also cover non-US citizens and permanent residents when personal data about them are processed by US federal institutions for scientific research purposes would solve the personal data transfer problem from the EEA to the FDA.[55] This could at least ease scientific collaboration between the EEA and one of its main research partners, the United States.

Conclusion

Both the legislation pertaining to human biological samples and personal data apply to organoid research. Organoids can currently be viewed as biotechnological artefacts created from stem cells (biological samples), from which personal data either about the donor (hiPSCs) or about the embryo's family (hESC) can be generated through analysis. As such, the existing legislation, though flawed, is still quite adequate to cover the current state of organoid research.

However, organoids are not mere things. Organoids are models. They model human development but may in the future become sufficiently similar to human embryos to trigger the question of why they should be regulated differently. Some scholars have already started posing that question, but often on faulty assumptions about the current state of research and similarity between model and reality. When we can implant an organoid into a human uterus and it will survive, or we can make organoids that develop consciousness and sentience, classifying organoids merely as artefacts or things or biological material will no longer adequately capture their nature. We will then likely need to consider that we are dealing with a hybrid category, between human biological material and personal data, and between a thing and a person. Sector-specific legislation may then become necessary, particularly if we need to consider the protection and rights of the hybrid itself.

Inspiration for legislation that may capture the hybrid element more adequately may be drawn, for instance, from confidentiality law and from privacy law. In contrast to data protection law more specifically, privacy law captures a wider scope than just data or information. And confidentiality law not only applies to living individuals; it goes beyond data protection law in time to continue to apply after death. One may say that data protection aids in the protection of both confidentiality and privacy. In confidentiality law and privacy law, human dignity is prominent, and a wider sphere than in data protection law is considered. Lifting the regulation of organoid research up a level in a similar sense may be useful to capture all hybrid elements worthy of protection. Protection may be justified also of non-living donors, such as deceased individuals from which hiPSCs have been derived, or from embryos from which hESCs were derived, particularly in situations where there will be transplantations into living human beings or if the scientific field advances so that creation of neural organoids generated from the hiPSCs or hESCs reach a stage of consciousness or sentience. Such protection can also draw on legislation related to protection of someone's honour. As relatives can also be identified through genetic analyses, considering only the individual may be regarded as insufficient. The "interdividual" aspects of the data should therefore also be considered, and to a wider extent than under data protection law, where only the data that also relate to a living individual is protected and the protection is then purely through the data being personal data about the living individual. Particularly when dealing with hESCs which some may consider as being derived under controversial circumstances, and where confidentiality is typically expected both by the mother and the father of the embryo, it should be considered if the scope of protected data is sufficiently wide. Drawing on privacy law and considering the right to respect for private and family life more generally may be helpful, akin to how reproductive rights are typically seen as an aspect of Article 8 of the European Convention on Human Rights in the case law of the European Court of Human Rights.

The strong legal divergence in the regulation of human embryonic stem cells across the EEA Member States suggests that finding a sufficiently harmonized common ground to ensure the necessary international collaboration in the field will be challenging. But there are strong incentives to initiating this difficult conversation: we can potentially save millions of animals from being used for scientific experiments, we can model early human development and bring light to the current black box of human development between days 14 and 28, we can model disease, screen drugs and toxins, personalize medical treatments, and, in time, hopefully create full-size organs for successful transplantation.

Acknowledgements

HBB is funded by the European Union, grant agreement IDs 101006012, 101006430, and 101071203, and the Research Council of Norway project number 322672.

Notes

1 Katie MacBride, "The Best Inventions of 2023. Studying Life: Human Embryo Model" Time Magazine (24 October 2023), available at: https://time.com/collection/best-inventions-2023/6324143/human-embryo-model/.
2 International Society of Stem Cell Research, "ISSCR Guidelines for Stem Cell Research and Clinical Translation" (Version 1.0, May 2021), available at: https://www.isscr.org/guidelines.
3 Ibid.
4 Ibid.
5 S.5002—117th Congress (2021–2022): FDA Modernization Act 2.0, S.5002, 177th Cong. (2022), available at: https://www.congress.gov/bill/117th-congress/senate-bill/5002; Jun-Ya Shoji and others, "Global Meta-Analysis of Organoid

and Organ-on-Chip Research" (2023) 2301067 *Advanced Healthcare Materials* e2301067, doi: 10.1002/adhm.202301067.

6 National Institutes of Health, "Complement Animal Research in Experimentation (Complement-ARIE) Program", available at: https://commonfund.nih.gov/complementarie.

7 Ibid.

8 Editorial, "Method of the Year 2023: Methods for Modeling Development" (2023) 20 *Nature Methods* 1831.

9 Lee A Bygrave, "The Body as Data? Biobank Regulation via the 'Back Door' of Data Protection Law" (2010) 2 *Law, Innovation and Technology* 1; Heidi B Bentzen, "Biologisk materiale som personopplysning" (2013) 115 *Lov & Data* 12.

10 Personvernnemnda PVN-2002-08 *Ullevål sykehus.*

11 Lee A Bygrave, "Forholdet mellom 'biologisk materiale' og 'personopplysning'. En utredning for Personvernnemnda" (The legal consideration is available as an appendix to the decision in PVN-2002-08), available at: https://www.personvernnemnda.no/sites/default/files/pdf/bygrave-bio-utredning.pdf.

12 Lov om supplerende bestemmelser til forordning om beskyttelse af fysiske personer i forbindelse med behandling af personoplysninger og om fri udveksling af sådanne oplysninger (databeskyttelsesloven) (Law No. 502 of 23 May 2018 § 10(3)(2)).

13 "Redegørelse om biobanker. Forslag til retlig regulering af biobanker inden for sundhedsområdet" (Betænkning 1414, May 2002), 49–53.

14 Ibid., 51.

15 Law No. 502 of 23 May 2018 (n 10) § 10(3)(2).

16 Jon Bing, "Legemet Som Data" (2005) 125 *Tidsskr Nor Laegeforen* 1128.

17 Dara Hallinan and Paul De Hert, "Many Have It Wrong—Samples Do Contain Personal Data: The Data Protection Regulation as a Superior Framework to Protect Donor Interests in Biobanking and Genomic Research" in Brent Mittelstadt and Luciano Floridi (eds), *The Ethics of Biomedical Big Data* (Springer 2016), 119–137.

18 Ibid., 120–121.

19 Article 29 Data Protection Working Party, "Opinion 4/2007 on the concept of personal data" (20 June 2007) *WP136* 9.

20 Convention for the Protection of Individuals with regard to Automatic Processing of Personal Data (ETS No. 108) [1981]; *S and Marper* v *United Kingdom*. The European Court of Human Rights—Grand Chamber, Strasbourg, 4 December 2008, no. 30562/04 and 30566/04.

21 Dag W Schartum and Lee A Bygrave, *Personvern i informasjonssamfunnet. En innføring i vern av personopplysninger* (2nd edn, Fagbokforlaget 2011), 108; Lee A. Bygrave, "The Body as Data?", n 7.

22 Personvernnemnda PVN-2013-01 *RMI internkontroll og informasjonssikkerhet.*

23 Politiregisterloven (Law 28 May 2010 number 16) § 2, politiregisterforskriften (Regulation 20 September 2013 number 1097) § 1–2 number 1.

24 Worku G Urgessa, "The Feasibility of Applying EU Data Protection Law to Biological Materials: Challenging 'Data' as Exclusively Informational" (2016) 7 *Journal of Intellectual Property, Information Technology and E-Commerce Law* 96, para 1.

25 Lee A Bygrave, "The Body as Data?", n 9, 16–17.

26 Article 288 of the Treaty on the Functioning of the European Union.

27 COM (2012) 11. Proposal for a regulation of the European parliament and of the Council on the protection of individuals with regard to the processing of personal data and on the free movement of such data (General Data Protection Regulation). 25 January 2012.

28 Bentzen, n 9.

29 Case C-418/18 P *Puppinck and Others* v *Commission* EU:C:2019:1113, para 76; Case C-156/21 *Hungary* v *Parliament and Council* ECLI:EU:C:2021:974, paras 191 and 332.
30 Case C-418/18 P *Puppinck and Others* v *Commission* EU:C:2019:1113, para 76.
31 Case C-10/18 P *Mowi ASA* v *European Commission* ECLI:EU:C:2020:149, para 44.
32 Lee A Bygrave, "Information Concepts in Law: Generic Dreams and Definitional Daylight" (2015) 35 *Oxford Journal of Legal Studies* 91–120, 97.
33 Nadya Purtova and Gijs van Maanen, "Data as an Economic Good, Data as a Commons, and Data Governance" (2024) 16 *Law, Innovation and Technology* 1.
34 *Trajkovski and Chipovski* v *North Macedonia*. The European Court of Human Rights—First Section, Strasbourg, 13 February 2020, no. 53205/13 and 63320/13.
35 *P.N.* v *Germany*. The European Court of Human Rights—Fifth Section, Strasbourg, 11 June 2020, no. 74440/17, para 84.
36 The Committee of Ministers adopted the Protocol amending the Convention for the Protection of Individuals with regard to Automatic Processing of Personal Data (CETS No. 223) 18 May 2018. The Amending Protocol requires 38 ratifications for entry into force. As of 31 January 2024, 31 States have ratified. See Council of Europe, "Chart of Signatures and Ratifications of Treaty 223", available at: https://www.coe.int/en/web/conventions/full-list?module=signatures-by-treaty&treatynum=223.
37 Recital 35 of the GDPR.
38 Lee A Bygrave and Luca Tosoni, *Article 4(13): Genetic Data*, in Christopher Kuner, Lee A Bygrave, Christopher Docksey, and Laura Drechsler (eds), *The EU General Data Protection Regulation (GDPR): A Commentary* (Oxford University Press 2020), 196–206, 202.
39 Sarah N Boers and others, "Organoids as Hybrids: Ethical Implications for the Exchange of Human Tissues" (2019) 45 *Journal of Medical Ethics* 131–139.
40 Andrea Lavazza and Federico G Pizzetti, "Human Cerebral Organoids as a New Legal and Ethical Challenge" (2020) 7 *Journal of Law and the Biosciences* lsaa005, doi: 10.1093/jlb/lsaa005; Masanori Kataoka and others, "The Legal Personhood of Human Brain Organoids" (2023) 10 *Journal of Law and the Biosciences* lsad007, doi: 10.1093/jlb/lsad007.
41 Article 27 of the Additional Protocol to the Convention on Human Rights and Biomedicine, concerning Biomedical Research (CETS No. 195).
42 Article 179 of the Treaty on the Functioning of the European Union.
43 Lov om supplerende bestemmelser til forordning om beskyttelse af fysiske personer i forbindelse med behandling af personoplysninger og om fri udveksling af sådanne oplysninger (databeskyttelsesloven) (Law No. 502 of 23 May 2018 § 2(5)).
44 TEHDAS Towards European Health Data Space, "Deliverable 5.2 Recommendations for European countries when planning national legislation on secondary use of health data" (1 March 2023), available at: https://tehdas.eu/results/tehdas-study-member-states-to-harmonise-national-legislation-to-enable-the-secondary-use-of-health-data/.
45 DG Health and Food Safety, "Assessment of the EU Member States' rules on health data in the light of GDPR" (Specific Contract No SC 2019 70 02 in the context of the Single Framework Contract Chafea/2018/Health/03. 2021), available at: https://health.ec.europa.eu/document/download/a7f11827-f4ca-4e4d-bd7a-c15c39664010_en; Fruzsina Molnár-Gábor and others, "Harmonization After the GDPR? Divergences in the Rules for Genetic and Health Data Sharing in Four Member States and Ways to Overcome Them by EU Measures: Insights from Germany, Greece, Latvia and Sweden" (2022) 84 *Seminars in Cancer Biology* 271.

46 European Commission, "Proposal for a Regulation on Substances of Human Origin", available at: https://health.ec.europa.eu/blood-tissues-cells-and-organs/overview/proposal-regulation-substances-human-origin_en.

47 Jonathan Lewis and Søren Holm, "HYBRIDA D6.1 Regulating organoid and organoid-related activities: An analysis of the regulatory gaps and areas of over-regulation" (14 October 2022), available at: https://hybrida-project.eu/deliverables/.

48 Sandra S-J. Lee and others, "'I Don't Want to be Henrietta Lacks': Diverse Patient Perspectives on Donating Biospecimens for Precision Medicine Research" (2019) 21 *Genetics in Medicine* P107.

49 Heather Messick, "How a European Data Law Is Impacting FDA" (U.S. Food and Drug Administration, 9 August 2022), available at: https://www.fda.gov/international-programs/global-perspective/how-european-data-law-impacting-fda.

50 Privacy Act of 1974, as amended, 5 U.S.C. § 552a.

51 Heidi B Bentzen, "Exchange of Human Data Across International Boundaries" (2022) 5 *Annual Review of Biomedical Data Science* 233.

52 Heidi B Bentzen and others, "Maximizing the GDPR Potential for Data Transfers: First in Europe" (2023) 27 *The Lancet Regional Health—Europe* 100600.

53 Isabelle Budin-Ljøsne and others, "Dynamic Consent: A Potential Solution to Some of the Challenges of Modern Biomedical Research" (2017) 18 *BMC Medical Ethics* 4.

54 European Data Protection Board, "Opinion 3/2019 concerning the Questions and Answers on the interplay between the Clinical Trials Regulation (CTR) and the General Data Protection regulation (GDPR) (art. 70.1.b))" (23 January 2019).

55 Heidi B Bentzen and others, "Remove Obstacles to Sharing Health Data with Researchers Outside of the European Union" (2021) 27 *Nature Medicine* 1329.

12

BALANCING THE RIGHT TO DATA PROTECTION WITH MANAGING THE CARE OF HIV PATIENTS

Experiences from the National Institute for Communicable Diseases, South Africa

Ciara Staunton, Ahmad Haeri Mazanderani, Tanya Murray, and Gayle Sherman

Introduction

South Africa is in the unenviable situation of having the largest HIV epidemic in the world, with an estimated 7.6 million adults and children in South Africa in 2022 living with HIV, which is almost 13% of the total population.[1] To its credit, South Africa also has the largest HIV treatment programme globally, with 75% of people living with HIV receiving antiretroviral therapy in 2022. This provision of HIV care occurs predominantly in the public healthcare system, often operating with less-than-optimal resources.

The South African National Health Laboratory Service (NHLS) is the provider of all diagnostic pathology services for the public health sector in South Africa and, in so doing, supports the national, provincial, and local departments in the delivery of healthcare. The NHLS is governed by the National Health Laboratory Service Act No 37 of 2000 (hereinafter referred to as the NHLS Act). It sets out the NHLS mandate as providing cost-effective health laboratory services, supporting health research, and providing training for health science education. In fulfilling this mandate, the NHLS plays a major role in screening, surveillance, treatment, and research, particularly for the priority national HIV programme.

The National Institute for Communicable Diseases (NICD) is a division of the NHLS with a focus on surveillance and reporting of communicable diseases such as HIV and TB, as well as on epidemiology and public health research. To enable the NICD to support individual patient care, fulfil its surveillance mandate, and meet its requirements under the national HIV

DOI: 10.4324/9781003394518-16

programme, it is essential that data held by the NICD can be used to track and trace individual patients. This is important for individual patient care, HIV surveillance, and improvements to the national HIV programme. An important contribution in this domain was the development of the "Results for Action (RfA) reports" by the NICD Paediatric HIV Surveillance Team (hereinafter generally abbreviated to the Team). The RfA reports are a mechanism to facilitate the tracking and follow-up of patients, and their use was recommended by the 2019 Department of Health National Consolidated Guidelines for the Management of HIV.[2]

The Protection of Personal Information Act (POPIA) No 4 of 2013 came into force in South Africa on 1 July 2020, with a one-year grace period granted to ensure compliance. Prior to this act coming into force, there was concern within the NICD that although the RfA reports are an essential part of South Africa's HIV programme, at that time, they would not be compliant with POPIA. To address this, over the following four years the Team embarked on a series of activities, procedures, and processes, with the result that the Team is now satisfied that the RfA reports are POPIA compliant. This was important to ensure that the NICD could continue to provide a crucial public health service to the South African population at a time when POPIA was coming into force and there was an increase in awareness of the rights to privacy and data protection. In so doing, the Team feels it is adequately balancing these with the right to health in how it processes personal information through the RfA reports.

In this chapter, we describe the challenges experienced and process followed to ensure that a public health initiative such as the RfA reports are in compliance with a national data protection regulation such as POPIA, and in so doing appropriately balance rights to privacy and protection of one's personal information with the wider public interest in delivering on a national HIV programme that protects and promotes public health.

We first set out POPIA, including its conditions and processes. We next turn to discuss the RfA reports and where the POPIA concerns arose, before turning to discuss how we embarked on a process of compliance by way of a concerted series of activities, procedures, and processes. Finally, we offer some comments on challenges we encountered and recommendations for other health institutions, including those situated outside South Africa, to overcome potentially similar challenges.

Protection of Personal Information Act (POPIA) 2013

POPIA is a general legal framework that regulates the processing of personal information in South Africa and affords a general right to the protection of one's personal information. Passed in 2013, most of its provisions only came into effect in 2020. The provisions on the Information Regulator came into force in 2014 and the delay for the Act coming into force was in part due to the need to give time for the Information Regulator to develop operational capacities. Subsequent to the 12-month grace period coming to an end in July 2021, POPIA violations can potentially carry a fine of up to R10 million (>$500,000 US Dollars) or ten years in jail. These punitive considerations have in part spurred a multi-sectoral review of data processing as well as engendering a restrictive approach to data sharing, including within the health sector.

POPIA was informed by the South African Law Reform Commission 2009 Report on Privacy and Data Protection, as well as earlier drafts of the EU General Data Protection Regulation (GDPR). Thus, like other data protection regulations that have been passed across Africa, it is quite similar in parts to the GDPR. This includes the overarching framework of regulating "personal information" or "personal data" based on automated "processing" activities and regulating such processing on a stricter scale when it involves certain categories of personal information, including health and genetic information.[3]

POPIA's preamble recognizes the right to privacy within South Africa's constitution and that this right to privacy "includes a right to protection against the unlawful collection, retention, dissemination and use of personal information". Section 2 explicitly states that one of the purposes of POPIA is to give effect to the right to privacy under the Constitution of South Africa. Indeed, throughout POPIA, reference is made to the right to privacy, particularly in the context of invoking any exceptions to the conditions of POPIA and the need to continue to guarantee the right of privacy to the data subject in this context. This right to privacy, however, is to be balanced against other important rights and interests. These other interests include the right of access to information and "the free flow of information within the Republic and across international borders". POPIA thus seeks to protect personal information, but also enable data sharing.[4] This is similar to the objective of the EU GDPR, which in Recital 10 speaks to "ensur[ing] a consistent and high level of protection of [individuals] and to remov[ing] the obstacles to flows of personal data within the [European] Union".

POPIA sets out eight conditions that must be met in the processing of personal information: accountability; processing limitation; purpose specification; further processing limitation; information quality; openness; security safeguards; and data subject participation. There is a general ban on the processing of "special" (i.e. sensitive) person information, which includes health information, unless the processing falls within one of the grounds for authorization concerning a data subject's health or sex life. Under Section 32, this includes if the processing is done by medical professionals, healthcare institutions, or social services if the processing is necessary for the proper care and treatment of the data subject. Equally, there is a general prohibition on the processing of personal information of children, unless the processing falls within the general authorization concerning the processing of personal information of children under Section 35. This includes if the processing is carried out with the consent of a competent person, such as a parent or legal guardian.

POPIA, like the EU GDPR, is an omnibus and general data protection legal framework that applies to the processing of all personal information and applies to all sectors. This said, the need for more tailored sector-specific guidance was foreseen and Chapter 7 of POPIA provides for the development of Codes of Conduct (this is similar to Article 40 of the GDPR). Codes of Conduct can be issued either by the Information Regulator or by a specific sector. The Information Regulator has provided further guidance on the development of Codes of Conduct and the prescribed form.[5] Any entity seeking to develop a Code of Conduct must satisfy the Information Regulator that they are sufficiently representative of a class of body, industry, professions, or vocation to which the Code will apply. The draft Code must be submitted to the Information Regulator, who will open it up to a period of public consultation, after which the Information Regulator must issue its decision within 13 weeks. Once approved, the Code of Conduct will be gazetted and will have the force of law.[6]

POPIA provides for exemptions from some of the conditions for the processing of personal data in Chapter 4, specifically at Section 37(1). The Information Regulator may grant an exemption to a Responsible Party (i.e. in this case for the discussion in this chapter, the CEO of the NHLS) to a condition on the processing of personal information if the Regulator is satisfied that the public interest, as defined under Section 37(2), to a substantial degree, outweighs any interference with the privacy of the data subject that could result from such processing, or, if the processing involves a clear interest to the data subject that outweighs, to a substantial degree, any interference with the privacy of the data subject or third party that could result from such processing. Section 37(1) does provide some examples of what the public interest exception could include. There is no explicit reference to health; thus, it would need to come under the ground of national security (e.g. in a pandemic situation) which would raise issues of securitization of health or research (for which normal clinical care would unlikely fall under), or else some other ground not listed would need to be argued for. Thus, exceptions for the health sector would have to rely on the benefit to the *individual*, which is relatively easy to prove in the context of clinical care, but may be much harder for treatment programmes. If exemptions are needed in such contexts, they will likely require a strong case for arguing for public interest that is not listed in POPIA.

Finally, Section 57 of POPIA also requires a Responsible Party to obtain prior authorization from the Information Regulator for certain processing activities. Any Responsible Party that intends to process unique identifiers of the data subject for a purpose for which the identifier was specifically intended at the time of processing, and is going to link that information together with information being processed by other responsible parties, must apply for prior authorization. This authorization must be obtained in advance of the processing activities. The delivery of care and the success of treatment programmes are in part contingent on different sections of the health sector, including the national Department of Health, the provincial Departments of Health, NGOs, and private hospitals sharing their personal information for the purposes of linking the data. The Team has experience that this section has had the effect of stopping the sharing of data due to POPIA-related concerns, which will be discussed later. Indeed, meeting the conditions of POPIA, identifying exemptions that may be required, and submitting an application for prior authorization became the core focus of the Team's work over the following four years, as we proceed to discuss below.

Results for Action Reports (RfA reports) in the NICD

Ordinarily, individual patient test results processed by the NHLS generate an electronic and hard copy report. The latter is physically delivered back to the healthcare facility from where the patient sample was submitted, to be checked and filed in the patient notes. Blood results that require intervention require that patients be recalled urgently. The ±260 NHLS laboratories are responsible for timeously returning patient results to around 4,000 public healthcare facilities situated nationally within 52 health districts. Yet, barriers exist at various levels for both hard copy (e.g. inaccurate sorting, delayed delivery or filing) and digital laboratory reports (e.g. lack of internet access or adequate computer equipment).

One of the solutions in place to overcome these barriers are the RfA reports. The RfA reports are an important tool to track and trace patients with or suspected of having HIV. They compile all recently completed and authorized HIV laboratory test results from multiple patients, either at facility or at healthcare district level, into a single report on a weekly or daily basis according to a particular user's requirements. These reports enable the easy identification of patient test results that require prompt clinical action for that week or day since they contain personal identifiers. RfA reports are particularly vital in the case of HIV-infected newborns, where guidelines recommend antiretroviral therapy be initiated within a week of diagnosis to reduce morbidity and mortality.[7] All babies born to HIV-infected women require an HIV PCR test at birth. However, the mother and baby are discharged shortly after birth, and the results must therefore be made available at a facility providing postnatal care, which is usually different from the birthing facility. The facility at which infants are scheduled to follow up is not known to the NHLS as there are no systems for the reporting and recording of such information, and the NHLS HIV PCR hard copy results are returned to the birthing facility. The RfA reports allow healthcare workers at the postnatal facility rapid access to these PCR results. They also provide for easy identification of the infants requiring urgent attention, without being hampered by the lack of a hard copy report or access to online results one specimen at a time. Hence, the RfA reports facilitate centralized monitoring and tracing to prevent HIV-infected newborns from falling through the gaps.

To access the RfA reports, all users register on a Self-Service Portal with their personal identifiers, namely, name, surname, contact number, email address, South African identity number or passport number, Health Professions Council of South Africa (HPCSA) or South African Nursing Council (SANC) registration number, their profession, and organization. Users are also required to accept the terms and conditions associated with using the RfA reports when they register on the portal. Once the report custodian has checked that the user's personal identifiers match a valid and active HPCSA/SANC number online, the user is approved to receive the RfA reports they requested. Prior to the commissioned legal opinion discussed below, RfA reports were distributed as a zipped, password-protected Excel file attachment via email. For ease of use, only two standard passwords were used for all the RfA reports by users.

Regardless of the quality and completeness of the data captured at the laboratory, the RfA reports always include identifiable personal information. This can include the patient's name and surname, date of birth, sex, address, mobile phone number, facility patient folder number, episode number (the unique laboratory number specific to a patient), and unique data warehouse identifier (unique number allocated by a patient linking algorithm in the data warehouse that links multiple tests belonging to a single patient).[8] If the RfA report concerns a newborn baby, the maternal details are often captured in lieu of or in association with the infant's details, and this may include the mother's name, surname, date of birth, mobile phone number, and folder number.

The RfA reports also contain the HIV test result and relevant previous HIV test results for that patient with all the personal identifiers associated with those previous tests. The RfA reports therefore can contain test results of HIV PCR (which detects HIV nucleic acid in the blood), HIV viral load (which quantifies the amount of nucleic acid, and hence virus, in the blood), HIV ELISA (which detects HIV antibodies in the blood), and CD4 count (which quantifies the CD4 cells in the blood). RfA reports thus always contain sensitive personal information and, if of a minor, may also contain the personal information of the mother.

The RfA reports currently only permit the cross-sectional follow-up of a patient (i.e. the status of a patient at one point in time). A new version has been developed, referred to as the "Results for Action Dashboard" (RfAD), which enables longitudinal follow-up of patients using bidirectional flow of data that remains stored within the NICD data warehouse providing a higher level of security. The RfAD provides HIV test results to assist in the identification of specific HIV-infected patients requiring clinical intervention, and allows healthcare workers in the field to enter clinical data (e.g. date of initiation of antiretroviral treatment, clinical action taken if a patient has a high viral load) pertaining to the patient on the RfAD. The enhanced information allows algorithms to flag patients more intelligently for interventions in a longitudinal manner (e.g. by identifying patients who have an overdue HIV viral load test based on the date of antiretroviral therapy initiation, as per national treatment guidelines).[9] Hence, the RfAD allows for detection of failed linkage to care, overdue viral load tests, lost to follow-up, and patients transferring between facilities and re-engaging in care. This is in addition to the RfA reports functions of providing collated laboratory results for action. Furthermore, the RfAD can provide near-real-time aggregated analytics for monitoring patient outcomes.

An additional function of improved HIV surveillance is longitudinal cohort monitoring. This requires linking the NHLS data with other datasets that are held outside of the NHLS to enhance the data per patient and ensure that the information held by the NHLS is accurate and up to date. However, the absence of a universally used, unique patient identifier in the South African health landscape requires that patient data be merged using demographic data. The National Digital Health Strategy for South Africa 2019–2024, published by the National Department of Health, sets out the need to digitalize health records and merge health data currently held in various repositories within health (such as pharmacy, laboratory, and radiology records) and more broadly (such as birth and death registries).[10] The Strategy is aiming to facilitate agile surveillance and research to improve health outcomes for the South African population. It is in accordance with the mandate as set out in the NHLS Act. Outside of this legal mandate, the benefits of improving health data are far-reaching, including allowing for strategic research to improve population health outcomes as well as allowing the clinical workforce to focus on managing patients rather than administrative functions such as manual data collection and transcription.

To improve individual patient care, HIV programme implementation, surveillance, and research, the NICD made several attempts to merge its data with external data sources. All were unsuccessful because of concerns and differing interpretations of the law from within the various external data sources as to whether this would be POPIA compliant. The focus of the legal opinion was on POPIA only as it was a new piece of legislation that was coming into force. The operation of the RfA reports had previously been deemed to be in compliance with other relevant legislation and principles of medical confidentiality to that point. The opinion sought to identify what processes needed to change to make the reporting system compliant with POPIA.

POPIA, Results for Action Reports, and proposals for compliance

In 2019, with permission from NHLS and NICD management, the NICD Paediatric HIV Surveillance Team sought a legal opinion[11] on the POPIA compliance status of the RfA reports. The opinion raised POPIA-related concerns on several grounds. It raised concerns that the email distribution was unlikely to be POPIA compliant due to the low levels of security. First, the registration process required the user's personal identifiers to match a valid and active health professions council number online, after which RfA reports' access was gained by entering a generic report-specific password, a password that was the same for all registered users. Second, the opinion had concerns with the lack of encryption of the zipped file. Overall, it found that the system of dissemination via email was vulnerable to breach and the Responsible Party was not taking all reasonable security precautions, particularly in relation to unlawful access to personal information.

Another issue raised by the opinion was the quantity of personal information in the reports. The RfA report users were receiving not only the results that they required but also the results of other patients in that district or facility. The users thus receive more personal information than necessary, and the legal opinion cautioned that this could be in breach of the condition of minimality under Section 10 of POPIA that states only personal information that is "adequate, relevant and not excessive" may be processed. The opinion recommended that user access should be restricted only to the personal information of patients that users required in the fulfilment of their duties. It went on to state that if it was not possible to introduce technical or organizational measures to restrict user access, the NICD should consider a POPIA Section 37 exemption application to this condition.

The legal opinion also noted that, under the old email system of RfA reports dissemination, there were challenges relating to government email accounts being unable to open zipped files, requiring many users to receive the files via their personal email accounts, including Gmail or Yahoo accounts. The opinion noted that the servers of these email accounts may not be in South Africa, and therefore this could constitute a transborder flow of information in a manner not compliant with POPIA.

The legal opinion also had several other recommendations for the RfA reports specifically and for the NICD generally. For the RfA reports, it recommended that the Team provide training for the healthcare professionals collecting the personal information to educate them on their duties and responsibilities under POPIA, including the importance of data quality when collecting personal information. The opinion further recommended training for all users of the RfA reports to ensure awareness of their responsibilities under POPIA.

For the NICD generally, the legal opinion drew attention to the need to appoint an NHLS Information Officer as mandated by POPIA. It also advised that NICD document all its processes and procedures, including the grounds for the processing of personal information, to enable the organization to demonstrate compliance with POPIA should the need arise. The legal opinion further recommended the NICD conduct a risk assessment of all foreseeable internal and external risks, including a security audit of all its systems to ensure no foreseeable risks of unauthorized access or security breaches. An NICD POPIA Code of Conduct was also recommended. Such a Code of Conduct would benefit the organization generally in ensuring POPIA compliance but would also provide additional guidance to the users of the RfA reports. Finally, the legal opinion recommended that all NICD processes, procedures, and standard operating procedures (SOPs) be updated to ensure they were POPIA compliant.

Working towards POPIA-compliant RfA Reports

Following this legal opinion, the Team embarked on a process over the ensuing four years to ensure that the RfA reports were POPIA compliant and in accordance with the recommendations from the opinion letter. The Team's focus can broadly be grouped into four areas of activity: development of an NHLS Code of Conduct; application for exemptions and prior authorization as required under POPIA; development of a new system to access the RfA reports, guidance, SOPs, and other documentation; and data protection-focused education for the NICD staff. Each of these areas will now be discussed in turn.

Code of conduct

During 2019, the Team hosted public lectures on POPIA attended by stakeholders within the NICD regarding the potential impact of POPIA on the operations of the NICD. Concerns centred on the impact that POPIA would have on the processing of personal health information and how to continue providing clinical care and a public health service while complying with the statute. The NICD processes vast amounts of sensitive personal data daily, and at the time there was a lack of clarity on how the NICD could comply with the strict provisions of POPIA and continue to operate, fulfilling its mandate of providing care to patients and protecting and promoting public health. The Team felt that guidance was critically needed on how to address the issues raised in the legal opinion relating to the RfA reports. In the absence of any forthcoming Code of Conduct for the health sector, the Team decided to begin the process of developing a POPIA Code of Conduct. As the NICD is not an independent legal entity, it was deemed that such a Code would need to apply to the NHLS as a whole, and thus be an NHLS Code rather than just an NICD Code.

Guidelines issued by the Information Regulator in February 2020 on the development of Codes of Conduct clarified the need for all stakeholders to be afforded the opportunity to comment on the Code of Conduct prior to submission to the Information Regulator for approval. Empirical work on conducting stakeholder engagement in South Africa has demonstrated the importance of three layers of engagement in policy development: high-level engagement (which includes funders, policymakers, and government officials); peer engagement (which includes healthcare professionals, scientists, and researchers); and community engagement (which includes patients and research participants).[12] Although not anticipated as stakeholder engagement at the time, NICD staff raised issues to be addressed on the NICD's road to POPIA compliance during open forum lectures organized by the Team in 2019 and 2020. Further engagement was deemed necessary to inform the development of a Code, particularly with stakeholders who do not work for, but engage with, the NICD. To further address this, the Team sought and obtained approval from NHLS management to conduct interviews with NHLS staff, draft a Code of Conduct, and apply for exemptions from the Information Regulator.

The findings of the stakeholder interviews have been reported elsewhere.[13] Overall, the participants emphasized the importance of striking a balance between privacy and data protection and the need to process personal information for continued patient care, success of HIV treatment programmes, and research. Participants clearly saw personal information as a resource to be protected, but equally a resource to be used, shared, and linked with other datasets for the delivery of individual care but also the wider public interest in treatment programmes.

Regarding the drafting of a Code of Conduct, the Team followed an iterative process of writing, review, and editing. Upon completion of a first draft, consultation began with others within the NICD and broader NHLS, specifically the legal officers, security, information technology, the data warehouse, and other divisions and personnel identified as having the ability to inform the development of the Code. However, subsequent to sharing the drafted Code of Conduct with NHLS management, no further engagement was received, thereby precluding further development. The requirements for broad consultation were deemed beyond the scope of the Team, and with the deadline for POPIA enforcement looming, this route was abandoned, and other measures were sought to ensure compliance for the RfA Reports.

Exemptions

With the stalling of the Code of Conduct, it was felt that there was a need to address some of the concerns expressed in the initial legal opinion, in the form of a POPIA Section 30 application for exemption to some of the processing activities and an application for prior authorization for the linking of datasets.

It is worth noting that the activities described in the exemption application were considered necessary and part of the normal, daily delivery of healthcare in South Africa. In the absence of a Code of Conduct or any sector specific guidance, it was, at the time of submitting the exemption application, unclear whether the Information Regulator would interpret POPIA strictly and find the NHLS in breach. It was due to this uncertainty that an exemption application was submitted. The exemption application made a request to be exempt from the conditions of processing limitation, information quality, and security safeguards for the RfA reports. The application had the support of NHLS management and was submitted by the NHLS Information Officer.

The exemption application described the process for registration to use the RfA reports, and the safeguards that had been introduced. The application noted that despite the improvements made to the reporting system, it was currently not technically possible to limit user access to receiving only the personal information of their own patients.

With regard to information quality, the application noted that the NHLS was aware that the data that it captured was not always accurate or complete. This was due in part to the pressures at the local healthcare facility and within the laboratory, and lack of digitized patient medical records and a unique patient identifier. Also, as people living with HIV continue to be stigmatized, it was noted that patients may give false or inaccurate information. Hence, the NHLS was aware that it was likely including false or inaccurate information in the RfA reports and thus requested an exemption to this ground.

Finally, the application noted that the NHLS had a robust, access-controlled system in place for accessing the RfA reports that guards against loss, damage, and unauthorized access to the RfA reports via the Self-Service Portal. It was essential that healthcare workers and community care workers received access to these reports. The reports are often saved and shared, whether via email and/or mobile phone apps, or printed and distributed.

As this sharing and storage at the facility and district level does not always meet the security requirements as per POPIA (e.g. risk of unauthorized access to personal information), the NHLS also sought an exemption to this ground.

After 12 months following the submission, the NHLS received a response from the Information Regulator, stating that the:

> NHLS met the requirements for section 37(1) (b) as a clear benefit to a data subject or third party in the processing of personal information outweighed, to a substantial degree, any interference with the privacy of data subjects that could result from the processing.[14]

The response also stated that it had assessed that the NHLS did not need to apply for a Section 30 exemption, as by its assessment, the NHLS already complied with the POPIA conditions. The Information Regulator did not provide any further explanation for this assessment, which differed from the assessment contained in the legal opinion discussed above. While under no obligation to provide such justification, the Team felt that such an explanation would have improved their understanding of how the Information Regulator interpreted and may continue to interpret POPIA in the context of health and could also be useful for other stakeholders who have similar POPIA-related concerns.

Prior authorization

As discussed, the linking of NHLS data with other datasets held outside of the NHLS is essential for providing individual patient care, HIV programme implementation, HIV surveillance, and HIV research, and to meet other activities set out in the NHLS Act. While there is a clear individual health need as well as a wider public benefit in linking these datasets, concerns that the linking of such datasets would not be compliant with POPIA has prevented Responsible Parties agreeing to the linking of such datasets.

To progress this further and address POPIA concerns, the Team decided to make a POPIA Section 57 prior authorization application to the Information Regulator. This was also recommended as part of the original legal opinion. The purpose of this application was to satisfy concerns, within both NICD and the Responsible Parties of external datasets, that such linking of datasets would be POPIA compliant. This should overcome legal concerns that were preventing further work that would essentially enhance the quality and use of the RfA reports, and, more broadly, strengthen HIV programme surveillance and research.

Similar to the POPIA Section 30 exemption application, the application for prior authorization set out the purpose of the RfA reports, the need to link with other datasets for individual care as well as public health, and the safeguards introduced. The response from the Information Regulator stated that "[I]t is the considered view of the Regulator that the application prior authorization is not required as the processing does not fall within the high-risk categories envisaged in section 57(1) of POPIA." Again, no further explanation was provided. Similar to the Section 30 exemption application, then, while not necessary, explanation could have informed the Team's understanding of the application of POPIA to the RfA reports and also inform the understanding of other Responsible Parties to whom the NICD wishes to link its datasets with.

Systems and documentation to support the operations of the RfA Reports and within the NICD

The RfA reports distribution system was upgraded after establishing the improvements that could be made with regard to POPIA. An online RfA portal was created, requiring a user to log in with a unique username and password and download the RfA reports for which they had registered. This replaced the previous system of directly emailing reports. A system to create a one-time user password (OTP) for a user to reset their own password was developed. Users who failed to download any RfA report for two months were automatically sent an email notifying them that continued disuse of the reports would result in their being unsubscribed as a user. After a third month of no downloading, the user was automatically unsubscribed. An unexpected advantage of this redevelopment was that NICD could easily monitor the usage of the reports since it was likely that users downloading the RfA reports each week were actually using them, whereas reports that landed in an email inbox may have never been opened.

To reflect new POPIA conditions, the Terms and Conditions (T&Cs) for the users of the RfA reports were updated and a User Privacy Policy was written. The updated T&Cs were vetted by the NHLS legal secretary. All registered RfA users were required to explicitly accept the User Privacy Policy and the updated T&Cs. Users who did not accept were unsubscribed and would be prompted to accept should they resubscribe for the RfA reports. Specific guidance was also developed for users of the RfA reports to understand the conditions of POPIA, and a user-friendly compliance checklist was developed and distributed via email on a weekly basis.

As the POPIA work of the Team became known, others within the NICD began to contact them for POPIA-related queries. Partly in response to this, it was decided to develop two SOPs for the wider NICD: (1) an SOP for ensuring POPIA-compliant research ethics committee (REC) applications, and (2) an SOP for the data warehouse to follow when they receive a request for access to data. However, subsequent to sharing these draft SOPs within the wider NICD, no further response was received from NICD management.

This work did not proceed any further, as organizational consultation and management approval for the implementation of these SOPs were required.

Ongoing education and training

Throughout the four-year period, there was ongoing education and training within the Team, as well as users of the RfA reports, and within the NICD generally. In June 2021, an online lecture was provided by Dr Ciara Staunton, who gave all the lectures throughout this process, to the users of the reports on "POPIA and the RfA reports". This was followed in March 2022 with the development of two training videos that all users of the reports are encouraged to watch that discuss POPIA generally, patient rights, and POPIA as it applies to the personal information held by the RfA reports.[15]

In addition to this, there was a real appetite within the NICD for further education and training on the implications of POPIA, in part due to the absence of detailed information from the Information Regulator on the impact of POPIA on the biomedical sector. Although the purpose of the project was to ensure POPIA compliance only in relation to the RfA reports, it was decided to have more general discussions on POPIA and health information. Between 2019 and 2022, additional lectures (both online and in-person) were delivered on POPIA and health information, POPIA and clinical care, and POPIA and the processing of personal information of children.

Lessons learned and conclusions

The period between 2019 and 2023 saw the Team undergo considerable activities to ensure the RfA reports complied with POPIA, while continuing to provide its core function of HIV reporting. During this time, several lessons were learned that could hold value not only for NICD but also for health organizations in South Africa and beyond.

Notably, POPIA compliance required a change of technical systems, change in processes, updated documentation, and local guidance to support the implementation of programmes. Two aspects of change were found to be particularly time-consuming. First, the technical change related to the RfA distribution system was both costly and time-consuming (e.g. supporting RfA users with navigating the RfA portal, the password reset function, and ensuring POPIA compliance while using the reports). Second, when the Team updated the T&Cs and privacy policy, this required all users of the reports to agree to the updated documents. Ensuring compliance required months of individual support from NICD staff. It is thus not just that on occasion, the systems change and development of documents take time, but also that additional support by personnel is required to ensure that the new systems are followed. Whereas the Team was supported by a Cooperative Agreement from the US

Centers for Disease Control and Prevention, the necessary resources and financial assistance are unlikely to be available in all such circumstances where there is concern regarding the potential conflict between data protection law on the one hand, and effective health service delivery on the other.

Public health institutions require both institutional and sectoral leadership to ensure a successful approach towards complying with new, complex data protection laws such as POPIA (or the GDPR for that matter). Complying with data protection law in the context of clinical care and public health requires a multi-stakeholder approach involving, at a minimum, clinicians, public health professionals, data security experts, information technology experts, lawyers, and human resources personnel. Compliance also comes at a cost in the context of personnel time, the possible need for additional personnel or external consultants, a change in systems, possible new technology and/or infrastructure, staff training, and any new guidance and/or documentation. A centralized approach to POPIA compliance from the NHLS leadership would mean that all departments and institutions can understand what is necessary to comply with a new law as well as supporting access to the necessary resources.

The Team found that despite its efforts to ensure an institutional approach towards POPIA compliance (i.e. not limited to just the RfA reports), the broad consultation required for this was beyond the scope of an individual team. Indeed, the lack of institutional buy-in meant that the Team's work developing a Code of Conduct for their organization, as well as data usage and REC application SOPs, stalled and still to date are not in place. Although the Team feels that this is was a missed opportunity, the draft Code is available to the NHLS, and indeed the wider health sector, and can potentially be used to guide the development of any code in the future. Despite the absence of institutional guidance, the Team continued its work to ensure that the RfA reports are compliant with POPIA. However, institutional support for POPIA compliance would not only likely have sped up the process, but would also have meant that stakeholders within the broader organization could have benefitted from the work.

Despite the lack of an overall institutional approach towards compliance, the Team has found that there was, and continues to be, a real appetite for education and information from staff on complying with POPIA in their day-to-day activities. There were high attendance rates, with up to 220 attendees, at the educational information webinars organized by the Team. The questions and feedback received demonstrated that staff are aware of numerous challenges pertaining to POPIA compliance and require ongoing further support in better understanding POPIA (as well as other relevant laws) and how it impacts their work making use of personal health information.

Outside of the NHLS, there is a clear need for sector-specific guidance in the delivery of healthcare and treatment programmes in South Africa.

Concerns from within the NHLS are almost certainly not isolated. In September 2021, the Information Regulator provided an online webinar on Section 57 prior authorization applications. In that webinar they noted that most applications they had received were not necessary. Indeed, the application for the linking of datasets with the NHLS data was deemed not to be necessary, despite the legal opinion advising NICD that it was necessary and other Responsible Parties declining to link their datasets due to concerns that the linking was not POPIA compliant. As the linking of these datasets requires the processing of sensitive personal information, including information that can lead to stigmatization and discrimination, it is reasonable that Responsible Parties are hesitant regarding this. However, the linking of these datasets would provide a public health service in a country with the world's greatest HIV burden. Essentially, the absence of guidance on the application of POPIA in the context of health has resulted in a restrictive interpretation of the law by health organizations at the expense of public health, even though this restrictive approach does not appear to be matched by the Information Regulator. As a result, privacy interests of patients and patients' data protection rights may be currently weighted too heavily and not appropriately balanced with the right to health and the state's obligation to protect and promote public health. This lack of statutory guidance has also meant that health organizations are being forced to make applications (such as prior authorization and exemption applications) that come at considerable time and personnel cost and may ultimately be deemed unnecessary. These applications can stall programmes, as teams stop data processing activities while they await the outcome of the applications. The uncertainty in the application of POPIA is not unique to the NICD or NHLS, but equally would apply to the broader health sector. Thus, a Code of Conduct for the entire health sector and not just NHLS is needed, but the development of such a code is likely best facilitated by the Department of Health, bringing together a wide array of stakeholders in healthcare and health research in South Africa.

Finally, national data protection authorities, in this case the Information Regulator, also have an important role to play. The Information Regulator has been proactive in having a series of public engagement exercises and webinars at a general level, describing the contours of POPIA, with none thus far focusing on the biomedical context. It is well documented that navigating data protection requirements in the biomedical context is challenging. Thus, targeted webinars and information sessions would be critical for this sector to ensure the ongoing delivery of care. The Team has found the Information Regulator to be considerably delayed with regard to response time, including responding to applications—with the NHLS exemption application taking almost one year to be processed. This was in part likely due to budgetary and staffing issues. However, as we have set out, compliance can come at a cost to the operation of public health programmes and clinical care. Additionally, the length of delays did little to offset concerns internally that the processes were not POPIA compliant. Governments have a responsibility to ensure these offices are adequately resourced at the outset to avoid any unnecessary delays in public health and clinical care.

In conclusion, the Team, and hopefully our users, have learnt the practical steps required to ensure better POPIA compliance while still maintaining robust clinical care and public health duties. It is reassuring and empowering for healthcare professionals to understand how to handle personal identifiable data despite the fear that can be engendered by legislation such as POPIA. These legal developments are necessary to ensure that the rights to privacy and protection of personal information are promoted, but the reality is that uncertainty in the application of POPIA in the context of health has likely impacted on the delivery of clinical care and public health programmes. Fear of the impact of non-compliance has resulted in restrictive interpretations of POPIA. Furthermore, the changes required to ensure compliance come with cost implications, raising concerns in a health system that is already resource-constrained. A cost-efficient approach to addressing these changes requires national and institutional leadership alike, and the buy-in of all staff to understand their role and responsibility in delivering clinical care and public health protection and promotion, while simultaneously respecting the rights to privacy and protection of one's personal information.

Funding

This project is supported by the President's Emergency Plan for AIDS Relief (PEPFAR) through the Centers for Disease Control and Prevention, under the terms of Cooperative Agreement Number [6 NU2GGH001934-04-07: Strengthening District Health Systems in support of the HIV and TB continuum of care].

Work on this article was supported by the US National Institute of Mental Health and the US National Institutes of Health (award number U01MH127690) under the Harnessing Data Science for Health Discovery and Innovation in Africa (DS-I Africa) programme. The content of this article is solely the authors' responsibility and does not necessarily represent the official views of the US National Institute of Mental Health or the US National Institutes of Health.

Notes

1 UNAIDS: https://www.unaids.org/en/regionscountries/countries/southafrica.
2 Department of Health (South Africa), *National Consolidated Guidelines for the Management of HIV in Adults, Adolescents, Children and Infants and the Prevention of Mother-to-Child Transmission* (February 2020), available at: https://knowledgehub.

health.gov.za/elibrary/national-consolidated-guidelines-management-hiv-adults-adolescents-children-and-infants.

3 Ciara Staunton and others, "Protection of Personal Information Act 2013 and Data Protection for Health Research in South Africa" (2020) 10 *International Data Privacy Law* 160; Edward S Dove and Jiahong Chen, "Should Consent for Data Processing Be Privileged in Health Research? A Comparative Legal Analysis" (2020) 10 *International Data Privacy Law* 117.

4 Ubuntu is an African philosophy that is particularly dominant in southern Africa. Generally speaking, it posits that it is through our connection with others that our humanity exists. Langa J, in *S v Makwanyane*, stated that the communal spirit of Ubuntu "places emphasis on communality and on the interdependence of the members of a community": see *S v Makwanyane* (CCT3/94) [1995] ZACC 3 at [224]. Reviglio and Alunge have also argued that understandings and protections of privacy in the contemporary digital and data-led paradigm can be advanced through notions of Ubuntuism. Specifically in relation to consent, the authors note:

> If the self is dependent on the community, then it can be argued that protecting the community amounts to protecting the individual, or that protecting the individual should start from protecting the community. In the big data context, Ubuntu would therefore support a top-down regulatory paradigm of privacy, as a right which protects an individual through principles and rules regulating the collection and sharing of data relating to entire communities or groups of individuals. Individual informed consent, for example, may not be sufficient at all. Ideally, "collective informed consent" may be much more appropriate.

See Urbano Reviglio and Rogers Alunge, "I Am Datafied Because We Are Datafied": An Ubuntu Perspective on (Relational) Privacy (2020) 33 *Philosophy and Technology* 595. For more on ubuntu and genomic data sharing, see Ciara Staunton and others, "A Framework to Govern the Use of Health data for Research in Africa: A South African Perspective", in Tomas Zima and David N. Weissub (eds), *Medical Research Ethics: Challenges in the 21st Century* (Springer 2023), 485–499.

5 Information Regulator (South Africa), Codes of Conduct, available at: https://inforegulator.org.za/codes-of-conducts/.

6 A Code to regulate the use of personal data for research was submitted to the Information Regulator for approval on 12 May 2023. For this proposed code and a list of all approved codes, see n 5.

7 Department of Health (South Africa), *National Consolidated Guidelines*, n 2.

8 Lebohang Radebe, Ahmad Haeri Mazanderani, and Gayle G Sherman, "Evaluating Patient Data Quality in South Africa's National Health Laboratory Service Data Warehouse, 2017–2020: Implications for Monitoring Child Health Programmes" (2022) 22 *BMC Public Health* 1266.

9 Department of Health (South Africa), *National Consolidated Guidelines*, n 2.

10 Department of Health (South Africa), *National Digital Health Strategy for South Africa 2019–2024* (2019), available at: https://www.health.gov.za/wp-content/uploads/2020/11/national-digital-strategy-for-south-africa-2019-2024-b.pdf.

11 This opinion was sought from Dr Ciara Staunton, lead author of this chapter. The opinion is not publicly available, but is on file with the authors and has been shared with others within the medical community to inform their work.

12 Ciara Staunton and others, "Rules of Engagement: Perspectives on Stakeholder Engagement for Genomic Biobanking Research in South Africa" (2018) 19 *BMC Medical Ethics* 13.

13 Ciara Staunton, Kathrina Tschigg, and Gayle Sherman, "Data Protection, Data Management, and Data Sharing: Stakeholder Perspectives on the Protection of Personal Health Information in South Africa" (2021) 16 *PLoS One* e0260341.

14 This response is not publicly available but is on file with the authors.

15 See training video from Dr Ciara Staunton, "POPIA, RfA Reports & RfA Dashboard", available at: https://mstrweb.nicd.ac.za/MicroStrategy/Images/ Video/RFAD/Training/RfA_RfAD_Training_Video.mp4.